Ultrasound and the Fetal Brain

PROGRESS IN OBSTETRIC
AND GYNECOLOGICAL
SONOGRAPHY SERIES

SERIES EDITOR: ASIM KURJAK

Ultrasound and the Fetal Brain

Edited by
F. A. CHERVENAK, A. KURJAK
and C. H. COMSTOCK

The Parthenon Publishing Group

International Publishers in Medicine, Science & Technology

NEW YORK   LONDON

British Library Cataloguing in Publication Data

Ultrasound and the Fetal Brain. –
(Progress in Obstetric & Gynecological
Sonography Series)
  I. Chervenak, Frank A. II. Series
618.3207543

  ISBN 1-85070-612-3

Library of Congress Cataloging-in-Publication Data

Ultrasound and the fetal brain / edited by F.A.
  Chervenak, A. Kurjak, and C.H. Comstock.
    p. cm. – (Progress in obstetric and
  gynecological sonography series)
    Includes bibliographical references and
    index.
    ISBN 1-85070-612-3
    1. Fetal brain–Ultrasonic imaging.
2. Fetal brain–Abnormalities. 3. Fetal
brain–Diseases. I. Chervenak, Frank A.
II. Kurjak, Asim. III. Comstock, C.H.
(Christine H.) IV. Series.
    [DNLM: 1. Fetal Diseases–ultrasonogra-
phy. 2. Brain Diseases–ultrasonography.
3. Brain–embryology. 4. Brain–pathology.
WQ 211 U47 1995]
RG629.B73U48 1995
618.3'26807543–dc20
DNLM/DLC   95-23988
for Library of Congress   CIP

Published in the UK and Europe by
The Parthenon Publishing Group Limited
Casterton Hall, Carnforth
Lancs. LA6 2LA

Published in North America by
The Parthenon Publishing Group Inc.
One Blue Hill Plaza
Pearl River
New York 10965, USA

Copyright © 1995 Parthenon Publishing Group Ltd

First published 1995

No part of this book may be reproduced in any form
without permission from the publishers, except for the
quotation of brief passages for the purposes of review

Composed by Keele University Press

Printed and bound in Great Britain by
Butler & Tanner Ltd, Frome and London

Contents

List of contributors

A. Achiron
Multiple Sclerosis Center
The Chaim Sheba Medical Center
Tel Hashomer 52621
Israel

R. Achiron
Department of Obstetrics and Gynecology
The Chaim Sheba Medical Center
Tel Hashomer 52621
Israel

Zs. Ádám
Department of Obstetrics and Gynecology
Semmelweis University Medical School
Budapest
Hungary

J. C. Birnholz
Diagnostic Ultrasound Consultants
120 Oak Brook Center
Oak Brook
Illinois 60521
USA

F. A. Chervenak
The New York Hospital–Cornell Medical Center
525 East 68th Street – M713
New York, New York 10021
USA

W. H. Clewell
Phoenix Perinatal Associates
1300 N. 12th Street
Suite 320
Phoenix, Arizona
USA

C. H. Comstock
Division of Fetal Imaging
Department of Obstetrics and Gynecology
William Beaumont Hospital
3601 West Thirteen Mile Road
Royal Oak, Michigan 48703
USA

V. D'Addario
Department of Obstetrics and Gynecology
University of Bari
Bari
Italy

P. Greco
Department of Obstetrics and Gynecology
University of Bari
Bari
Italy

G. Gunnarssón
Department of Obstetrics and Gynecology
University Hospital MAS
S-21401 Malmö
Sweden

M. Imanishi
Department of Pediatrics and NICU
Seirei Hospitals
Hamamatsu
Japan

M. Judaš
Section of Neuroanatomy
Croatian Institute for Brain Research
School of Medicine, University of Zagreb
Šalata 3, 41000 Zagreb
Croatia

P. Kirkinen
Department of Obstetrics and Gynecology
University of Kuopio
Finland

I. Kostović
Croatian Institute for Brain Research
School of Medicine, University of Zagreb
Šalata 3
41000 Zagreb
Croatia

S. Kupesic
Ultrasonic Institute
School of Medicine, University of Zagreb
'Sveti Duh' Hospital
Sveti Duh 64
41000 Zagreb
Croatia

A. Kurjak
Ultrasonic Unit
Department of Obstetrics and Gynecology
University of Zagreb
'Sveti Duh' Hospital
Sveti Duh 64
41000 Zagreb
Croatia

R. N. Laurini
Division of Developmental & Pediatric Pathology
Institute of Pathology
Rue du Bugnon 25
1011 Lausanne
Switzerland

K. Maeda
Department of Obstetrics and Gynecology
Seirei Hospitals
Hamamatsu
Japan

A. Maesel
Department of Obstetrics and Gynecology
University Hospital MAS
University of Lund
S-21401 Malmö
Sweden

K. Maršál
Department of Obstetrics and Gynecology
University Hospital MAS
University of Lund
S-21401 Malmö
Sweden

L. B. McCullough
Baylor College of Medicine
Center for Ethics, Medicine and Public Issues
Houston
USA

A. Monteagudo
Department of Obstetrics and Gynecology
Sloane Hospital for Women
Columbia Presbyterian Medical Center
622 West 168th Street
New York
NY 10032
USA

Z. Papp
Department of Obstetrics and Gynecology
Semmelweis University Medical School
Budapest
Hungary

M. Resta
Department of Neuroradiology
Institute of Neurology
University of Bari
Bari
Italy

M. Ryynänen
Department of Obstetrics and Gynecology
University of Kuopio
Finland

M. Smith-Levitin
Department of Obstetrics and Gynecology
Division of Maternal–Fetal Medicine
The New York Hospital–Cornell Medical Center
New York
USA

P. Spagnolo
Department of Neuroradiology
Institute of Neurology
University of Bari
Bari
Italy

I. E. Timor-Tritsch
Department of Obstetrics and Gynecology
Sloane Hospital for Women
Columbia Presbyterian Medical Center
622 West 168th Street
New York
NY 10032
USA

M. Utsu
Department of Obstetrics and Gynecology
Seirei Hospitals
Hamamatsu
Japan

D. Zudenigo
Ultrasonic Institute
School of Medicine, University of Zagreb
'Sveti Duh' Hospital
Sveti Duh 64
41000 Zagreb
Croatia

Progress in Obstetric and Gynecological Sonography Series

An ongoing series documenting recent advances in key subject areas, with a new volume scheduled for publication approximately every 3 months.

Titles currently planned in the Series include:

From an exciting novelty, ultrasound has now become the best single diagnostic technique available in obstetrics and gynecology. The original excitement is, of course, still felt by many of us. One cannot stop wondering how many applications of this relatively simple invention the future will hold. On the other hand, the wave of interest created by the present possibilities is spreading rapidly through almost all major journals. Any interested individual will find it difficult to read or even scan all of these articles, although he might wish to do so. The purpose of this newly conceived series of books is to overcome the problem by providing expert, up-to-date analyses of current advances in each specialized topic.

This new series is dedicated to the in-depth evaluation of the latest developments and advances in an area where progress is on a wide front and where diagnostic potential changes so rapidly. Each book contains critical reviews by leading experts, backed up by the best bibliographical information available. Unique and contemporary in concept, design and content, the new series provides a timely and continuing resource of expert information in a highly readable, consistent format.

It is hoped that this unique series will promote current awareness and help clinicians and research workers to keep abreast of today's most significant research and current developments.

Therefore titles in this series will be produced accurately, concisely and rapidly over a short time period. The chapters provide not only essential new data, but also serve as guides for interpretation of the literature and to the repercussions for clinical practice. In other words, the objective of each book is to inform our colleagues of the evidence and data available on the topic concerned, how reliable this information appears to be and what conclusions may be drawn from it. It should be a tool for distinguishing facts from fiction.

We believe that these new volumes will prove to be major sources of innovative ideas and effective solutions for the practice of obstetric and gynecological sonography.

Asim Kurjak
Series Editor

COLOR PLATES

Color Plate A Ultrasound scan (left), showing vein of Galen aneurysm (G) in the center, with a large straight and signoid sinus posteriorly (arrows). On the right is the same view with color Doppler

Color Plate B Color flow imaging and flow velocity waveforms of the fetal aorta at 9/10 weeks' gestation. End-diastolic flow is absent

Color Plate C Flow velocity waveforms obtained from the umbilical artery at 9/10 weeks' gestation. Note the absence of end-diastolic blood flow velocity

Color Plate D Transvaginal color Doppler scan of the fetal head in the same patient as in Color Plate C (9/10 weeks' gestation). Blood flow velocity waveforms of the middle cerebral artery demonstrate constant end-diastolic flow

Color Plate E Transverse scan of the fetal head. At the inner edge of the choroid plexus, a pulsed signal was obtained. Note the moderate systolic and relatively high end-diastolic components of blood flow

Color Plate F Circulus arteriosus (circle of Willis) of a healthy fetus at 36 weeks of gestation, visualized by means of color Doppler

Color Plate G Energy Doppler displays of the circle of Willis at different gestational ages. The posterior cerebral arteries are typically absent before 12 weeks' gestational age and appear early in the second trimester

Color Plate H Regional coronal views of a small, intensely vascular choroid glomus with ventriculomegaly and relatively thin cortex in a third-trimester case of trisomy 21

Color Plate I Sagittal cranial views at the start of the second trimester. The anterior cerebral artery circulation outlines a rudimentary, vertical corpus callosum

Color Plate J Subependymal and lenticulostriate venous patterns in coronal, energy Doppler views

Color Plate K Sagittal energy Doppler sections of a developed anterior cerebral artery circulation. The magnification view (bottom) includes the recurrent artery of Heubner

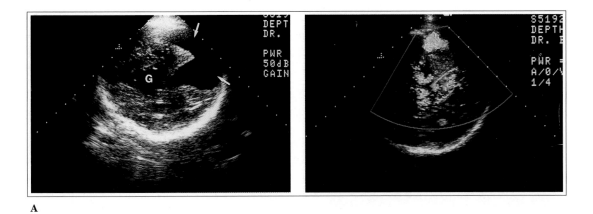

A

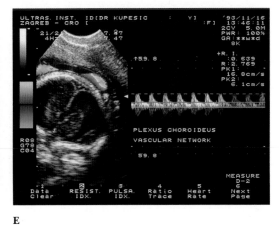

B

C

D

E

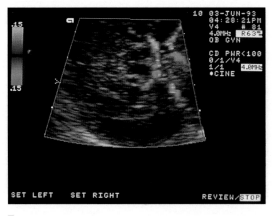

F

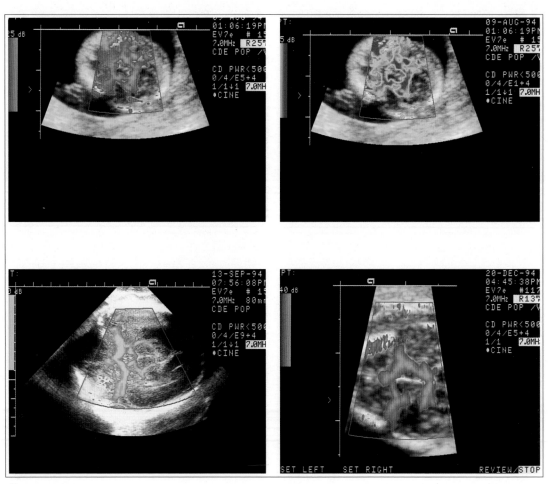

G

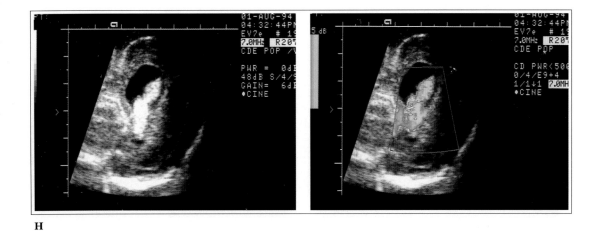

H

I

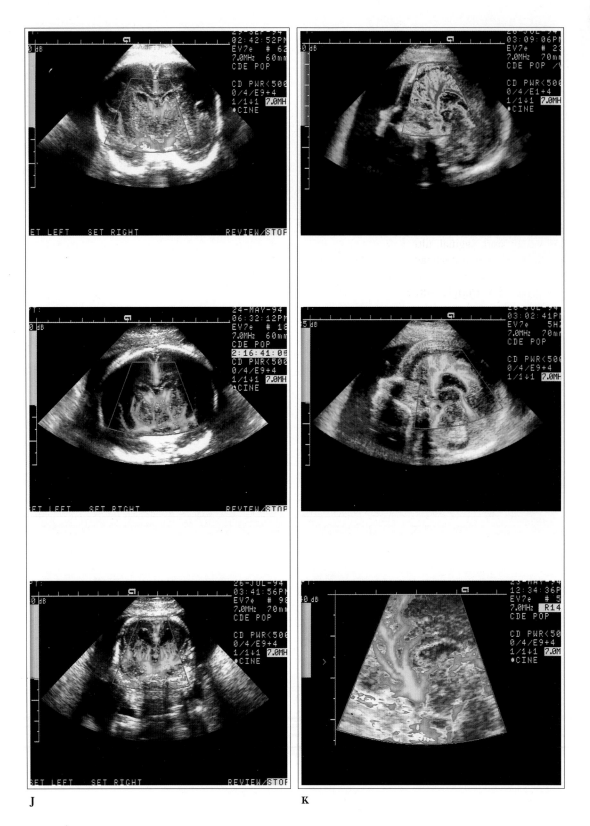

J

K

Foreword

Understanding the structure and function of the fetal brain has long challenged the medical profession. With the development of modern obstetric ultrasound, evaluation of the fetal brain is now possible. Our book describes the state of the art of ultrasound and the fetal brain. A background of neuroanatomical development and pathology of the fetal brain is invaluable to ultrasound diagnosis. Abdominal and vaginal ultrasound permit the definition of the minute details of normal anatomy and the accurate diagnosis of virtually all anomalies. Color flow Doppler ultrasound is a safe and effective tool to study cranial circulation while magnetic resonance imaging is an alternative imaging technique of adjunctive value in special circumstances. The powerful diagnostic tools of imaging and Doppler ultrasound enable an *in vivo* evaluation of fetal neurology and brain damage. Genetic and prognostic considerations permit the physician to counsel patients regarding management options including fetal shunting for hydrocephalus and cephalocentesis.

The Editors hope that this comprehensive, multidisciplinary international work will help all physicians dedicated to the care of fetal patients and to the provision of accurate counsel to their parents.

Frank A. Chervenak
Asim Kurjak
Christine H. Comstock

Prenatal development of the cerebral cortex 1

I. Kostović and M. Judaš

INTRODUCTION

In this review, we summarize our current views and evidence on the key role of the transient fetal subplate zone in the prenatal and perinatal development and reorganization of the human cerebral cortex. The review is based on two decades of continuous and systematic research, during which we applied different techniques for demonstrating the cytoarchitectonics (Nissl staining), neuronal morphology (Golgi impregnation), synaptogenesis (electron-microscopic analysis), growing pathways (acetylcholinesterase (AChE) histochemistry) and transmitter-related properties of developing neuronal populations (immunocytochemistry and histochemistry) on a number of human brains of the Zagreb Neuroembryological Collection[1]. The decision to focus on the subplate zone was prompted by several reasons.

Early quantitative electron-microscopic studies demonstrated that the initial synapses in the cerebral cortex of fetal dog[2], cat[3] and human[4,5] are concentrated in two strata that lie above and below the cortical plate. The correlation of this bilaminar pattern of synaptogenesis with Nissl- and Golgi-architectonics has led to a new interpretation of the morphological characteristics and the extent (in depth) of the human fetal cortex and the delineation of a hitherto unrecognized and essential compartment within the cortical anlage[5]. This compartment, initially termed the subplate layer[5] and at present widely recognized as the subplate zone[6], reaches its greatest prominence in humans, and represents the thickest part of the human fetal cortex as well as the major site of early synaptogenesis and neuron maturation[4,5]. Its prominence and significance in the developing monkey cortex were recognized early and subjected to the systematic series of experimental studies by Rakic, Goldman-Rakic and colleagues

at Yale University[6–13]. Furthermore, the long-term collaborative research of teams from Zagreb and Yale has revealed the comparative aspects of the subplate development in human and monkey brain and thus strengthened the initial interpretations[14–17]. Finally, these results were accepted and confirmed by other leading research groups studying the developing monkey and human cortex[18–24].

In a series of excellent experimental studies on fetal cats and kittens, Shatz and her collaborators collected a wealth of data concerning the role of the subplate zone in the developing carnivore cortex[25–32] and stressed the role of the subplate in the development of thalamocortical connectivity[33–35] as well as the development of initial corticofugal projections[36]. Similar results were obtained in other studies of the developing cat[37–42] and ferret brain[43,44] as well as in a number of studies of the rodent brain[45–55].

At present, the subplate zone is widely recognized as an essential compartment of the developing mammalian cortex[16,35,49]. Furthermore, on the basis of available data, it is reasonable to conclude that the enlargement of the subplate zone occurs relatively late in evolution and reaches its greatest prominence in the primate, especially the human, brain[16]. Therefore, we have recently proposed[16] that the highest elaboration of the subplate zone in primates may serve as a substrate for the competition of a large contingent of corticocortical connections and thus participate in the three-dimensional modelling of the cortical architecture during the formation of cerebral convolutions and parcellation of cytoarchitectonic areas.

However, a different view concerning the neocortical development has been put forward, based on the concept of the 'primordial plexiform layer' (PPL). The concept of the PPL was originally proposed by Marin-Padilla[56] with the name 'the primordial neocortical organization', and subsequently elaborated in a series of his Golgi studies of developing rodent, cat and human neocortex[57-62]. Recently, Marin-Padilla carefully summarized his views and proposed 'a unifying developmental cytoarchitectonics theory of the mammalian neocortex'[63]. Since, on the one hand, this concept of PPL has been widely accepted by those studying the cortical development in the rodent and carnivore brain[35,45] and, on the other hand, our views derived from the long-term research of developing human and monkey brain are significantly different[6,8,16], some general comments seem appropriate before the detailed exposition of our own views.

There is no doubt that Marin-Padilla's work represents the major contribution to the study of neocortical development; his early studies were instrumental in shaping the current views on the initial development of the neocortical anlage. Furthermore, the concept of primordial plexiform layer seems useful for the description of early cortical development in rodent and especially cat brain. However, the extension of that concept to the much more complex monkey and human cortex seems less warranted, for the following reasons.

First, with respect to the classical staging system of neocortical development (i.e. the system of Poliakov as modified by Sidman and Rakic[64]), three periods proposed by Marin-Padilla are not sufficient to encompass satisfactorily the series of complex transformations of the prenatal cortical anlage. Second, while our staging system (see below) relies heavily upon the existence of transient and reorganizational phenomena, in his account of neocortical development Marin-Padilla almost completely ignores 'regressive' and reorganizational events. Third, Marin-Padilla stresses the key developmental role of layer I (marginal zone) and pyramidal neurons and ignores the role of the subplate zone, although he himself claims that both the marginal and subplate zones are descendants of the PPL; this suggests that the subplate zone is not regarded as an essential compartment of the cortical anlage. On the other hand, all other authors, who otherwise accept the concept of PPL, insist on the crucial role of the subplate zone in neocortical development[35,45,49,54,55].

Finally, Marin-Padilla explicitly insists on the structural and organizational similarities between the embryonic mammalian and adult amphibian or reptilian cortex and claims that the marginal and subplate zones represent vestigial elements of a pre-mammalian cortical organization. This view has a strong flavor of classical recapitulation theory, which was at first accepted by early comparative neuroanatomists[65-67], but was subsequently disproved and rejected by modern students of the relationships between phylogeny and ontogeny[68,69]. As we have already pointed out, all evidence from the current literature clearly shows that the subplate zone progresses along the phylogenetic scale; the enlargement of the subplate occurs relatively late in evolution and reaches its greatest prominence in the primate and human brain[16].

HISTOGENETIC EVENTS AND THE STAGING OF CORTICAL DEVELOPMENT

In addition to the embryonic zones common to the whole central nervous system, the developing cerebral (telencephalic) wall contains a number of special zones characteristic of the development of the cerebral cortex. Since all cellular events (proliferation, migration, differentiation, growth of fiber pathways, synaptogenesis, cell death as well as initial overproduction and subsequent elimination of axonal collaterals, dendritic spines and synapses) take place in one or more of these zones, it is logical to divide the whole prenatal histogenesis into a series of subsequent stages on the basis of complex cytoarchitectonic transformations of embryonic zones.

Therefore, to enhance the understanding of the developmental history and role of the subplate zone, in this section we shall first briefly describe our staging system and summarize the major histogenetic events during the embryonic and early fetal (preceding the appearance of the subplate zone), mid-fetal, late fetal and newborn periods. At the end of this section, we shall summarize the major differences between isocortical and allocortical development. For a more detailed exposition, the reader should consult our recent review[70].

Table 1 Relative intensity and timing (in gestational weeks) of major histogenetic processes leading to the formation of the human neocortex

Histogenetic processes	Embryonic period (4–7 weeks)	Early fetal period (8–12 weeks)	Mid-fetal period (13–24 weeks)	Late fetus and premature infant (25–38 weeks)	Newborn
Proliferation	+	+++	+	+–	–
Migration	+	+++	+++	+	–
Differentiation	–	+	+++	+++	+++
Growth of afferents	–	+	+++	+++	+++
Growth of efferents	–	–+	+	+	+
Synaptogenesis	–	+	+	+++	+++
Cell death	–	+–	+–	?	?
Plasticity	–	?	?	?	?

Staging system

In a way, our staging system (see also Tables 2 and 3) may be regarded as an updated and elaborated version of the system of Poliakov[71] and Sidman and Rakic[64, 72]. However, the main advantage and originality of our system lie in the fact that it fully recognizes the importance of two major developmental phenomena which were not taken into consideration in previous classifications: (1) the developmental history of the subplate zone, and (2) the transient and reorganizational processes in the developing human brain.

On the basis of multiple structural features as well as the relative intensity of different histogenetic events (Table 1), we have divided the whole prenatal cortical development into six developmental phases containing 11 distinct stages (Table 2). However, to enhance the correlation with physiological and clinical data, these stages and phases can be easily brought into correspondence with five more plausible periods of human prenatal development: embryonic (first 2 months), early fetal (9–12 weeks of gestation), mid-fetal (13–24 weeks of gestation), late fetal and preterm (25–38 weeks of gestation) and newborn periods (Table 3).

Embryonic and early fetal period

During the 3rd and 4th weeks of gestation, the thin wall of telencephalic vesicles consists solely of the *ventricular zone*, composed of immature, elongated neuroepithelial (ventricular) cells arranged into the pseudostratified epithelium. One end of these elongated cells is attached to the ventricular (ectodermal or inner) surface while the other stretches towards the superficial, mesodermal surface covered by the basal lamina. These cells proliferate intensively. During the 5th week of gestation, the superficial process of ventricular cells together with processes of the first post-mitotic neurons form a new pale layer – the *marginal zone* – so that the wall of the telencephalic vesicle now consists of two embryonic zones, marginal and ventricular (our stage 1 of cortical development). The major histogenetic event of this period is proliferation within the ventricular zone, which leads to the increase in number of neuroepithelial cells and gradual growth of the telencephalon.

During the 6th week of gestation, post-mitotic cells generated within the ventricular zone detach from the ventricular surface and migrate away from it, thus forming a new *intermediate zone* at the interface between the marginal and ventricular zones. The telencephalic wall now consists of three embryonic zones characteristic for the development of all parts of the central nervous system: the marginal, intermediate and ventricular zones (Figure 1, left). Therefore, we designated the whole embryonic period as the phase of universal embryonic zones (phase I) and this particular stage as stage 2 of cortical development.

By the end of the 6th week of gestation, another zone, the *subventricular zone*, develops at the interface between the ventricular and intermediate zones. This zone, characteristic for the developing

Table 2 Developmental phases and stages of human neocortical histogenesis during prenatal and perinatal life

Period	Gestational age (weeks)	Phase		Stage		Lamination pattern
Embryonic	4–7	I	universal embryonic zones	S1	two embryonic zones	VZ, MZ
				S2	three embryonic zones	VZ, IZ, MZ
				S3	four embryonic zones	VZ, SV, IZ, MZ
Early fetal	8–9	II	formation of CP	S4	formation of CP	VZ, SV, IZ, CP, MZ
	10–12			S5	primary consolidation of CP	VZ, SV, IZ, CP, MZ
Mid-fetal	13–15	III	formation of typical fetal transitory compartments	S6	subplate formation	VZ, SV, IZ, SP, CP, MZ
	16–18			S7	secondary consolidation of CP	VZ, SV, IZ, SP, CP, MZ
	19–24	IV	typical fetal lamination pattern	S8	developmental peak of SP	VZ, SV, IZ, SP, CP, MZ
Late fetal	25–34	V	transformation of fetal lamination pattern	S9	initial lamination of CP, local resolution of SP	VZ, SV, IZ, SP, CP (layers II–VI), MZ
	35–38			S10	general resolution of SP, six-layered *Grundtypus*	VZ, WM, SP, layers I–VI
Newborn		VI	immature adult-like lamination	S11	immature six-layered cortex	

VZ, ventricular zone; SV, subventricular zone; IZ, intermediate zone; CP, cortical plate; SP, subplate zone; MZ, marginal zone; WM, white matter

telencephalon, is a site of intensive proliferation and generates a substantial number of neurons destined for the future neocortex. Thus, in this stage (stage 3), the lateral cerebral wall consists of the following four zones: the ventricular, subventricular, intermediate and marginal zones (Figure 1, right). The subventricular zone becomes very thick within the basolateral part of the telen-

cephalic wall, thus leading to the formation of the *ganglionic eminence*. Although the ganglionic eminence generates primarily the future neurons of the basal ganglia, it may contribute to the population of cortical neurons as well.

During the 7th week of gestation, characterized by a significant increase in the size of cerebral vesicles, an intensive proliferation continues within

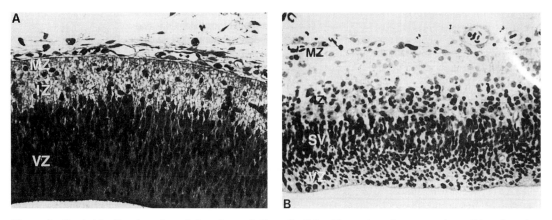

Figure 1 Semi-thin (1 µm) section of the telencephalic wall of the 16-mm-long human embryo (A) and section through the rostrobasal pallium of 24-mm-long human embryo (B), before the formation of the cortical plate. VZ, ventricular zone; SV, subventricular zone; IZ, intermediate zone; MZ, marginal zone. Nissl staining, magnification 20×

Table 3 Basic features of the histogenesis of the pallium and cerebral cortex during prenatal and perinatal life

Period	Gestational age (weeks)	Phase	Main features
Embryonic	4–7	I	universal embryonic zones
Early fetal	8–12	II	formation of the cortical plate
Mid-fetal	13–15	III	formation of typical fetal transitory compartments
	16–24	IV	typical fetal lamination pattern, developmental peak of the subplate zone
Late fetus and premature infant	25–38	V	transformation of fetal lamination pattern (initial lamination within the cortical plate, resolution of the subplate zone)
Newborn		VI	immature adult-like six-layered cortex

the ventricular zone and a number of cells migrate towards the subventricular and intermediate zones. The development of the subventricular zone and the establishment of regional differences in the thickness of the pallium indicate the end of the phase of universal embryonic zones and foreshadow the incipient development of specific fetal cortical zones.

The most important event for the delineation of a new developmental period is the appearance of the *cortical plate* within the basolateral pallium towards the end of the 8th week of gestation. After being generated within the ventricular–subventricular zone, young post-mitotic neurons migrate through the intermediate zone and finally form a cortical plate – a characteristic layer of tightly packed and vertically aligned immature neurons situated at the interface of the intermediate and marginal zones. With the formation of the cortical plate, a true laminar cortical anlage is established. As a result of the proliferation and migration during the 8th and 9th weeks of gestation, new neurons are continuously added to the cortical plate of the lateral pallium. The cortical plate gradually spreads throughout the dorsomedial and rostrocaudal regions of the cerebral vesicle. With this process, the formation of the cortical plate in the neopallial anlage is completed by 9 weeks of gestation (Figure 2).

In summary, during the embryonic period (first 2 months of gestation), the wall of cerebral vesicles (telencephalic wall) is at first very thin (less than 1mm) and consists of the same zones as in other parts of the neural-tube derivatives: the ventricular–subventricular, intermediate and marginal zones. This initial period of cytoarchitectonic development (4–7 weeks of gestation) can be described as a phase of universal embryonic zones (phase I, stages 1 to 3). The proliferation is the dominant event during early histogenesis and the first migratory wave of young (post-mitotic) neurons destined to form the cortical plate appears at the very end of the embryonic period. Therefore, the cortical plate develops at the end of this period and during the subsequent early fetal period (phase II, stages 4 and 5).

Mid-fetal, late fetal and newborn period

Another zone characteristic for the development of the cerebral cortex, the *subplate zone*, appears next and marks the beginning of the mid-fetal period (phase III, stages 6 and 7). After the formation of two cortex-specific zones (cortical plate and subplate), the mid-fetal cerebral pallium displays a typical fetal pattern of lamination (phase IV, stage 8) consisting of the following zones (starting from pia to ventricle): marginal zone (MZ), cortical plate (CP), subplate zone (SP), intermediate (IZ), subventricular (SV) and ventricular zone (VZ). Three of these fetal zones (MZ, CP and SP) represent the anlage of the future adult cerebral cortex (Figure 3, right; Figure 4, right). It is essential to emphasize that these cortical fetal zones are specific fetal elements: their neuronal content is permanently changing; they contain transient elements and have no direct relationship with layers of the adult cortex.

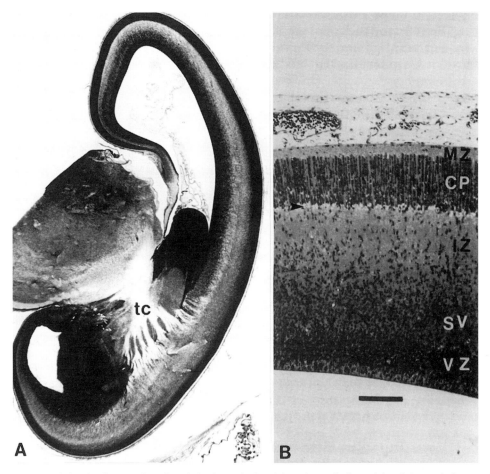

Figure 2 (A) Nissl-stained coronal section (left) through the right telencephalic vesicle of the early human fetus (10th week of gestation, crown–rump length 55mm), during the stage of primary consolidation of the cortical plate; tc, thalamocortical fibers penetrating from diencephalon into the telencephalic wall. (B) Nissl-stained 1-μm plastic section (right) showing mid-lateral cortex of a 10-week-old human fetus. Pre-subplate zone is pale narrow band indicated by arrowhead. Bar=100μm. MZ, marginal zone; CP, cortical plate; IZ, intermediate zone; SV, subventricular zone; VZ, ventricular zone

The last part of the mid-fetal period, i.e. at 19–24 weeks of gestation, is characterized by the developmental maximum of the fetal pattern of lamination in the neocortex and the developmental peak of the transient subplate zone; this is accompanied by the initial, transitory lamination within the cortical plate.

The late fetal period (25–38 weeks of gestation, the period of low-birth-weight premature infants) is the period of transformation of the fetal pattern of lamination characterized by the gradual resolution of the subplate zone (Figure 5), the onset of areal differentiation, the appearance of the defini-

tive adult-like six-layered pattern of lamination within the cortical plate (*Grundtypus* of Brodmann[65]), transient expression of neurotransmitter properties and laminar shifts and relocation of cortical afferents (phase V, stages 9 and 10).

Accordingly, the definitive pattern of cortical lamination is already outlined in the newborn infant (phase VI, stage 11). However, the immaturity of the newborn cortex clearly indicates that histogenetic processes continue during the early postnatal period. Therefore, the newborn stage can be appropriately described as the stage of immature and transient neocortical organization.

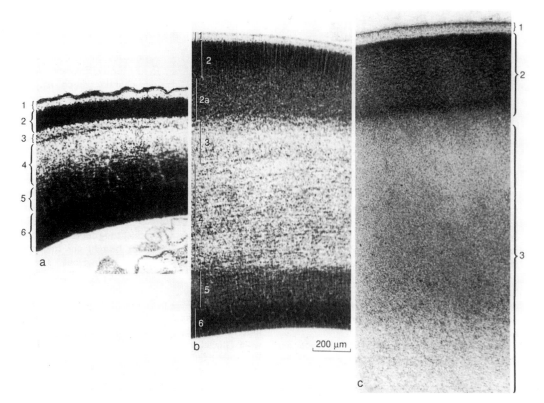

Figure 3 Development of the cortical plate, subplate zone and the typical fetal lamination pattern, for (a) 9.5-week-old human fetus, at the stage of the primary condensation of the cortical plate (phase II, stage 5); (b) 12.5-week-old human fetus with the formation of the bilaminar cortical plate and the subplate zone (phase III, stage 6); (c) 21-week-old human fetus, with typical fetal lamination pattern (phase IV, stage 8). 1, marginal zone; 2, cortical plate; 2a, 'secondary' cortical plate; 3, pre-subplate (left), subplate in formation (middle) and subplate zone (right); 4, intermediate zone; 5, subventricular zone; 6, ventricular zone. From reference 146, with permission

Isocortical vs. allocortical development

Already during the 5th week of gestation, morphogenetic cell death occurs along the midline, within the thin wall of the telencephalon medium (impar), thus contributing to its morphogenetic shaping. During the 6th week, as a reflection of general histogenetic gradients, all three embryonic zones are significantly thicker in the basal mid-lateral than in the more dorsal, rostral, caudal or medial portions of the telencephalic wall. Furthermore, a special lamination pattern occurs in the most medial part of the telencephalic vesicle (the anlage of the limbic allocortex); the telencephalic wall is here slightly curved and the marginal zone is significantly enlarged. This is the site of the future formation of the hippocampus. From this hemispheric edge ('limbus') the cerebral wall continues

as a thin epithelial lamina (area epithelialis, lamina tectoria) stretching from one hemispheric vesicle to the other. After the formation of the cortical plate throughout the largest part of the cerebral pallium during the 8th and 9th weeks of gestation, clear differences appear between the lateral (neocortical), limbic (archicortical) and mediobasal (paleocortical) parts of the telencephalic pallium.

Although basic histogenetic processes are essentially the same in all these three major types of cortex, they occur with different time schedules, spatial relationships and laminar patterns. Thus, the lateral neocortex develops a prominent cortical plate and (later) the subplate zone; the limbic archicortex develops an exceptionally wide marginal zone and thin, convoluted cortical plate, while the mediobasal paleocortex never develops a true cortical plate.

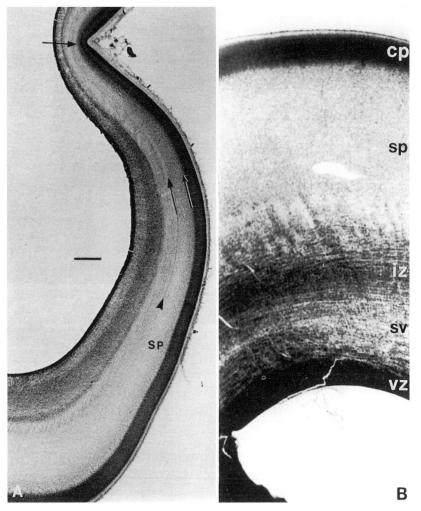

Figure 4 (A) Visual cortex of a 15-week-old human fetus during formation of the subplate zone. Different stages in the formation of the subplate zone can be seen along the curvature of the caudomedial occipital cortex. At the depth of the calcarine fissure (arrow), there is a thin pre-subplate zone, while at the borders of the calcarine cortex, formation of the second cortical plate is seen as a gradual decrease in cell density (between arrows). The interface between the subplate zone and underlying 'white' matter is seen as a sharp line (arrowhead). The prestriate occipital neocortex, which is situated close to the basal cerebral surface, already shows the true subplate zone (sp). Bar = 1 mm. From reference 16, with permission. (B) Nissl-stained section of the neocortical pallium of a 21-week-old human fetus showing typical fetal lamination pattern. Note that at this stage the subplate zone is the thickest compartment of the neocortical anlage (4× thicker than the cortical plate!). VZ, ventricular zone; SV, subventricular zone; IZ, intermediate zone; sp, subplate zone; cp, cortical plate

THE SUBPLATE ZONE AS A CYTOARCHITECTONIC COMPARTMENT

In this section, we shall describe the timetable of development and extent of the subplate zone, as well as cytological criteria for its definition and delineation of its boundaries. This description is based primarily on the detailed comparative study performed on human and monkey brains by Kostović and Rakic[16], who divided the development of the subplate zone into five major stages:

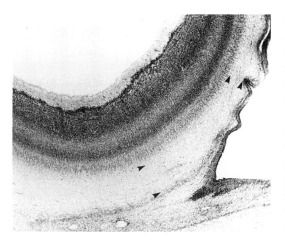

Figure 5 Low-power photomicrograph of a Nissl-stained coronal section of the primary visual cortex (area 17) of a 30-week-old human fetus during the period of dissolution of the subplate zone. Typical adult-like lamination is already present within the immature cortex, while the subplate zone is reduced to the thin layer situated between arrowheads; furthermore, the subplate is thinner towards the bottom of the sulcus (upper right corner) than below the gyral wall (figure bottom)

1 Stage I   Presubplate stage (10–12 weeks);

2 Stage II   Subplate formation stage (13–15 weeks);

3 Stage III   Subplate stage (15–35 weeks);

4 Stage IV   Subplate dissolution stage; and

5 Stage V   Postsubplate stage.

In general, the subplate zone can be recognized by its position below the developing cortical plate and by its content of sparsely distributed polymorphic neurons scattered among abundant neuropile.

Presubplate stage

During the 10th, 11th and 12th weeks of gestation, the cortical plate increases in thickness and becomes densely packed with post-migratory cells. The cortical plate is thickest in the mid-lateral part of the neocortical anlage, above the level of the ganglionic eminence. Below the cortical plate, at the interface to the intermediate zone, there is a narrow, cell-sparse tissue band (Figure 2, right; Figure 3, left) containing large extracellular spaces and some large cell bodies with round, pale cell nuclei. This zone can be regarded as a part of the cortical anlage and as a forerunner of the subplate zone, thus a term *pre-subplate zone* is appropriate. In this developmental phase, the cortical anlage consists of three layers (from the pia to the ventricle): the marginal zone, cortical plate and pre-subplate zone. The cortical plate is the thickest part of the cortical anlage. The pre-subplate zone is already rich in dendritic and axonal processes, which belong mostly to the bipolar, radially orientated neurons situated in the deep part of the cortical plate. The pale cells in this zone are polymorphic neurons with well-pronounced dendrites, and they have pale, relatively homogeneous heterochromatin, indicating a higher level of differentiation than cells in the cortical plate. Furthermore, electron microscopy of the pre-subplate zone reveals a loose arrangement of neuronal processes of variable orientation that stands in contrast to the radial, geometrically regular arrangement of processes within the cortical plate and predominantly tangential arrangement of fiber bundles in the underlying intermediate zone.

Subplate formation stage

During a relatively short period, between the 12th and 13th post-ovulatory weeks, in the deep part of the cortical plate, the cell-packing density decreases and the border between the cortical plate and the pre-subplate zone becomes obscured. The whole cortical plate shows bilaminar organization: its superficial part is cell-dense, while its deep part is characterized by low cell-packing density (Figure 3, middle). Simultaneously, there is an enlargement of the pale, cell-poor zone below the cortical plate which merges with the deep part of the cortical plate. This broad but poorly delineated zone, interposed between the cortical plate above and the intermediate zone below, replaces the thin pre-subplate zone of the previous stage. Instead of the thin pre-subplate zone of the earlier stage, there now appears the permanently enlarging new layer, the *subplate zone*. So, the fetal cerebral wall at this age contains seven embryonic zones: the relatively acellular marginal zone, cell-dense cortical plate, fiber- and cell-rich upper subplate zone, cell-sparse lower subplate zone (subplate zone proper), intermediate fiber-rich zone, and densely cellular subventricular and ventricular zones (Figure 3, middle).

From the above description, it is clear that the subplate zone can be subdivided into two strata: the upper and the lower subplate. The upper subplate gives the impression of being a 'loose' part of the cortical plate – therefore, it was earlier designated as the 'second' cortical plate[64, 71]. However, we consider it as a subplate in formation for the following reasons: (a) unlike the cortical plate, the upper subplate zone has no strict radial arrangement of cell bodies and contains neurons with variable shapes and tinctorial properties; (b) both upper and lower subplate contain cell bodies orientated obliquely or parallel to the pia, and many of these cells have relatively elaborate dendritic trees; (c) synapses are present in both upper and lower subplate at this stage, but are absent from the cortical plate; (d) the gradual increase in width and the spread of the upper subplate zone suggests its transformation into the subplate zone proper; and (e) by the beginning of the next stage, there is only a single, uniformly populated cell-loose layer below the cortical plate. Finally, it should be noted that during this period different stages in the formation of the subplate zone can be seen in different parts of the telencephalic wall (Figure 4, left).

In summary, the major histogenetic events contributing to this enlargement of the deep, fibrous cortical anlage and the formation of the subplate zone are: ingrowth of axons, loss of radial cell orientation in the deep part of the cortical plate and growth of dendrites with intensive synaptogenesis.

Subplate stage

This stage lasts about 3 months in humans and 2 months in the monkey[16], and is characterized by the developmental maximum of the fetal lamination pattern[70]. At this stage, the neocortical anlage consists of the following three compartments: the marginal zone, cortical plate and subplate zone (Figure 3, right). Below the subplate zone, there are other transient pallial compartments: the intermediate, subventricular and ventricular zones. The main features of the lamination pattern are a thick cortical plate, which undergoes 'secondary' consolidation (at 16–18 weeks) and a very large, prominent, fibrous, synapse-rich subplate zone, which is the thickest zone of the cortical anlage during this period (Figure 4, right).

It is useful to subdivide the subplate stage into two distinct phases[16]: the phase of the increase in subplate thickness (during which the subplate dramatically expands) and the stationary phase of the subplate zone (in which the thickness of the subplate remains constantly high).

During the phase of increase in the subplate thickness (16–18 weeks), the overall thickness of the cerebral wall increases rapidly. The growth is mainly the result of a large influx of axons into this zone during midgestation[6, 7], rather than acquisition of new cells[6, 14, 16]. Toward the end of this period, the width of the subplate zone in humans is four times greater than that of the cortical plate, while in the monkey it is about three times thicker[16]. Three major types of cell can be distinguished in the subplate zone during this period[14, 16, 73, 74]: (1) immature bipolar post-mitotic migrating neurons, with dark, spindle-shaped nucleus, relatively thin trailing process and a more voluminous leading process; (2) immature astrocytes with multipolar stellate processes; and (3) large multipolar and pyramid-like neurons with round or oval nuclei, dispersed chromatin, and abundant cytoplasm rich in rough endoplasmatic reticulum. Furthermore, the subplate zone contains numerous axons and growth cones, as well as the thick shafts of radial glial cells; synapses are present throughout the entire thickness of the subplate and are predominantly of asymmetrical type associated with thick post-synaptic membrane densities and clear, round vesicles[4, 14, 16].

During the stationary phase (19–34 weeks), there are relatively few changes in the thickness of the subplate zone, although considerable changes occur in the other embryonic zones. The subplate zone remains the thickest and most easily delineated (Figure 6) stratum of the cerebral wall, but its thickness reveals significant regional variations, with the greatest size in the mid-lateral neocortical regions. Furthermore, the variations in the thick-

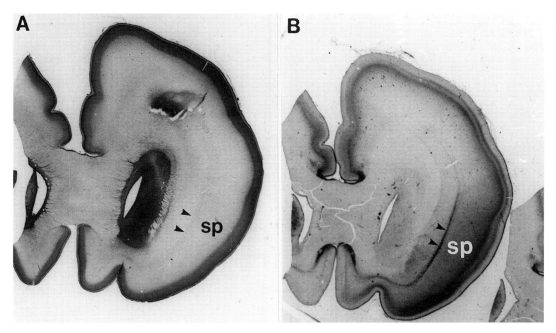

Figure 6 Low-power micrograph of the coronal sections across the frontal lobe in a 26-week-old human fetus, showing that the subplate zone (sp) can easily be delineated in both Nissl-stained (A) and acetylcholinesterase (AChE) histochemistry stained (B) preparations. Arrowheads mark the strongly AChE-reactive capsula externa (B) situated at the lower border of the subplate zone (A)

ness of the subplate zone are directly proportional to the amount of fiber tracts that accumulate below the cortical plate; the largest accumulation of such fibers (i.e. the thickest subplate) occurs preferentially at the places where gyri become pronounced[16].

Another remarkable change during the stationary phase concerns the level of cytological differentiation of the subplate neurons: the nuclei contain fine, dispersed chromatin and a large nucleolus, the volume of cytoplasm increases significantly and elaborate endoplasmic reticulum is present. Therefore, during this period, together with Cajal–Retzius cells of the marginal zone, subplate neurons are the most differentiated neurons in the neocortical areas (Figure 7).

One of the most prominent features of the subplate zone during the peak period of its thickness is that it maintains a loose, plexiform character (Figure 8). On the other hand, axons situated deeply in the intermediate zone begin to form large, densely packed fiber bundles, which segregate into axonal strata of preferential orientations[75].

Subplate dissolution stage

After 35 weeks of gestation, the subplate zone diminishes and eventually disappears at a relatively slow rate, during the prolonged period in which the external configuration of the cerebrum is dramatically changing, due to deepening of the primary fissures and emergence of secondary and tertiary sulci. In other words, the subplate dissolution stage coincides with the period when the final external configuration of the cerebral hemisphere is being formed. The dissolution of the subplate begins at the bottom of the sulci before it begins at the summit of the gyri, and this difference in time may be up to 8 weeks in the human and 4 weeks in the monkey[16]. For example, in the occipital lobe of the 7-day-old monkey and 1-month-old human infant, the subplate zone no longer exists as a distinct cytoarchitectonic entity[16]. In general, the subplate zone is resolved around the end of the first postnatal week in monkeys and the first postnatal month in humans, but (at least in the prefrontal cortex) a trace of it can be found until 2 months in monkeys and 6 months in humans[16].

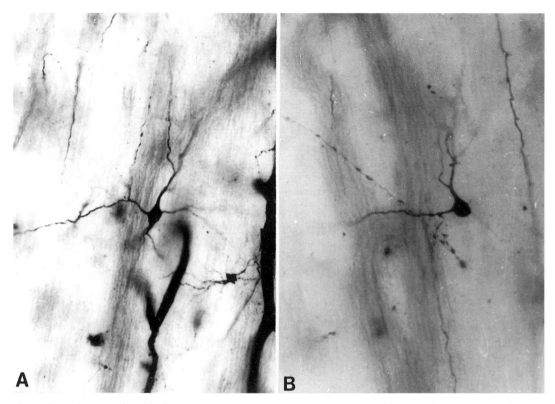

Figure 7 Golgi-stained multipolar neurons of the subplate zone in a 21-week-old human fetus. Typical multipolar neurons (A) or their varieties (B) are, together with Cajal–Retzius neurons of the marginal zone, the most differentiated neurons of the neocortical anlage at this stage

During this stage, the subplate zone contains large, mature cell bodies of random orientation, the growth cones become rare and the large extracellular space that characterizes the earlier period becomes drastically reduced; below the gradually diminishing subplate zone lies a large territory, which consists mainly of axonal bundles and several types of glial cells, i.e. the developing white matter. However, it should be noted that many subplate neurons survive beyond that period and become incorporated in the white matter as so-called interstitial cells[14].

In summary, neurons, growing cortical afferents and their synapses in the fetal human cerebrum form a sizeable transient tissue compartment situated below the developing cortical plate. This compartment is termed the subplate zone, represents an essential part of the cortical anlage, undergoes changes throughout the last two-thirds of gestation and gradually disappears during early

infancy. This subplate zone is characterized by the plexiform neuropil, numerous synapses, enlarged extracellular space and a 'waiting' complement of cortical afferents (see below); therefore, it can be considered to represent a continuously changing interface between incoming afferents and subplate cells situated below the developing cortical plate[16].

MORPHOLOGICAL, CHEMICAL AND CONNECTIONAL DIVERSITY OF SUBPLATE NEURONS

The subplate zone contains a heterogeneous population of neurons with a variety of connections and transmitters[16,35]. Furthermore, different developmental stages are characterized by both different types and different proportions of morphological types of subplate neurons[14,16,73,74].

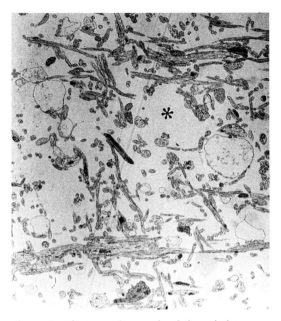

Figure 8 Electron micrograph of the subplate zone situated below the somatosensory cortical anlage in a 24-week-old human fetus. Note the loose, plexiform character and a prominent extracellular space (asterisk)

In the pre-subplate stage (10–12 weeks of gestation), the relatively few neurons in the presubplate zone are more differentiated than those in the cortical plate itself. These neurons can be distinguished as polymorphous and bipolar. Polymorphous neurons have horizontally or obliquely orientated oval or irregularly shaped cell bodies, from which two or three dendrites protrude in all directions and then branch several times. The bipolar neurons of the pre-subplate zone are orientated vertically; they have larger cell bodies than those in the cortical plate and their apical dendrites can be seen to reach the marginal zone, in which they branch[73].

In the subplate formation stage (13–15 weeks of gestation), the neurons in the subplate zone are more differentiated and possess a larger number of dendrites than the neurons in the cortical plate; they are polymorphous and with variable orientation. In addition to polymorphous neurons, bipolar vertically orientated migrating neurons and horizontal bipolar or unipolar neurons are frequently observed throughout the subplate and intermediate zones.

At the beginning of the subplate stage (16 weeks), three major types of cell can be distinguished in the subplate zone[16]: immature bipolar (post-mitotic) migrating neurons, immature astrocytes, and large multipolar and pyramid-like subplate neurons. Different types of subplate neuron can be observed for the first time at 17 weeks of gestation[73]: fusiform-like neurons, inverted pyramidal neurons, pyramidal neurons with their usual shape and orientation, and polymorphous neurons. An additional cell type, the large multipolar neuron, is found in the subplate zone between 19 and 23 weeks of gestation[73]. The axons of fusiform neurons either ascend toward the cortical plate or descend into the intermediate zone; characteristic ascending axons of inverted pyramidal neurons probably project to the cortical plate, while the axons of 'normally' orientated subplate pyramidal neurons usually descend toward the intermediate zone. The axons of multipolar neurons extend into a horizontal, a descending or an ascending direction[73]. During this period, the subplate zone also contains migrating neurons, numerous immature neurons with small cell bodies and horizontal or oblique dendrites, radial glia fibers and immature astrocytes[16].

In accordance with these, during the developmental peak (stationary phase) of the subplate zone, there are five well-differentiated types of subplate neuron[16]: (1) giant multipolar neurons with an asymmetrical stellate orientation of long smooth dendrites that run randomly for about 1 mm; (2) a pyramidal neuron with the main apical dendrite directed towards the pia, which, in contrast to the pyramids of the cortical plate, have fewer basal dendritic branches; (3) a large, fusiform neuron with a long main dendrite having few side branches; (4) a pyramidal neuron with apical dendrite orientated away from the pia; and (5) a polymorphous neuron with a pear-shaped body and polarized orientation of dendritic branching.

At this stage of development, most axons of the subplate neurons ascend toward the cortical plate, while the remaining axons run into the deep part of the pallium or remain in the subplate zone. The highest frequency of ascending axons is observed in inverted pyramidal neurons (about 90%) and in polymorphous neurons (about 60%); approximately equal numbers of axons of the multipolar and fusiform neurons follow either an ascending or a descending course[73]. Furthermore, some spine-like protrusions on the cell bodies and dendrites of multipolar, polymorphous and fusiform subplate neurons appear at this stage of development[73].

In the late prematurus (32–34 weeks of gestation), subplate neurons show further dendritic differentiation, especially approximately 1.5 mm below the fetal layer VI[74]. One can observe varicosities and growth-cone-like terminal tips on dendrites and short, newly formed branches arising from the main dendrites of subplate neurons. About half the population of all types of subplate neurons have ascending axons and the other half have axons descending toward the subcortical anlage. At the end of the preterm infant period (36 weeks of gestation) another interneuron type appears in the subplate zone – a small type of neuron with strictly local axonal arborization which probably corresponds to the 'neurogliaform cell' of Cajal[74]. These small interneurons, which in the preterm infant are only found in the subplate zone, are already present in the cortical layers during the first 3 postnatal months.

In the newborn, the subplate zone has mainly disappeared from the bottom of the sulci, but it is still present in the summit of the gyri. However, the same classes of subplate neurons as at previous stages are nevertheless observed, and their orientation varies from horizontal to perpendicular and oblique with respect to the pial surface. The dendrites of the subplate neurons extend as much as those observed in the previous stage (the dendritic extent of some fusiform neurons is 0.6–1 mm), and a substantial number of short dendritic spines was observed on the dendrites of subplate (especially the fusiform-like) neurons[73]. The axons of subplate neurons have a number of collaterals within the subplate zone. It should be noted that during the early postnatal period fusiform neurons with very long dendrites are the most frequently encountered subplate cell type in the white matter fiber bundles, and a constant increase of spine number can be observed in these neurons between 1 and 7 months of age[74]. A rich morphological diversity of subplate neuronal types has also been documented in the monkey[10, 12, 14, 16, 76–80], carnivore[27–30, 37, 38, 40–42, 56, 58, 81] and rodent brain[47, 53, 54, 82–84].

The neurochemical diversity of subplate neurons even surpasses the diversity of their morphological types. For example, in only the human cortex, the following neurotransmitters, neuropeptides, transmitter-related enzymes and other specific molecular markers have thus far been demonstrated in the subplate neurons or their descendants in the adult brain, interstitial neurons: GABA[85, 86], substance P[86, 87], somatostatin[88, 89], neuropeptide Y[86, 90, 91], AChE[14, 92, 93], NADPH diaphorase[94, 95], MAP2[23], p75 low affinity nerve growth factor (NGF) receptor[96], NCAM[96], Alz-50, a putative degeneration marker[74, 98], and plasma proteins albumin, prealbumin, transferrin and α-fetoprotein[99].

GABAergic neurons were demonstrated in the subplate zone of the human[85, 86], monkey[12, 21], cat[27, 31, 81], ferret[100] and rodent brain[46, 47, 53, 101, 102]. Furthermore, GABA-A receptors are present in the monkey subplate[12, 103] and benzodiazepine binding sites were noted beneath the developing rat cortical plate[104]. It is interesting to note, however, that GABA labelling in neurons beneath the cortical plate appears very early[27, 47, 53, 102], as early as embryonic days E45–E50 in the monkey[105, 106] or 14th week of gestation in the human[85]. Therefore, GABA and GABA-A receptors may also be involved in trophic processes in the early cortical anlage[12]. It should also be noted that GABA-positive fibers and even somata have been detected in the cortical white matter of adult monkeys[107, 108]. Finally, choline acetyltransferase-immunoreactive subplate neurons were observed in fetal monkey cortex[78] as well as in rat cortex[82]. Furthermore, a variety of neuropeptides are present in subplate neurons of monkeys, carnivores and rodents: neuropeptide Y[21, 27, 29, 30, 40, 79], cholecystokinin[29, 30, 78], somatostatin[21, 27, 29–31, 42, 75], substance P[42, 76, 80, 84], and vasoactive intestinal peptide[41].

Since GABAergic neurons are interneurons, and most neuropeptides are co-localized in subpopulations of GABAergic neurons or are otherwise shown to be present exclusively in local circuit neurons, it is not surprising that local functional synaptic connections were successfully demonstrated in the subplate zone of cats[27, 31, 32, 109] and ferrets[31]. Axons of subplate cells also terminate within the developing cortical plate[27, 31, 32, 38, 40, 41, 73].

However, a subpopulation of subplate neurons are undoubtedly long-projection neurons: subplate axons terminate in the thalamus of the cat[36], ferret[31], rat[48] and monkey[110]; in the superior colliculus of the cat[36]; and in the contralateral hemisphere in the cat[27], ferret[31] and monkey[9, 10, 111, 112]. Accordingly, the uptake of excitatory amino acids (as major transmitters of cortical projection neurons) was demonstrated in the subplate neurons of the cat and ferret[31].

Finally, it has been demonstrated that subplate neurons receive synaptic input from other subplate neurons[31, 32, 109], from developing cortical plate neurons[113, 114] and from thalamic axons[115].

THE 'WAITING' COMPARTMENT FOR GROWING CORTICAL AFFERENTS

The complement of axons, which wait in the subcortical position prior to entering the cortical plate, were discovered following injection of radioactive tracers into the fetal eye that pass transneuronally to thalamocortical afferents[7]. Since thalamocortical fiber systems remain in the subcortical position for a considerable period of time before entering the cortex, it was proposed that this entire zone should be considered a 'waiting' compartment[7]. This 'waiting' compartment is, in fact, the subplate zone[6], which in the primate and human brain serves as a temporary target not only for growing thalamocortical[7, 15–17, 116], but also for basal forebrain[117], ipsilateral and callosal corticocortical[9, 10, 112] and probably monoaminergic afferents[24]. The 'waiting period' was also demonstrated in developing carnivore and rodent brain[34, 44, 49, 50–52, 118–123], although a recent study questioned its existence in the rat[124].

With respect to the sequential ingrowth of various cortical afferents, it is generally considered that monoaminergic afferents are first to enter the subplate zone, while cholinergic afferents originating from the basal forebrain seem to be a second class of afferents that enter the subplate zone before the thalamocortical fibers[16, 117]. However, the growth of both basal forebrain and thalamocortical systems significantly overlaps within the subplate zone[16]. The ipsilateral and contralateral corticocortical connections arrive last and

remain the longest in the subplate zone; they also represent the largest proportion of axons in the subplate in both the monkey and the human brain[16].

In the human fetus at 15–24 weeks of gestation, ingrowing afferents of basal forebrain and thalamic origin 'wait' in the subplate zone[15–17, 117] (see Figures 9; 10; 11, left). This transient deep concentration of pre-synaptic axons, synapses and post-synaptic elements within the subplate zone changes dramatically between 24 and 28 weeks of gestation, when thalamocortical fibers penetrate the cortical plate (see Figures 9, middle; 11, right). During this period, thalamocortical fibers display transient intensive AChE reactivity and columnar distribution[17, 125]. The appearance of thalamocortical afferents in the prestriate visual[15], auditory[126, 127] and somatosensory[16] cortices correlates well with the development of synapses in the cortical plate after the 23rd week[4]. Furthermore, the elaboration of terminal fields of thalamocortical axons within the prospective layer IV of the cortical plate parallels the intensive development of dendrites of layer III pyramidal neurons[73, 74] and in some parts of the cortical anlage one can see the initial vertical segregation of the thalamocortical fibers[17]. In the monkey visual cortex, geniculocortical axons are present in layer 4 at embryonic day E124, while by E144 ocular dominance columns begin to form[7, 128] and are complete by 6–10 postnatal weeks[129, 130].

Experimental studies in the monkey have shown that commissural corticocortical fibers reside in the subplate zone between embryonic days E100 and E123[9]. Ipsilateral corticocortical fibers also 'wait' in the subplate zone for several weeks before entering the cortical plate[10, 111]. In addition, some subplate neurons transiently send their axons through the corpus callosum[10]. In the monkey, callosal axons are at birth three times more numerous than in the adult[131] and the final number is achieved by the process of competitive elimination during the early postnatal period[19, 131]. These data point to the considerable postnatal reorganization of corticocortical connectivity. Since in the human cortex, 'waiting' associative and commissural pathways are major constituents of the subplate zone after 28 weeks of gestation[16], and since the development proceeds in humans more slowly than in the monkey, we expect that

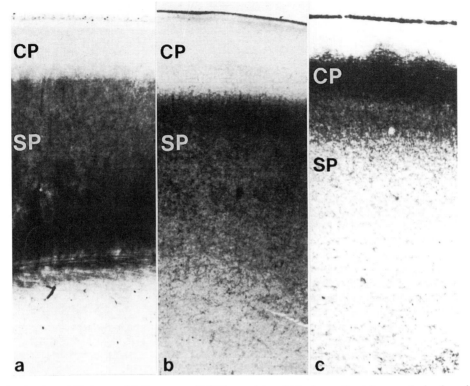

Figure 9 Laminar shifts in acetylcholinesterase (AChE)-reactivity within the prefrontal neocortical anlage during the mid-fetal and late fetal periods. The subplate zone contains strongly AChE-reactive thalamocortical afferents from the mediodorsal nucleus in an 18-week-old (a) and 22-week-old (b) human fetus, while at 28 weeks (c), AChE reactivity has shifted towards the cortical plate and appears to be particularly dense in prospective layer III. CP, cortical plate; SP, subplate zone

this protracted postnatal reorganization of cortico-cortical connectivity is even more pronounced in the human brain.

THE SITE OF TRANSIENT SYNAPSES AND A SUBSTRATE OF NEURONAL INTERACTIONS

The development of synapses in the human cortical anlage begins after the formation of the cortical plate at the end of the 8th week of gestation. There are very few synapses in the cortical anlage during this period and they are distributed in bilaminar fashion: a superficial synaptic lamina is within the boundaries of the marginal zone, whereas the deep synaptic lamina is situated below the cortical plate and corresponds to the pre-subplate zone[4,5,16].

Furthermore, the earliest post-synaptic elements, dendrites, also develop in bilaminar fashion above and below the cortical plate, in the marginal and pre-subplate zone, respectively. Deep dendrites distributed within the pre-subplate zone belong to the basal dendritic arborizations of neurons in the cortical plate as well as to early maturing neurons of the pre-subplate zone[16].

The number of synapses increases significantly within the newly formed subplate zone between the 13th and 15th weeks of gestation[4,16]. Between the 16th and 19th weeks of gestation, many axons grow into the subplate zone and this zone becomes the most significant site of synaptogenesis in the cortical anlage (the other zone with intensive early synaptogenesis is the marginal zone). Significant numbers of synapses develop within the cortical plate only after the 19th week of gestation, but

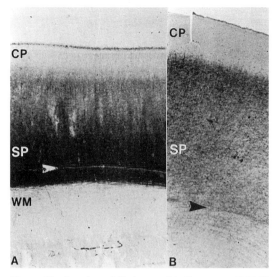

Figure 10 Laminar shifts in acetylcholinesterase (AChE) reactivity within the somatosensory neocortical anlage during the mid-fetal period. (A) Strongly AChE-reactive subplate zone (SP) (left) is situated between AChE-negative cortical plate (CP) and AChE-positive fiber bundles of the external capsule (arrowhead) in 18-week-old human fetus, while the fiber systems lying within the fetal 'white matter' (WM) are AChE-negative. (B) At 22 weeks of gestation (right), the overall AChE reactivity within the subplate zone has decreased (arrowhead marks the border between the subplate zone and fetal white matter). Note the shift in AChE reactivity from deep (in A) to superficial (in B) subplate zone, probably reflecting the outward relocation of 'waiting' thalamocortical afferents before their penetration into the cortical plate

intensive synaptogenesis occurs between the 24th and 28th weeks of gestation, when thalamocortical fibers leave the subplate zone and penetrate the cortical plate[4, 16, 132]. After the 24th week of gestation, synaptogenesis within the cortical plate occurs in a deep-to-superficial fashion. The same pattern of synaptogenesis has been documented for the corresponding stages of the developing monkey cerebral cortex[13, 16, 133–139].

These studies have clearly demonstrated that the subplate zone is a major site of synaptogenesis in the developing cortical anlage. However, since the subplate neurons are transient fetal populations of cells, it is important to know whether the subplate neurons directly participate in transient synaptic circuits and what is the role of these transient synapses.

As already mentioned above, the subplate neurons are both projection and local circuit neurons. The presence of synaptic contacts on the subplate neurons has been demonstrated by the localization of synaptic vesicle antigens[140] and electron-microscopic analysis[14, 16, 140]. Subplate neurons receive synaptic input from other subplate neurons[31, 32, 109], from developing cortical plate neurons[113, 114] and from thalamic axons[115].

Many of the synapses in the subplate have typical symmetric membrane junctions[16], suggesting that they may be GABAergic in nature[12]. As many subplate neurons are GABAergic[12, 31, 47, 85] and GABA-A receptors are found on the dendrites of subplate cells[12], at least some of the targets of GABAergic subplate axons are likely to be dendrites of other subplate neurons.

Some synapses remain on the interstitial neurons as the surviving remnants of the subplate neurons[14], but most of them are transient and are eliminated during the subsequent development. One logical explanation for the loss of synapses from the subplate zone is the relocation of the thalamocortical afferents to the cortical plate[6, 7, 16, 128]. The possible role of subplate neurons in transient fetal circuits will be discussed in the last section of this chapter.

THE FORMATION OF CEREBRAL CONVOLUTIONS AND CORTICAL PARCELLATION

Experimental studies in developing monkeys suggest that the pattern and amount of thalamocortical and corticocortical connections may play a major role in the formation of cerebral convolutions[8, 141]. Furthermore, the marked regional differences in subplate thickness occur in association with the emergence of sulci and gyri and the developmental peak of the subplate zone coincides with the establishment of the gyral pattern in the monkey and human brain[16]. It has recently been proposed that the highest elaboration of the subplate zone in primates may serve as a substrate for the competition of a large contingent of corticocortical connections during parcellation of cytoarchitectonic areas and the formation of cerebral convolutions[8, 16]; this proposal is based on the following lines of evidence:

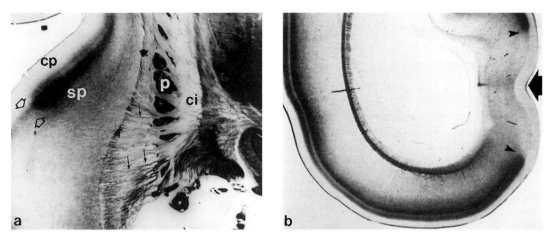

Figure 11 Acetylcholinesterase (AChE)-reactivity of 'waiting' thalamocortical afferents within the subplate zone can serve as a marker of an early areal parcellation within the neocortex. (a) Low-power micrograph (left) of the superior temporal cortex in a 22-week-old human fetus (AChE staining). Note boundaries of the prospective auditory cortex (empty arrowheads), approaching thalamocortical fibers (arrows), and capsula externa (black arrowhead). cp, cortical plate; sp, subplate zone; p, putamen, ci, capsula interna. (b) Section across the occipital lobe (right) in a 26-week-old human fetus, demonstrating AChE-labelled projections from the pulvinar to the prestriate visual cortex. By this fetal age, positively stained fibers are present in the cortical plate itself. The calcarine fissure is indicated by a thick arrow. Note the rather abrupt fall-off in AChE staining in the cortex at the borderline between prospective areas 17 and 18 (arrowheads)

(1) The subplate zone is considerably thinner in species with a lissencephalic brain, such as rodents[142–144], than in species with a gyrencephalic brain, such as the cat[25, 26, 37, 38] and ferret[43];

(2) The subplate zone expands further in primates and reaches the largest size in the human fetus[14, 16];

(3) There is a progressively larger increase in the relative size of the subplate zone in comparison with the increase in thickness of the cortical plate as the cerebrum becomes convoluted – for example, the ratio between the thickness of the subplate zone and that of the cortical plate in the lateral neocortex is approximately 4:1 in the human, 3:1 in the monkey, 1:1 in the cat, and 1:2 in mice and rats[16];

(4) Both temporal and spatial parameters indicate that the content and size of the subplate zone in primates reflects the overlapping, but sequential ingrowth of afferents from the brainstem, basal forebrain and thalamus as well as a large contingent of callosal and association fibers[9, 10, 15–17, 117];

(5) The ipsilateral and contralateral cortico-cortical connections arrive last and remain the longest in the subplate zone; they also represent the largest proportion of axons in this transient zone in both monkey and human brain[9, 10, 16, 111, 112, 131, 145];

(6) The thickness of the subplate zone is proportional to the number of contributing cortico-cortical fiber systems[146] – for example, the subplate zone situated below the somatosensory area, which is abundant in callosal and association fibers, is thicker than the subplate zone in the visual area where these fibers are less numerous[14,16]. Likewise, the hippocampal region, which receives a small contingent of thalamic and commissural inputs, also has a thin subplate zone[147, 148];

(7) The subplate zone reaches its maximal size and lasts the longest in the human association cortex; and

(8) The postnatal shaping of tertiary gyri in the frontal cortex is accompanied by the more prolonged existence of the subplate zone in this region[74, 132, 147, 149].

In conclusion, information from the literature indicates that the duration of the subplate zone may expand in evolution to allow the genesis of a larger number of corticocortical fibers, which in turn may be responsible for the shaping of cerebral gyral and the sulcal pattern. In other words, the subplate zone may participate in the three-dimensional modelling of the cortical architecture during gyral formation[16].

CORTICAL PLASTICITY AFTER THE PERINATAL LESIONS

The subplate zone may serve as a substrate for cortical repair following neonatal injuries. For example, the resection of the cortex in the fetal and perinatal monkey, which leaves intact the subplate zone, results in milder abnormalities than when the ablation involves the subplate itself or is conducted after its resolution[8, 141, 150]. Moreover, as the subplate zone is the thickest part of the prenatal human cortex and contains fetal neurons, 'waiting' axons and synapses, it is logical to assume that the variety of transiently arranged, growing neuronal elements and transmitter-related substances of the subplate zone participate in the plastic changes and reconstitutive processes after perinatal brain damage in humans.

Therefore, we correlated neuroanatomical developmental parameters with sequential ultrasonography scans to reveal the structural basis of functional recovery after early focal hypoxic lesions of the human frontal lobe in premature infants[146]. We studied two groups of live-born infants: (1) younger (lesion occurred between 26 and 34 weeks of gestation) and (2) older (lesion occurred between 37 weeks and term). Indeed, ultrasonography revealed remarkable structural rearrangements of the cerebral wall when the hypoxic lesion occurred during the developmental peak of the subplate zone (i.e. in low-birth-weight infants). Anechoic cavities ('cysts') developed rapidly (within 3 weeks) in premature brains, the rebuilding of these lesions continued after birth, and cavities disappeared around the 11th month[146]. More specifically, these structural rearrangements in premature infants were present in eight of 17 cases in the younger vs. eight of 56 cases in the older group.

Among all cerebral compartments, the subplate zone shows the greatest proportion of the extracellular space and, thus, the plexiform, loose arrangement of its cellular elements may contribute substantially to the vigorous development of cavities in the brains of premature infants characterized by the prominent subplate zone. Both waiting afferents and fetal cells residing in the subplate zone probably recover from the hypoxic episode and may participate in the structural reconstitution and plastic changes occurring after the perinatal developmental lesion. Furthermore, after the lesion has occurred, subplate neurons and axons may be more readily rerouted than other cortical cells, which show a strict modular arrangement and more rigid connectivity. Finally, changes in the connectivity after perinatal lesion may promote the survival of some subplate neurons.

In conclusion, although further studies of this topic are certainly warranted, we propose that the transient population of 'waiting' axons and cells of the subplate zone participate in structural and functional plasticity of the human cerebral cortex after perinatal brain damage.

THE DEVELOPMENTAL FATE OF SUBPLATE NEURONS

The subplate neurons are cogenerated with the Cajal–Retzius neurons of the marginal zone, and both types of cell represent the earliest generated cell of the cortical anlage which are born before neurons destined for future cortical layers II–VI[25, 26, 30, 43, 45, 55, 83].

While a significant proportion of subplate neurons is eliminated by cell death[14, 25, 26, 37, 38, 40, 54], a certain population survives and becomes incorporated into the adult white matter as interstitial neurons[14, 29, 54]. In addition, the extent of subplate neuron death is almost certainly not the same in all species, nor is it likely to be uniform between cortical areas or among the different subplate neuron phenotypes in a given species[14, 16, 30, 35, 73, 74, 80]. For example, a substantial proportion of subplate neurons in rodents survive in adults, as part of layer VIb[54, 83], while about 90% of subplate neurons in the cat die during the first postnatal month[29, 30].

On the other hand, a conservative semiquantitative estimate indicates that at least 5 million subplate neurons survive as interstitial cells in the 2-month-old rhesus monkey and many more in the human infant[14]. Thus, the total number of interstitial cells in the primate telencephalon probably approaches the number of neurons in the inferior olive, red nucleus, medial geniculate and lateral geniculate nucleus combined[14].

Those subplate neurons which do degenerate display the features of dying mature neurons: a swelling of the endoplasmic reticulum and Golgi apparatus followed by a progressive darkening of the cytoplasm[14,38,40]. While the mechanism by which subplate neurons die is unknown, several molecular changes accompanying subplate neuron death have been described[39,98,151,152]. For example, an antibody termed SP-1 labelled transiently and exclusively the subplate neurons of the cat at a time that corresponded to the peak of cell death[151]. Another monoclonal antibody, Alz-50, which is thought to be a general marker for dying neurons, labelled the subplate neurons in the rat[152], cat[39] and human[74,97] during a period of active cell death.

Although immunoreactive neurons labelled with the Alz-50 in the human brain are occasionally present in the subplate as early as 25 weeks of gestation, a large increase in their number is observed in the preterm infant period around 34 weeks, when members of all types of subplate neurons are stained with Alz-50 antibody[74]. In the preterm infant, Alz-50-immunoreactive neurons are present exclusively in the subplate zone, and some of these neurons have swollen and patchily stained dendrites[74]. The highest frequencies of Alz-50-immunoreactive neurons have been observed from 34 weeks of gestation until birth; however, it should be noted that Alz-50-immunoreactive subplate neurons nevertheless represent only a minority of all subplate neurons present in the preterm infant and newborn.

Survival and death of subplate neurons may be under the control of neurotrophic factors. For example, subplate neurons express the low-affinity NGF receptor p75 soon after they become post-mitotic[153] and expression of this receptor remains high during maturation of the subplate neurons and the waiting period for thalamic axons[153,154]; however, just before the subplate neurons begin to die, they lose p75 NGF receptor immunoreactivity[153]. It is fair to say that these topics still need further investigation and that the exact mechanisms of subplate neuron death or survival are still unknown.

THE POSSIBLE FUNCTIONAL ROLES OF THE SUBPLATE ZONE AND NEURONS

In the previous sections we have discussed the role of the subplate zone in the formation of cerebral convolutions and cytoarchitectonic parcellation of the cerebral cortex, as well as the role of the subplate in cortical plasticity after perinatal lesions. Furthermore, we have stressed the significance of the subplate zone as the 'waiting' compartment for various cortical afferents and as the major site of synaptogenesis in the early cortical anlage; finally, we have pointed out that subplate neurons are involved in transient fetal circuits. Obviously, the subplate neurons display a variety of morphological, neurochemical types, act both as projection and local circuit neurons, and receive a variety of synaptic inputs. It is not surprising, therefore, that a number of investigators have proposed diverse roles for subplate neurons in cortical development. Since the major part of this chapter has expressed our views, in order to provide the reader with wider scope, we will conclude by listing the major concepts emerging from the current literature on the role of the subplate in cortical development.

(1) The connection between the marginal and subplate zone constitutes the first functional circuit identified in the developing mammalian cortex and can be recognized at early stages prior to the maturation of the cortical plate[16,32,56,58];

(2) Subplate neurons act as intermediate links between white matter axons and cells of the cortical plate, and thus mediate the differentiation of the neurons and connectional circuits of the cortical plate[32,83];

(3) The subplate zone serves as a compartment for transient cellular interactions with 'waiting'

cortical afferents and provides trophic support prior to their invasion of the cortical plate [16, 27, 32, 120];

(4) At later developmental stages, subplate neurons may provide a crucial link required for the normal segregation of geniculocortical axons into ocular dominance columns [122,123];

(5) Subplate neurons may locally regulate neurite outgrowth [28, 53];

(6) By expression of inhibitory neurotransmitters, subplate neurons may protect developing cortical plate cells prior to the elaboration of intracortical inhibitory circuits from possible excitotoxic effects induced by the excitatory transmitters of the afferent projection systems [40, 41]; and

(7) 'Pioneer' axons of subplate neurons may play a critical role in establishing cortical efferent projections [35, 36, 48].

ACKNOWLEDGEMENTS

This work was supported by a grant awarded through the Croatian Ministry of Science. The excellent technical assistance of Zdenka Cmuk, Danica Budinšćak and Božica Popović is cordially appreciated.

References

1. Kostović, I., Judaš, M., Kostović-Knežević, Lj., Šimić, G., Delalle, I., Chudy, D., Šajin, B. and Petanjek, Z. (1991). Zagreb Research Collection of human brains for developmental neurobiologists and clinical neuroscientists. *Int. J. Dev. Biol.*, **35**, 215–30

2. Kostović, I., Molliver, M.E. and Van der Loos, H. (1973). The laminar distribution of synapses in neocortex of fetal dog. *Anat. Rec.*, **175**, 362

3. Cragg, B.G. (1972). The development of synapses in cat visual cortex. *Invest. Ophthalmol.*, **11**, 377–85

4. Molliver, M.E., Kostović, I. and Van der Loos, H. (1973). The development of synapses in cerebral cortex in the human fetus. *Brain Res.*, **50**, 403–7

5. Kostović, I. and Molliver, M.E. (1974). A new interpretation of the laminar development of cerebral cortex: synaptogenesis in different layers of neopallium in the human fetus. *Anat. Rec.*, **178**, 395

6. Rakic, P. (1982). Early developmental events: cell lineages, acquisition of neuronal positions, and areal and laminar development. *Neurosci. Res. Prog. Bull.*, **20**, 439–51

7. Rakic, P. (1977). Prenatal development of the visual system in the rhesus monkey. *Phil. Trans. R. Soc. (London) B.*, **278**, 245–60

8. Rakic, P. (1988). Specification of cerebral cortical areas. *Science*, **241**, 170–6

9. Goldman-Rakic, P.S. (1982). Neuronal development and plasticity of association cortex in primates. *Neurosci. Res. Prog. Bull.*, **20**, 520–32

10. Schwartz, M.L., Rakic, P. and Goldman-Rakic, P.S. (1991). Early phenotype expression of cortical neurons: evidence that a subclass of migratory neurons have callosal axons. *Proc. Natl. Acad. Sci. USA*, **88**, 1354–8

11. Lidow, M., Goldman-Rakic, P.S. and Rakic, P. (1991). Synchronized development of neurotransmitter receptors in diverse regions of the primate cerebral cortex. *Proc. Natl. Acad. Sci. USA*, **88**, 10218–21

12. Meinecke, D.L. and Rakic, P. (1992). Expression of GABA and GABA-A receptors by neurons of the subplate zone in developing primate occipital cortex; evidence for transient local circuits. *J. Comp. Neurol.*, **317**, 91–101

13. Bourgeois, J.P. and Rakic, P. (1993). Changes of synaptic density in the primary visual cortex of the macaque monkey from fetal to adult stage. *J. Neurosci.*, **13**, 2801–20

14. Kostović, I. and Rakic, P. (1980). Cytology and time of origin of interstitial neurons in the white matter in infant and adult human and monkey telencephalon. *J. Neurocytol.*, **9**, 210–42

15. Kostović, I. and Rakic, P. (1984). Development of prestriate visual projections in the monkey and human fetal cerebrum revealed by transient cholinesterase staining. *J. Neurosci.*, **4**, 25–42

16. Kostović, I. and Rakic, P. (1990). Developmental history of the transient subplate zone in the visual and somatosensory cortex of the macaque monkey and human brain. *J. Comp. Neurol.*, **297**, 441–70

17. Kostović, I. and Goldman-Rakic, P.S. (1983). Transient cholinesterase staining in the mediodorsal nucleus of the thalamus and its connections in the developing human and monkey brain. *J. Comp. Neurol.*, **219**, 431–47

18. Burkhalter, A. (1993). Development of forward and feedback connections between areas V1 and V2 of human visual cortex. *Cerebral Cortex*, **3**, 476–87

19. Chalupa, L.M. and Killackey, H.P. (1989). Process elimination underlies ontogenetic change in the distribution of callosal projection neurons in the postcentral gyrus of the fetal rhesus monkey. *Proc. Natl. Acad. Sci. USA*, **86**, 1076–9

20. Hendrickson, A.E., Van Brederode, J.F., Mulligan, K.A. and Celio, M.R. (1991). Development of the calcium-binding protein parvalbumin and calbindin in monkey striate cortex. *J. Comp. Neurol.*, **307**, 626–46

21. Huntley, G.W., Hendry, S.H.C., Killackey, H.P., Chalupa, L.M. and Jones, E.G. (1988). Temporal sequence of neurotransmitter expression by developing neurons of fetal monkey visual cortex. *Dev. Brain Res.*, **43**, 69–96

22. Kennedy, H. and Dehay, C. (1993). Cortical specification of mice and men. *Cerebral Cortex*, **3**, 171–86

23. Sims, K.B., Crandall, J.E., Kosik, K.S. and Williams, R.S. (1988). Microtubule-associated protein 2 (MAP2) immunoreactivity in human fetal neocortex. *Brain Res.*, **449**, 192–200

24. Verney, C., Milošević, A., Alvarez, C. and Berger, B. (1993). Immunocytochemical evidence of well-developed dopaminergic and noradrenergic innervations in the frontal cerebral cortex of human fetuses at midgestation. *J. Comp. Neurol.*, **336**, 331–44

25. Luskin, M.B. and Shatz, C.J. (1985). Neurogenesis of the cat's primary visual cortex. *J. Comp. Neurol.*, **242**, 611–31

26. Luskin, M.B. and Shatz, C.J. (1985). Studies of the earliest generated cells of the cat's visual cortex: cogeneration of subplate and marginal zones. *J. Neurosci.*, **5**, 1062–75

27. Chun, J.J.M., Nakamura, M.J. and Shatz, C.J. (1987). Transient cells of the developing mammalian telencephalon are peptide-immunoreactive neurons. *Nature (London)*, **325**, 617–20

28. Shatz, C.J., Chun, J.J.M. and Luskin, M.B. (1988). The role of the subplate in the development of the mammalian telencephalon. In Peters, A. and Jones, E.G. (eds.) *Cerebral Cortex*, vol. 7; *Development and Maturation of Cerebral Cortex*, pp. 35–58. (New York and London: Plenum Press)

29. Chun, J.J.M. and Shatz, C.J. (1989). Interstitial cells of the adult neocortical white matter are the remnant of the early-generated subplate neuron population. *J. Comp. Neurol.*, **282**, 555–69

30. Chun, J.J.M. and Shatz, C.J. (1989). The earliest-generated neurons of the cat cerebral cortex: characterization by MAP2 and neurotransmitter immunohistochemistry during fetal life. *J. Neurosci.*, **9**, 1648–67

31. Antonini, A. and Shatz, C.J. (1990). Relation between putative transmitter phenotypes and connectivity of subplate neurons during cerebral cortical development. *Eur. J. Neurosci.*, **2**, 744–61

32. Friauf, E., McConnell, S.K. and Shatz, C.J. (1990). Functional synaptic circuits in the subplate during fetal and early postnatal development of cat visual cortex. *J. Neurosci.*, **10**, 2601–13

33. Ghosh, A., Antonini, A., McConnell, S.K. and Shatz, C.J. (1990). Requirement for subplate neurons in the formation of thalamocortical connections. *Nature (London)*, **347**, 179–81

34. Ghosh, A. and Shatz, C.J. (1993). A role of subplate neurons in the patterning of connections from thalamus to neocortex. *Development*, **117**, 1031–47

35. Allendoerfer, K.L. and Shatz, C.J. (1994). The subplate, a transient neocortical structure: its role in the development of connections between thalamus and cortex. *Annu. Rev. Neurosci.*, **17**, 185–218

36. McConnell, S.K., Ghosh, A. and Shatz, C.J. (1989). Subplate neurons pioneer the first axon pathway from the cerebral cortex. *Science*, **245**, 978–82

37. Valverde, F. and Facal-Valverde, M.V. (1987). Transitory population of cells in the temporal cortex of kittens. *Dev. Brain Res.*, **32**, 283–8

38. Valverde, F. and Facal-Valverde, M.V. (1988). Postnatal development of interstitial (subplate) cells in the white matter of the temporal cortex of kittens: a correlated Golgi and electron microscopic study. *J. Comp. Neurol.*, **269**, 168–92

39. Valverde, F., Lopez-Mascaraque, L.I. and DeCarlos, J.A. (1990). Distribution and morphology of Alz-50 immunoreactive cells in the developing visual cortex of kittens. *J. Neurocytol.*, **19**, 662–71

40. Wahle, P. and Meyer, G. (1987). Morphology and quantitative changes of transient NPY-ir neuronal populations during early postnatal development of the cat visual cortex. *J. Comp. Neurol.*, **261**, 165–92

41. Wahle, P. and Meyer, G. (1989). Early postnatal development of vasoactive intestinal polypeptide- and peptide histidine isoleucine-immunoreactive structures in the cat visual cortex. *J. Comp. Neurol.*, **282**, 215–48

42. Wahle, P. (1993). Differential regulation of substance P and somatostatin in Martinotti cells of the developing cat visual cortex. *J. Comp. Neurol.*, **329**, 519–38

43. Jackson, C.A., Peduzzi, J.D. and Hickey, T.L. (1989). Visual cortex development in the ferret. I. Genesis and migration of visual cortical neurons. *J. Neurosci.*, **9**, 1242–53

44. Johnson, J.K. and Casagrande, V.A. (1993). Prenatal development of axon outgrowth and connectivity in the ferret visual system. *Vis. Neurosci.*, **10**, 117–30

45. Bayer, S.A. and Altman, J. (1990). Development of layer I and the subplate in rat neocortex. *Exp. Neurol.*, **107**, 48–62

46. Cobas, A., Fairen, A., Alvarez-Bolado, G. and Sanchez, M.P. (1991). Prenatal development of the

intrinsic neurons of the rat neocortex: a comparative study of the distribution of GABA-immunoreactive cells and GABA receptor. *Neuroscience*, **40**, 375–97

47. Del Rio, J.A., Soriano, E. and Ferrer, I. (1992). Development of GABA-immunoreactivity in the neocortex of the mouse. *J. Comp. Neurol.*, **326**, 501–26

48. DeCarlos, J.A. and O'Leary, D.D.M. (1992). Growth and targeting of subplate axons and establishment of major cortical pathways. *J. Neurosci.*, **12**, 1194–211

49. O'Leary, D.D.M., Schlaggar, B.L. and Tuttle, R. (1994). Specification of neocortical areas and thalamocortical connections. *Annu. Rev. Neurosci.*, **17**, 419–39

50. Kageyama, G.H. and Robertson, R.T. (1993). Development of geniculocortical projections to visual cortex in rat: evidence for early ingrowth and synaptogenesis. *J. Comp. Neurol.*, **335**, 123–48

51. Agmon, A., Yang, L.T., O'Dowd, D.K. and Jones, E.G. (1993). Organized growth of thalamocortical axons from the deep tier of terminations into layer IV of developing mouse barrel cortex. *J. Neurosci.*, **13**, 5365–82

52. Kristt, D.A. (1989). Acetylcholinesterase in immature thalamic neurons: relation to afferentation, development, regulation and cellular distribution. *Neuroscience*, **29**, 27–43

53. Van Eden, C.G., Mrzljak, L., Voorn, P. and Uylings, H.B.M. (1989). Prenatal development of GABAergic neurons in the neocortex of the rat. *J. Comp. Neurol.*, **289**, 213–27

54. Woo, T.U., Beale, J.M. and Finlay, B.L. (1991). Dual fate of subplate neurons in a rodent. *Cerebral Cortex*, **1**, 433–43

55. Wood, J.G., Martin, S. and Price, D.J. (1992). Evidence that the earliest generated cells of the murine cerebral cortex form a transient population in the subplate and marginal zone. *Dev. Brain Res.*, **66**, 137–40

56. Marin-Padilla, M. (1971). Early prenatal ontogenesis of the cerebral cortex (neocortex) of the cat (Felis domestica): a Golgi study. *Ztschr. Anat. Entwicklungsgesch.*, **134**, 117–45

57. Marin-Padilla, M. (1972). Prenatal ontogenetic history of the principal neurons of the neocortex of the cat (*Felis domestica*): a Golgi study. II. Developmental differences and their significance. *Ztschr. Anat. Entwicklungsgesch.*, **136**, 125–42

58. Marin-Padilla, M. (1978). Dual origin of the mammalian neocortex and evolution of the cortical plate. *Anat. Embryol.*, **152**, 109–26

59. Marin-Padilla, M. (1983). Structural organization of the human cerebral cortex prior to the appearance of the cortical plate. *Anat. Embryol.*, **168**, 21–40

60. Marin-Padilla, M. (1988). Early ontogenesis of the human cerebral cortex. In Peters, A. and Jones,

E.G. (eds.) *Cerebral Cortex*, vol. 7; *Development and Maturation of Cerebral Cortex*, pp. 1–34. (New York and London: Plenum Press)

61. Marin-Padilla, M. (1990). Three-dimensional structural organization of layer I of the human cerebral cortex. A Golgi study. *J. Comp. Neurol.*, **299**, 89–105

62. Marin-Padilla, M. and Marin-Padilla, M.T. (1982). Origin, prenatal development and structural organization of layer I of the human cerebral (motor) cortex: a Golgi study. *Anat. Embryol.*, **164**, 161–206

63. Marin-Padilla, M. (1992). Ontogenesis of the pyramidal cells of the mammalian neocortex and developmental cytoarchitectonics: a unifying theory. *J. Comp. Neurol.*, **321**, 223–40

64. Sidman, R.L. and Rakic, P. (1982). Development of the human central nervous system. In Haymaker, W. and Adams, R.D. (eds.) *Histology and Histopathology of the Nervous System*, pp. 3–145. (Springfield: Thomas)

65. Brodmann, K. (1909). *Vergleichende Lokalisationslehre der Grosshirnrinde in ihren Prinzipien dargestellt auf Grund des Zellenbaues*. (Leipzig: Barth)

66. Rose, M. (1926). Ueber das histogenetische Prinzip der Einteilung der Grosshirnrinde. *J. Psychol. Neurol. (Lpz)*, **32**, 97–160

67. Kappers, C.U.A. (1928). The development of the cortex and the functions of its different layers. *Acta. Psychiat. (Kbh)*, **3**, 115–32

68. Gould, S.J. (1977). *Ontogeny and Phylogeny*. (Cambridge, Massachusetts and London, England: The Belknap Press of Harvard University Press)

69. Finlay, B.L., Wikler, K.C. and Sengelaub, D.R. (1987). Regressive events in brain development and scenarios for vertebrate brain evolution. *Brain Behav. Evol.*, **30**, 102–17

70. Kostović, I. and Judaš, M. (1994). Prenatal and perinatal development of the human cerebral cortex. In Kurjak, A. and Chervenak, F.A. (eds.) *Fetus as a Patient*, pp. 35–55. (Casterton, UK: Parthenon Publishing)

71. Poliakov, G.N. (1979). *Entwicklung der Neuronen des menschlichen Grosshirnrinde*. (Leipzig: VEB Georg Thieme)

72. Sidman, R.L. and Rakic, P. (1973). Neuronal migration, with special reference to developing human brain: a review. *Brain Res.*, **62**, 1–35

73. Mrzljak, L., Uylings, H.B.M., Kostović, I. and Van Eden, C.G. (1988). Prenatal development of neurons in the human prefrontal cortex: I. A qualitative Golgi study. *J. Comp. Neurol.*, **271**, 355–86

74. Mrzljak, L., Uylings, H.B.M., Van Eden, C.G. and Judaš, M. (1990). Neuronal development in human prefrontal cortex in prenatal and postnatal stages. *Progr. Brain Res.*, **85**, 185–222

75. Kostović, I., Uylings, H.B.M., Van Eden, C.G. and Judaš, M. (1991). Axonal strata and fibre systems

in the frontal lobe of the human fetal and infant brain. *Soc. Neurosci. Abstr.*, **17**, 1132

76. Yamashita, A., Hayashi, M., Shimizu, K. and Oshima, K. (1989). Ontogeny of somatostatin in cerebral cortex of macaque monkey: an immuno-histochemical study. *Dev. Brain Res.*, **45**, 103–11

77. Yamashita, A., Shimizu, K. and Hayashi, M. (1990). Ontogeny of substance P-immunoreactive structures in the primate cerebral neocortex. *Dev. Brain Res.*, **57**, 197–207

78. Hendry, S.H., Jones, E.G., Killackey, H.P. and Chalupa, L.M. (1987). Choline acetyltransferase-immunoreactive neurons in fetal monkey cerebral cortex. *Brain Res.*, **465**, 311–17

79. Hayashi, M., Yamashita, A., Shimizu, K. and Oshima, K. (1989). Ontogeny of cholecystokinin-8 and glutamic acid decarboxylase in cerebral neo-cortex of macaque monkey. *Exp. Brain Res.*, **74**, 249–55

80. Mehra, R.D. and Hendrickson, A.E. (1993). A comparison of the development of neuropeptide and MAP2 immunocytochemical labeling in the macaque visual cortex during pre- and postnatal development. *J. Neurobiol.*, **24**, 101–24

81. Wahle, P., Meyer, G., Wu, J.Y. and Albus, K. (1987). Morphology and axon terminal pattern of glutamate decarboxylase-immunoreactive cell types in the white matter of the cat occipital cortex during early postnatal development. *Dev. Brain Res.*, **36**, 53–61

82. Parnavelas, J.G. and Dori, I. (1986). A transient population of cholinergic neurons in the devel-oping rat cerebral cortex. *Neurosci. Lett. (Suppl.)*, **24**, S47

83. Valverde, F., Facal-Valverde, M.V., Santacana, M. and Heredia, M. (1989). Development and differentiation of early generated cells of sublayer VIb in the somatosensory cortex of the rat: a correlated Golgi and autoradiographic study. *J. Comp. Neurol.*, **290**, 118–40

84. Del Rio, J.A., Soriano, E. and Ferrer, I. (1991). A transitory population of substance P-like immuno-reactive neurones in the developing cerebral cortex of the mouse. *Dev. Brain Res.*, **64**, 205–11

85. Yan, X.X., Zheng, D.S. and Garey, L.J. (1992). Prenatal development of GABA-immunoreactive neurons in the human striate cortex. *Dev. Brain Res.*, **65**, 191–204

86. Masood, F., Wadhwa, S. and Bijlani, V. (1993). An immunohistochemical study of neurotransmitter profiles in developing human visual cortex. *Int. J. Dev. Neurosci.*, **11**, 387–97

87. Mehra, R.D. and Hendrickson, A.E. (1993). A comparison of the development of neuropeptide and MAP2 immunocytochemical labeling in the macaque visual cortex during prenatal and post-natal development. *J. Neurobiol.*, **24**, 101–24

88. Kostović, I. and Fučić, A. (1985). Distribution of somatostatin immunoreactive neurons in frontal neocortex and underlying 'white' matter of the human fetus and preterm infant. *Soc. Neurosci. Abstr.*, **11**, 352

89. Kostović, I., Štefulj-Fučić, A., Mrzljak, L., Jukić, S. and Delalle, I. (1991). Prenatal and perinatal development of the somatostatin-immunoreactive neurons in the human prefrontal cortex. *Neurosci. Lett.*, **124**, 153–6

90. Delalle, I. and Kostović, I. (1991). Laminar distribution of NPY-immunoreactive neurons in the human prefrontal cortex during prenatal and postnatal development. *Eur. J. Neurosci. (Suppl. 4)*, **132**

91. Delalle, I., Uylings, H.B.M. and Kostović, I. (1993). Developmental differences in the laminar distribution of NPY-ir neurons between prefrontal and visual human cortex during prenatal period. *Soc. Neurosci. Abstr.*, **19**, 731

92. Kostović, I. (1984). Prenatal development of interstitial neurons in the 'white' matter of the human telencephalon. *Soc. Neurosci. Abstr.*, **10**, 47

93. Kostović, I., Kelović, Z., Mrzljak, L. and Kračun, I. (1981). Distribution and morphology of interstitial acetylcholinesterase (AChE) reactive neurons in the fiber bundles of the human fetal telen-cephalon. *Neurosci. Lett. (Suppl.)*, **7**, S288

94. Meyer, G., Wahle, P., Castaneyra-Perdomo, A. and Ferres-Torres, R. (1992). Morphology of neurons in the white matter of the adult human neocortex. *Exp. Brain Res.*, **88**, 204–12

95. Akbarian, S., Bunney, W.E., Potkin, S.G., Wigal, S.B., Hagman, J.O., Sandman, C.A. and Jones, E.G. (1993). Altered distribution of nicotinamide adenine dinucleotide phosphate-diaphorase cells in frontal lobe of schizophrenics implies dis-turbances of cortical development. *Arch. Gen. Psychiatry*, **50**, 169–77

96. Kordower, J.H. and Mufson, E.J. (1992). Nerve growth factor receptor-immunoreactive neurons within the developing human cortex. *J. Comp. Neurol.*, **323**, 25–41

97. Terkelsen, O.B., Stagaard, J.M., Bock, E. and Mollgard, K. (1992). NCAM as a differentiation marker of postmigratory immature neurons in the developing human nervous system. *Int. J. Dev. Neurosci.*, **10**, 505–16

98. Wolozin, B.A., Scicutella, A. and Davies, P. (1988). Re-expression of a developmentally regulated antigen on Down's syndrome and Alzheimer's disease. *Proc. Natl. Acad. Sci. USA*, **85**, 6202–6

99. Mollgard, K. and Jacobsen, M. (1984). Immuno-histochemical identification of some plasma proteins in human embryonic and fetal forebrain with particular reference to the development of the neocortex. *Dev. Brain Res.*, **13**, 49–63

100. Peduzzi, J.D. (1988). Genesis of GABA-immuno-reactive neurons in the ferret visual cortex. *J. Neurosci.*, **8**, 920–31

101. Wolff, J.R., Bottcher, R., Zetzsche, T., Oertel, W.H. and Chronwall, B.M. (1984). Development of gabergic neurons in rat visual cortex as identified by glutamate decarboxylase-like immunoreactivity. *Neurosci. Lett.*, **47**, 207–12

102. Lauder, J.M., Han, V.K.M. and Henderson, P. (1986). Prenatal ontogeny of the GABAergic system in the rat brain: an immunocytochemical study. *Neuroscience*, **19**, 465–93

103. Huntley, G.W., deBlas, A.L. and Jones, E.G. (1990). GABA-A receptor immunoreactivity in adult and developing monkey sensory-motor cortex. *Exp. Brain Res.*, **82**, 519–35

104. Schlumpf, M., Richards, J.G., Lichtensteiger, W. and Mohler, H. (1983). An autoradiographic study of the prenatal development of benzodiazepine-binding sites in rat brain. *J. Neurosci.*, **3**, 1478–87

105. Schwartz, M.L. and Goldman-Rakic, P.S. (1988). Early development of GABA immunoreactive neurons in cerebral cortex of fetal monkeys. *Soc. Neurosci. Abstr.*, **14**, 1021

106. Meinecke, D.L. and Rakic, P. (1989). The temporal relationship between GABA and GABA-A/benzodiazepine receptor expression in neurons of the visual cortex of the developing rhesus monkeys. *Soc. Neurosci. Abstr.*, **15**, 1335

107. Hendrickson, A.E., Hunt, S.P. and Wu, J.Y. (1981). Immunocytochemical localization of glutamic acid decarboxylase in monkey striate cortex. *Nature (London)*, **292**, 605–7

108. Schwartz, M.L., Zheng, D.S. and Goldman-Rakic, P.S. (1988). Periodicity of GABA-containing cells in primate prefrontal cortex. *J. Neurosci.*, **8**, 1962–70

109. Friauf, E. and Shatz, C.J. (1991). Changing patterns of synaptic input to subplate and cortical plate during development of visual cortex. *J. Neurophysiol.*, **66**, 2059–71

110. Giguere, M. and Goldman-Rakic, P.S. (1988). Mediodorsal nucleus: areal, laminar and tangential distribution of afferents and efferents in the frontal lobes of rhesus monkey. *J. Comp. Neurol.*, **277**, 195–213

111. Schwartz, M.L. and Goldman-Rakic, P.S. (1982). Single cortical neurones have axon collaterals to ipsilateral and contralateral cortex in fetal and adult primates. *Nature (London)*, **299**, 154–6

112. Schwartz, M.L. and Goldman-Rakic, P.S. (1991). Prenatal specification of callosal connections in rhesus monkey. *J. Comp. Neurol.*, **307**, 144–62

113. Callaway, E.M. and Katz, L.C. (1992). Development of axonal arbors of layer 4 spiny neurons in cat striate cortex. *J. Neurosci.*, **12**, 570–82

114. Lowenstein, P.R. and Shering, A.F. (1992). Synaptic input to subplate neurons in the cat: infragranular neurons provide synaptic input to underlying subplate cells during early postnatal neocortical development. A light and electron microscopical study. *J. Anat.*, **180**, 383

115. Herrmann, K., Antonini, A. and Shatz, C.J. (1991). Thalamic axons make synaptic contacts with subplate neurons in cortical development. *Soc. Neurosc. Abstr.*, **17**, 899

116. Darian-Smith, C. and Darian-Smith, I. (1993). Thalamic projections to areas 3a, 3b, and 4 in the sensorimotor cortex of the mature and infant macaque monkey. *J. Comp. Neurol.*, **335**, 173–99

117. Kostović, I. (1986). Prenatal development of nucleus basalis complex and related fiber systems in man: a histochemical study. *Neuroscience*, **17**, 1047–77

118. Lund, R.D. and Mustari, M.J. (1977). Development of the geniculocortical pathway in rats. *J. Comp. Neurol.*, **173**, 289–306

119. Wise, P.S. and Jones, E.G. (1978). Developmental studies of thalamocortical and commissural projection of rat somatic sensory cortex. *J. Comp. Neurol.*, **168**, 313–43

120. Shatz, C.J. and Luskin, M.B. (1986). The relationship between the geniculocortical afferents and their cortical target cells during development of the cat's primary visual cortex. *J. Neurosci.*, **6**, 3655–68

121. Innocenti, G.M. (1986). General organization of callosal connections in the cerebral cortex. In Jones, E.G. and Peters, A. (eds.) *Cerebral Cortex*, vol. 5, pp. 291–353. (New York: Plenum Publishing Corporation)

122. Ghosh, A. and Shatz, C.J. (1992). Involvement of subplate neurons in the formation of ocular dominance columns. *Science*, **255**, 1441–3

123. Ghosh, A. and Shatz, C.J. (1992). Pathfinding and target selection by developing geniculocortical axons. *J. Neurosci.*, **12**, 39–55

124. Catalano, S.M., Robertson, R.T. and Killackey, H.P. (1991). Early ingrowth of thalamocortical afferents to the neocortex of the prenatal rat. *Proc. Natl. Acad. Sci. USA*, **88**, 2999–3003

125. Kostović, I., Škavić, J. and Strinović, D. (1988). Acetylcholinesterase in the human frontal associative cortex during the period of cognitive development: early laminar shifts and late innervation of pyramidal neurons. *Neurosci. Lett.*, **90**, 107–12

126. Krmpotić-Nemanić, J., Kostović, I., Kelović, Z. and Nemanić, -D. (1980). Development of acetylcholinesterase (AChE) staining in human fetal auditory cortex. *Acta Otolaryngol. (Stockh.)*, **89**, 388–92

127. Krmpotić-Nemaniić, J., Kostović, I., Kelović, Z., Nemanić, -D. and Mrzljak, L. (1983). Development of the human fetal auditory cortex: growth of afferent fibers. *Acta Anat.*, **116**, 69–73

128. Rakic, P. (1976). Prenatal genesis of connections subserving ocular dominance in the rhesus monkey. *Nature (London)*, **261**, 589–91

129. Hubel, D.H., Wiesel, T.N. and LeVay, S. (1977). Plasticity of ocular dominance columns in monkey

striate cortex. *Phil. Trans. R. Soc. London B.*, **278**, 377–409

130. LeVay, S., Wiesel, T.N. and Hubel, D.H. (1980). The development of ocular dominance columns in normal and visually deprived monkeys. *J. Comp. Neurol.*, **191**, 1–51

131. LaMantia, A.S. and Rakic, P. (1990). Axon overproduction and elimination in the corpus callosum of the developing rhesus monkey. *J. Neurosci.*, **10**, 2156–75

132. Kostović, I., Petanjek, Z., Delalle, I. and Judaš, M. (1992). Developmental reorganization of the human association cortex during the perinatal and postnatal life. In Kostović, I., Knežević, S., Wisniewski, H.M. and Spillich, G.J. (eds.) *Neurodevelopment, Aging and Cognition*, pp. 3–17. (Boston, Basel, Berlin: Birkäuser)

133. Rakic, P., Bourgeois, J.P., Eckenhoff, M.F., Zečević, N. and Goldman-Rakic, P.S. (1986). Concurrent overproduction of synapses in diverse regions of the primate cerebral cortex. *Science*, **232**, 232–5

134. Bourgeois, J.P., Jastreboff, P.J. and Rakic, P. (1989). Synaptogenesis in visual cortex of normal and preterm monkeys: evidence for intrinsic regulation of synaptic overproduction. *Proc. Natl. Acad. Sci. USA*, **86**, 4297–301

135. Mates, S.L. and Lund, J.S. (1983). Developmental changes in the relationship between type 1 synapses and spiny neurons in the monkey visual cortex. *J. Comp. Neurol.*, **221**, 91–7

136. Mates, S.L. and Lund, J.S.(1983). Developmental changes in the relationship between type 2 synapses and spiny neurons in the monkey visual cortex. *J. Comp. Neurol.*, **221**, 98–105

137. Zečević, N. and Rakic, P. (1991). Synaptogenesis in the primary somatosensory cortex of the rhesus monkey during fetal and postnatal life. *Cerebral Cortex*, **1**, 510–23

138. Zečević, N., Bourgeois, J.P. and Rakic, P. (1989). Changes in synaptic density in motor cortex of rhesus monkey during fetal and postnatal life. *Dev. Brain Res.*, **50**, 11–32

139. Zielinski, B.S. and Hendrickson, A.E. (1992). Development of synapses in macaque monkey striate cortex. *J. Vis. Neurosci.*, **8**, 491–504

140. Chun, J.J.M. and Shatz, C.J. (1988). Distribution of synaptic vesicle antigens is correlated with the disappearance of a transient synaptic zone in the developing cerebral cortex. *Neuron*, **1**, 297–310

141. Goldman-Rakic, P.S. and Rakic, P. (1984). Experimental modification of gyral patterns. In Geschwind, N. and Galaburda, A.N. (eds.) *Cerebral Dominance: The Biological Foundation*, pp. 179–92. (Cambridge, MA: Harvard University Press)

142. Crandall, J.E. and Caviness, V.E. (1984). Axon strata of the cerebral wall in embryonic mice. *Dev. Brain Res.*, **14**, 185–95

143. Goffinet, A.M. (1984). Events governing organization of postmigratory neurons: studies on brain development in normal and reeler mice. *Brain Res. Rev.*, **1**, 261–96

144. Van Eden, C.G. and Uylings, H.B.M. (1985). Cytoarchitectonic development of the prefrontal cortex in the rat. *J. Comp. Neurol.*, **241**, 253–67

145. Goldman-Rakic, P.S. (1987). Development of cortical circuitry and cognitive function. *Child Dev.*, **58**, 601–22

146. Kostović, I., Lukinović, N., Judaš, M., Bogdanović, N., Mrzljak, L., Zečević, N. and Kubat, M. (1989). Structural basis of the developmental plasticity in the human cerebral cortex: the role of the transient subplate zone. *Metabol. Brain Dis.*, **4**, 17–23

147. Kostović, I. (1990). Entwicklung des Zentralnervensystems. In Hinrichsen, K. (ed.) *Humanembryologie – Lehrbuch und Atlas der vorgeburtlichen Entwicklung des Menschen*, pp. 381–448. (Berlin: Springer-Verlag)

148. Kostović, I., Seress, L., Mrzljak, L. and Judaš, M. (1989). Early onset of synapse formation in the human hippocampus: a correlation with Nissl–Golgi architectonics in 15- and 16.5-week-old fetuses. *Neuroscience*, **30**, 105–16

149. Kostović, I. (1990). Structural and histochemical reorganization of the human prefrontal cortex during perinatal and postnatal life. *Progr. Brain Res.*, **85**, 131–47

150. Goldman-Rakic, P.S. and Galkin, T.W. (1978). Prenatal removal of frontal association cortex in the rhesus monkey: anatomical and functional consequences in postnatal life. *Brain Res.*, **52**, 451–85

151. Naegele, J.R., Barnstable, C.J. and Wahle, P.R. (1991). Expression of a unique 56-kDa polypeptide by neurons in the subplate zone of the developing cerebral cortex. *Proc. Natl. Acad. Sci. USA*, **88**, 330–4

152. Al-Ghoul, W.M. and Miller, W.M. (1989). Transient expression of Alz-50 immunoreactivity in developing rat neocortex: a marker for naturally occurring neuronal death? *Brain Res.*, **481**, 361–7

153. Allendoerfer, K.L., Shelton, D.L., Shooter, E.M. and Shatz, C.J. (1990). Nerve growth factor receptor immunoreactivity is transiently associated with the subplate neurons of the mammalian telencephalon. *Proc. Natl. Acad. Sci. USA*, **87**, 187–90

154. Meinecke, D.L. and Rakic, P. (1993). Low-affinity p75 nerve growth factor receptor expression in the embryonic monkey telencephalon: timing and localization in diverse cellular elements. *Neuroscience*, **54**, 105–16

Fetal brain pathology and ultrasound

2

R. N. Laurini

INTRODUCTION

Modern fetomaternal surveillance has drawn attention to antepartum events that contribute to subsequent neurological handicap in children[1]. Moreover, there is a growing body of evidence to show that defects in neurological development may be the consequence of prenatal brain damage[2]. Therefore, we need to ascertain the fetal condition before delivery in order to understand the possible influence of prenatal events on the perinatal and postnatal periods.

The new non-invasive techniques of modern fetal surveillance allow for the structural and functional evaluation of the fetus *in utero*. Nowadays, fetal neurosonography represents an important part of obstetric ultrasound. The introduction of high-frequency sonography, including transvaginal sonography, has resulted in detailed imaging of the normal anatomy of the central nervous system (CNS) and its pathology. Nevertheless, there is still a need for better definition of parameters in use, as illustrated by the ongoing discussion of fetal ventriculomegaly[3].

In this context, I believe there is much to gain from a routine correlation between the morphological patterns seen with sonography and those encountered at postmortem. Furthermore, there is a need to correlate the fetal behavioral patterns obtained with real-time ultrasound imaging and the recordings on Doppler ultrasound with the findings at postmortem.

Therefore, the main aim of this chapter is to illustrate the possible contribution of developmental neuropathology to imaging techniques in the context of fetal brain pathology. This chapter will be based on the pathology of the fetal period up to 24 weeks' gestation.

METHODS IN DEVELOPMENTAL NEUROPATHOLOGY

It must be emphasized that the morphological examination of the CNS, peripheral structures and muscle is an integral part of a complete developmental postmortem. As for any other organ or system, the interpretation of the neuropathological findings will depend on the available clinical data together with the findings in the rest of the postmortem[2]. The etiological heterogeneity of neural tube defects and fetal hydrocephalus are good examples of the need for a careful evaluation of sonographic and postmortem findings[4,5].

The final aim of a fetal neuropathological examination is to assess the findings in the context of the degree of maturity and growth of the individual case, and to attempt to differentiate between a primary maldevelopment and brain damage secondary to an environmental cause (e.g. asphyxia). This can be achieved only if a qualified subspecialist follows a comprehensive standard protocol, consisting of a detailed gross examination including selected biometry combined with the absolutely necessary histological evaluation. The latter is essential, since significant changes (e.g. pathological gliosis) are not seen on gross examination or neurosonography.

Morphological assessment

The very first priority of any assessment in developmental medicine is to determine the developmental stage and growth pattern, in order to interpret the structural and/or functional findings.

The introduction of prenatal neurosonology and postnatal neurosonography, computerized tomography (CT) and magnetic resonance

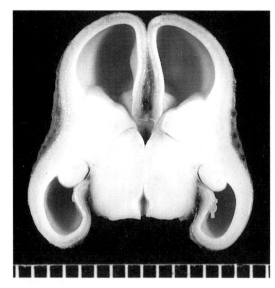

Figure 1 Coronal section at the level of the third ventricle from a psychosocial termination at 12 weeks' gestation. Transverse cerebellar diameter at postmortem was 8.9 mm

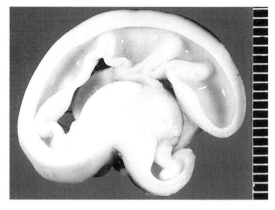

Figure 2 Parasagittal plane showing cortical folding along the internal aspect of the lateral ventricle wall adjacent to the interhemispheric fissure. Termination of pregnancy at 15 weeks' gestation. Transverse cerebellar diameter was 12.9 mm

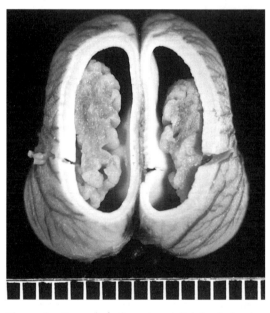

Figure 3 Coronal section at occipital level showing choroid plexus that occupied >50% of the lateral ventricles. Psychosocial termination at 12 weeks' gestation

imaging (MRI) for the assessment of brain development and damage has resulted in an increased interest in the morphological examination of the fetal, perinatal and post-neonatal brain. In view of this, we have modified the traditional method for brain cutting to follow the coronal, sagittal and parasagittal planes used with brain imaging[2]. Following the introduction of transvaginal sonography (TVS), the protocols for neurosonography are now very similar to those used for the macroscopic examination of the fetal brain. This includes the assessment of structures (e.g. macroscopic appearance of choroid plexus) as well as biometry. Figures 1, 2 and 3 illustrate the gross appearance of a fetal brain in early pregnancy.

Table 1 shows the main parameters used at postmortem. There is an excellent correlation between the nomograms established from sonographic and postmortem evaluation of skeletal development[6] and transverse cerebellar diameter[7] (and R. N. Laurini, unpublished data). Furthermore, the gyral pattern observed on gross examination corresponds well to that seen on ultrasound[8] (and R.N. Laurini, unpublished data). In addition, there is a relationship between gyral and renal development in the human[9].

From 1993, we have routinely measured the distance from the thalamus to the internal tip of the occipital pole (Figure 4), and the depth of the lateral ventricle on a midline coronal plane at the level of the third ventricle. These measurements correlate well with the detailed charts of ventricular size recently published by Monteagudo and co-workers[10]. Our measurement of the distance

Table 1 Main parameters for assessment of developmental stage at postmortem

Postmortem radiology	skeletal development
Gross examination	foot length
	brain gyral pattern
	transverse cerebellar diameter
Histology	renal development
	cerebellar development

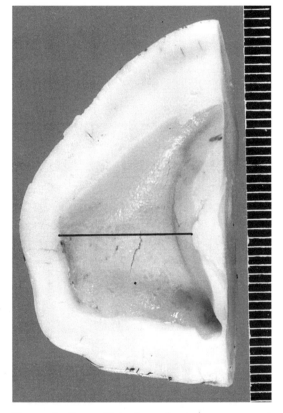

Figure 4 Parasagittal plane showing measurement (black line) from thalamus to internal tip of occipital horn (16.5 mm). Termination of pregnancy at 18 weeks' gestation for trisomy 18

from the thalamus to the tip of the occipital pole (internal aspect) corresponds to theirs of the choroid plexus thickness, while the depth of the lateral ventricle is identically measured. Nevertheless, our experience shows that it is difficult to correlate sonographic and postmortem measurements for size of lateral ventricles when the coronal plane is used.

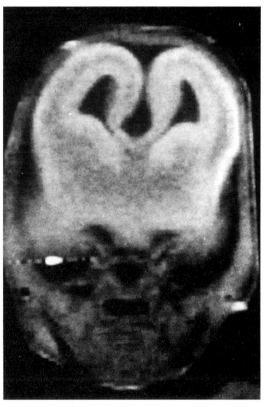

Figure 5 Magnetic resonance image showing coronal plane of the head from a psychosocial termination at 16 weeks' gestation. The crown–rump length was 105 mm

Our recent trials with MRI to assess brain morphology at postmortem has given promising results (M. Erzen and colleagues, in preparation). The image illustrated by Figure 5 allows not only study of ventricular size *in situ* but also delineation of the germinal, intermediate and cortical areas within the fetal brain parenchyma[11]. This capacity for better defintion of parenchymatous structure can be extremely helpful to diagnose neuronal heterotopias with or without abnormal cortication. Moreover, other more subtle brain lesions, as in tuberous sclerosis[12], can also benefit from this increased imaging capacity. Nevertheless, as for many other pathologies, there are cases of tuberous sclerosis with normal MRI and gross examination, where lesions were revealed only after histological examination[13] (and R. N. Laurini, unpublished data). Therefore, routine histological examination including immunoreactivity to glial

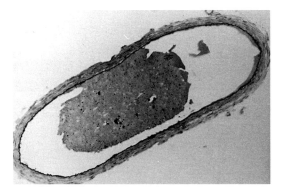

Figure 6 Cross-section from dilated anterior cerebral artery of a fetus (20 weeks' gestation) with a chorioamnionitis and hemorrhage of the falx and tentorium. Elastin van Gieson, ×88

fibrillary acidic protein (GFAP) should be performed in all cases. Sampling for histology must be carried out on standard blocks from selected areas that are helpful for estimation of development and represent target areas associated with hypoxic–ischemic changes[2].

Functional cerebral vascular morphology

The morphological findings of the fetus, placenta and uteroplacental circulation can be related to both intrauterine structure and function. This dynamic rendering is defined as functional morphology[14]. This concept is of particular relevance in understanding fetal and neonatal cerebral hemodynamics in the context of the cerebral macro- and microcirculation and their possible role in autoregulation.

Systematic postmortem examinations of fetal and neonatal cerebral vessels show that, in the presence of asphyxia, there is a variable dilatation of *both* cerebral arteries (Figure 6) and veins. These findings are usually accompanied by a considerable dilatation of the vein of Galen (see Figure 21). Histological examination demonstrates that these extracerebral arteries have only an internal elastic lamina and a significantly thinner wall than extracranial muscular arteries of the same caliber (Figure 6).

Our preliminary findings suggest that extracerebral arteries function in a manner similar to veins. In the presence of hypoxia and hypercapnia

and/or with changes in perfusion, vasodilatation reduces the vasomotor capacity of arteries for further adaptation ('vessel paralysis'). The initial arterial vasodilatation is probably a part of the phenomenon of redistribution of blood flow, the known fetal response to stress. Further distress increases the vasodilatation to the point where these particular arteries lose their ability to dilate and constrict, and, consequently, autoregulation is impaired or lost[15].

Furthermore, these particular anatomical characteristics are already present as early as 12 weeks' gestation (R. N. Laurini, unpublished data). In this context, it is of interest to note that cerebral arteries from late first-trimester fetuses show the presence of end-diastolic velocities in blood flow velocity waveforms. This finding suggests a lower vascular resistance at the cerebral level than in the placenta or in splachnic organs in early gestation[16]. Such lower resistance can be explained by the specific anatomical characteristics of the arterial wall that readily allow for vasodilatation.

The vascularization of the choroid plexus may represent a further example of this specific cerebral vascular morphology. Figure 7 illustrates the thin, capillary-like vessels that enter the choroid plexus at 9 weeks' gestation. In comparison, Figure 8 shows the well-established arterial and venous vascularization at 12 weeks' gestation. Once again, we observe the characteristic appearance of a cerebral artery, where the relationship between the diameter of the lumen and the thickness of the wall clearly favors the diameter of the vessel. Indeed there is a structural resemblance between the arteries and neighboring veins. As was the case for extracerebral arteries, this change in arterial morphology is associated with a decreasing resistance to flow velocity. Recent work by Kurjak and associates[17] on color flow ultrasonography of the choroid plexus demonstrated that there is a steady decline in resistance from 11 weeks' gestation.

MALFORMATIONS AND CHROMOSOMAL ANOMALIES

Maldevelopment of the CNS represents a typical example of etiological heterogeneity. During the fetal period, the brain undergoes considerable

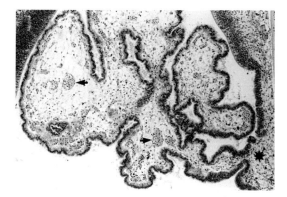

Figure 7 Histological image of a choroid plexus and its vascularization from a psychosocial termination at 9 weeks' gestation. Note capillary-like vascular supply at the hilus (star) and in the interstitium (arrows). Hematoxylin–eosin, ×45

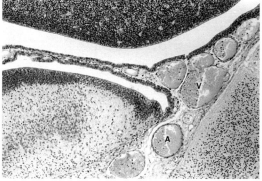

Figure 8 Histological image of a choroid plexus and its vascularization from a psychosocial termination at 12 weeks' gestation. Note well-developed arterial (A) and venous (V) circulation at the hilus. Hematoxylin–eosin, ×45

developmental changes. This process can be affected by anomalies in cellular programming (e.g. genetic etiology) and/or insults from the environment (e.g. vascular etiology). The former can be considered a primary form of maldevelopment, while the latter represents an example of secondary maldevelopment. Therefore, the same anomaly revealed by imaging and/or postmortem can differ in etiology and in relevance for genetic and/or obstetric counselling. An abnormal cortication (e.g. polymicrogyra) can represent an inherited disorder of neuronal migration[18] or be secondary to a pathological gliosis that affects the radial glia with ensuing migration defect (see Figures 28 and 29). In fact, there is a significant overlapping in the etiology of the different morphological patterns of brain damage.

Chromosomal anomalies are frequently associated with mental retardation, but their relation to CNS malformations is less specific. This applies even to the association between trisomy 13 and holoprosencephaly[19]. Nevertheless, with the introduction of high-resolution techniques, previously unidentifiable minute chromosomal defects have been detected in the Miller–Dieker syndrome (microcephaly, lissencephaly and dysmorphic changes), consisting of a partial monosomy of chromosome 17[20].

Neural tube defects are a well-known example of etiologic heterogeneity[4], but the precise mechanism of formation is still unknown. Among this group, exencephaly and anencephaly represent different stages of the same developmental anomaly. Figure 9 illustrates a case of exencephaly in which histology of the 'cerebral hemispheres' confirmed the presence of a severe dysplasia associated with a marked hypoplasia of the adrenal glands.

Abnormal cortication can be associated with chromosomal disorders, genetic disease, malformation syndromes, defects in perfusion, infections and toxic agents. An abnormal development of the temporal lobes has been reported in cases of fetal thanatophoric dysplasia[14]. In Figure 10, we can observe a similar developmental anomaly in a case of triploidy, confirming the heterogeneity of most developmental defects.

There is a large spectrum of developmental defects related to failure of neural tube growth that ranges from aprosencephaly to isolated arhinencephaly. Figures 11 and 12 (right) illustrate two of the more common examples of this group of developmental defects. Figure 12 (left) shows a normal brain at 18 weeks' gestation, when the anterior part of the corpus callosum and the cavum septi pellucidi can be recognized. Total or partial agenesis of the corpus callosum is rarely an isolated event. More commonly it is associated with holoprosencephaly, absent septum pellucidum, Dandy–Walker syndrome and the Arnold–Chiari malformation[21]. Nevertheless, anomalies of the septum pellucidum can be observed in the presence of a normal corpus callosum[22].

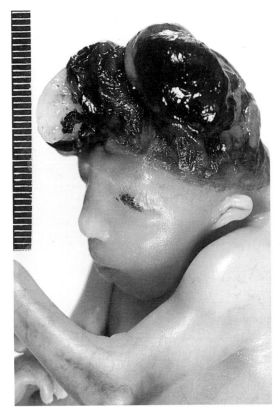

Figure 9 Gross appearance of an exencephalic fetus. Termination of pregnancy at 18 weeks' gestation

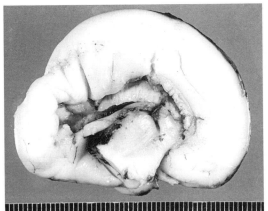

Figure 10 Left brain hemisphere from a 19-week fetus with triploidy showing an abnormal temporo-occipital lobe

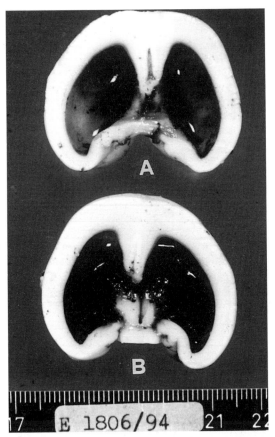

Figure 11 Interruption of pregnancy at 20 weeks for trisomy 13, showing coronal sections of a semilobar holoprosencephaly. Note incomplete interhemispheric division with continuity of frontal cortex (A) and partial fusion of thalamus–striatum (B)

Failure of growth can also affect the cerebellum in a great variety of situations, including several chromosomal anomalies. Figure 13 portrays a hypoplasia of the right hemisphere with a reduced transverse cerebellar diameter.

Choroid plexus cysts are a frequent finding in fetal postmortems (Figure 14). Routine use of antenatal ultrasonography has shown that choroid plexus cysts can be transient, perhaps even a normal aspect of fetal brain development[23]. Nevertheless, large choroid plexus cysts have been reported in association with trisomy 18[24].

Fetal ventriculomegaly represents an important morphological change in both primary and secondary forms of CNS maldevelopment. Many cerebral anomalies are thought to arise from early fetal ventriculomegaly[25] and the development of neurohandicap is significantly associated with white matter lesions related to ventriculomegaly.

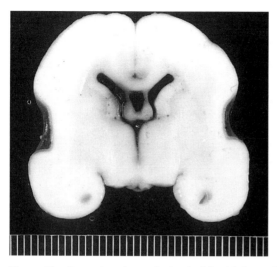
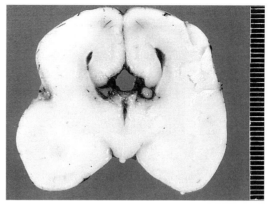

Figure 12 Coronal section at the level of the third ventricle at 18 weeks' gestation from a psychosocial termination (left) and from a case of trisomy 18 (right), showing total agenesis of the corpus callosum

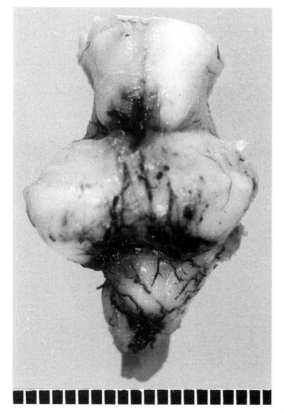

Figure 13 Posterior view of the cerebellum showing slight hypoplasia of the right lobe. Transverse cerebellar diameter at postmortem was 17.1 mm. Termination of pregnancy at 20 weeks' gestation for trisomy 21

Despite this recognition of fetal ventriculomegaly as a marker of abnormal brain development, its diagnosis remains a major challenge. In our experience, this is particularly the case for fetuses with a mild ventriculomegaly at less than 22 weeks' gestation. A ventricular dilatation, as in Figure 15, will pose no problems on imaging or post-mortem examination.

Routine morphological examination of fetal brains suggested that dilatation of the caudal portion was the earliest and most reliable morphological sign of ventriculomegaly (R.N. Laurini, unpublished data). This postmortem finding has been recently confirmed by the work of Monteagudo and colleagues[10,26] on *in utero* detection of ventriculomegaly by TVS. Figure 16 illustrates the difference between a normal and a dilated caudal portion in two cases of trisomy. The cases portrayed in Figures 4 and 12 (right) also revealed a ventriculomegaly limited to the posterior aspect of the lateral ventricles.

The fetal Dandy–Walker malformation represents another brain defect in which careful assessment of ventricular size is important. This malformation is characterized by a posterior fossa cyst, hypoplasia or agenesis of the cerebellar vermis and dilatation of the fourth ventricle, and the degree of ventriculomegaly is very variable[27]. The use of TVS allows for very early sonographic

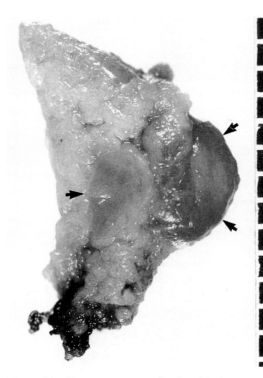

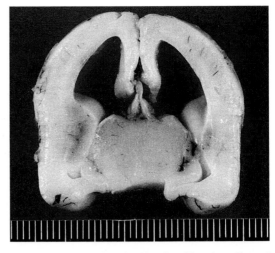

Figure 15 Coronal section showing dilatation of lateral ventricles in a case of lumbosacral spina bifida with Arnold–Chiari malformation at 18 weeks' gestation

Figure 14 Gross appearance of a choroid plexus cyst (arrows) from a psychosocial termination of pregnancy at 19 weeks' gestation

diagnosis, as is shown in Figure 17. In this case, it represented the sole malformation, as can often be found[27].

In addition, I have seen two cases of trisomy 13 (a holoprosencephaly and an isolated arhinencephaly with hydrocephaly) with only a dilatation of the fourth ventricle associated with a mild inferior vermis hypoplasia (Figure 18). Such cases may be considered as examples of Dandy–Walker variant[27].

HEMORRHAGIC PATHOLOGY

There are two main forms of fetal CNS damage: hemorrhagic and hypoxic–ischemic pathology. A more comprehensive approach to this subject has recently been published[2]. In this chapter, the morphological appearance of the most common lesions is stressed.

Table 2 summarizes the main hemorrhagic lesions observed in the fetal CNS. These changes are mainly secondary to acute intrauterine asphyxia

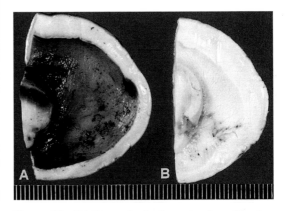

Figure 16 (A) Parasagittal plane showing dilatation of caudal portion of the right lateral ventricle. The measurement from thalamus to internal tip of occipital horn at postmortem was 20 mm. Termination of pregnancy at 19 weeks' gestation for trisomy 21. (B) Parasagittal view in a case with normal size for comparison. The measurement from thalamus to internal tip of occipital horn at postmortem was 10 mm. Termination of pregnancy at 18 weeks' gestation for trisomy 18

and are commonly associated with chorioamnionitis and/or abruptio placenta in the fetal stage. Identical findings are observed in psychosocial termination of pregnancy with the use of prostaglandins[2].

Meningeal congestion (Figure 19) represents an early morphological marker of fetal asphyxia. More severe fetal distress is frequently associated

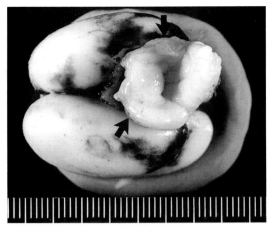

Figure 17 Basal view of a Dandy–Walker malformation, showing a hypoplasia of the vermis and a cyst of the fourth ventricle with the rest of the membranes (arrows). Termination of pregnancy at 16 weeks' gestation

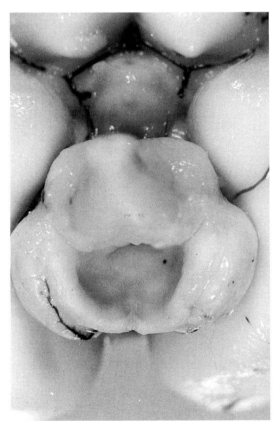

Figure 18 Basal view of the brain showing only moderate dilatation of the fourth ventricle and mild inferior vermis hypoplasia in a case of trisomy 13 with an isolated arhinencephaly and hydrocephaly

Table 2 Main hemorrhagic lesions

Meningeal congestion
Falx and/or tentorium hemorrhage
Subarachnoidal hemorrhage
Periventricular radial congestion
Periventricular radial hemorrhage
Germinal matrix hemorrhage
Intraventricular hemorrhage
Choroid plexus hemorrhage
Other hemorrhages

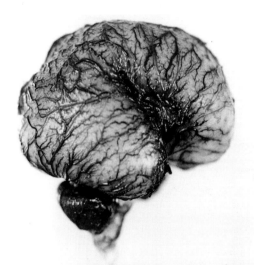

Figure 19 Marked meningeal congestion and subarachnoid hemorrhage of the cerebellum. Intrauterine death at 20 weeks' gestation with important signs of fetal asphyxia. Placenta showed a funiculitis, vasculitis and ischemic lesions associated with fresh and ancient marginal hematomas

with extensive subarachnoidal and falx/tentorium hemorrhages (Figures 19, 20 and 21). Germinal matrix hemorrhage, with or without intraventricular hemorrhage, is frequently associated with chorioamnionitis and a fetal abruptio placenta (Figure 22). In fact, many cases of chorioamnionitis also show a marginal placental hematoma as morphological expression of fetal abruptio placenta[2]. Periventricular radial congestion or hemorrhage represents another characteristic lesion seen in fetal asphyxia (Figure 23). It is very difficult to determine the origin of these vascular

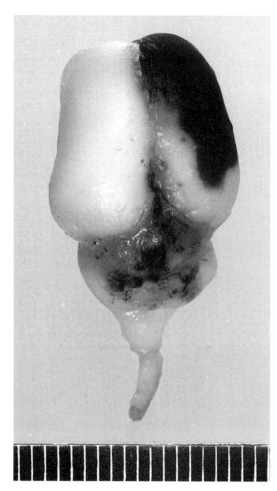

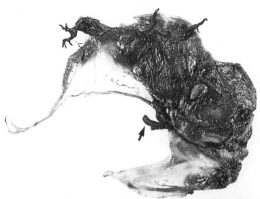

Figure 21 Massive hemorrhage of the falx in a case of intrauterine death at 20 weeks' gestation. The fetus showed lesions of acute asphyxia and the placenta revealed a chorioamnionitis. Note congestion of the vein of Galen (arrow)

Figure 20 Extensive subarachnoid hemorrhage in a case of intrauterine death at 12 weeks' gestation. The fetus showed lesions of acute asphyxia associated with ischemic pathology of the placenta

changes, but there is good evidence to believe that they represent lesions of the venous system. In this context, it should be stressed that all these hemorrhagic lesions are frequently associated with a marked congestion of the vein of Galen (Figure 21). Hemorrhagic lesions can be seen in other brain structures, such as the choroid plexus (Figure 24) and the pons (Figure 25).

HYPOXIC–ISCHEMIC PATHOLOGY

Careful histological examination of the CNS from fetal deaths associated with ischemic and, occasionally, hemorrhagic pathology of the placenta

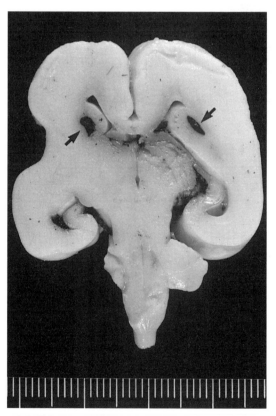

Figure 22 Coronal section, showing a bilateral germinal matrix hemorrhage (arrows) from an intrauterine death at 21 weeks' gestation. Twin pregnancy with acute fetal asphyxia and a large retroplacental hematoma

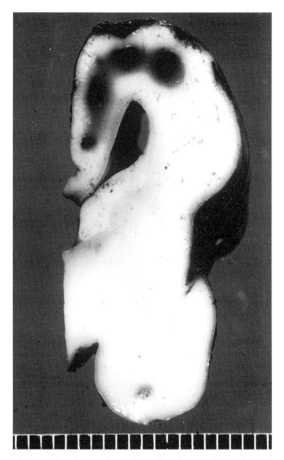

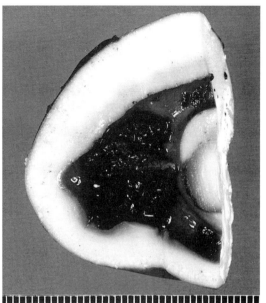

Figure 24 Parasagittal plane of caudal portion of left lateral ventricle, showing a choroid plexus hemorrhage. Termination of pregnancy at 21 weeks' gestation for malformations

Figure 23 Coronal section, showing multiple foci of periventricular venous congestion and hemorrhage. Intrauterine death at 15 weeks' gestation with fetal asphyxia and marginal hematoma associated with ischemic lesions of the placenta

revealed the presence of hypertrophic astrocytes, foci of periventricular leukomalacia and areas of abnormal cortication. GFAP staining in these cases confirmed the presence of pathological gliosis[2].

In the context of this chapter, it is of great relevance to emphasize that the vast majority of these forms of brain damage are not seen on either sonographic or gross examination of the fetal brain. Neuronal heterotopias and abnormal cortication (microgyria, polymicrogyria) can be best observed with MRI. Therefore, *all* fetal CNS should undergo a comprehensive neuropathological examination with the inclusion of a detailed histological evaluation. The following examples are included in order to illustrate this point further.

Routine morphological assessment of the fetal brain frequently reveals the presence of focal abnormal cortication (Figure 26). In a number of cases there is an explanation of this finding, as in the case of Figure 27. In cytomegalovirus infection, the anomaly may be of vascular origin. In a significant number of other cases of abnormal cortication, histological evaluation sometimes depicts a normal cortex, whereas in other cases, it shows a cortical dysplasia without obvious causes. Although its significance is still a matter of controversy, I have found a relationship between pathological gliosis of white matter and these foci of abnormal cortication. My working hypothesis is that the pathological gliosis affects the radial glia and impairs the migration of neuroblasts from the germinal matrix to the cortex.

The brain damage present in a termination of pregnancy at 22 weeks' gestation for HELLP syndrome and pre-eclampsia clearly illustrates this hypothesis. Moreover, the placenta showed extensive ischemic changes and acute atherosis of the decidual portion of spiral arteries. Figures 28 and 29 display a severe pathological gliosis associated

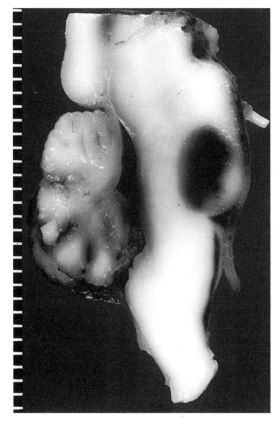

Figure 25 Standard block of brainstem and cerebellum, showing a pontine hemorrhage. Intrauterine death at 22 weeks' gestation with chorioamnionitis

with an impaired neuroblast migration depicted by multiple groups of neuroblasts that remained in the vicinity of the ependyma. In addition, Figure 30 shows the characteristic appearance of

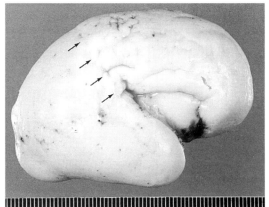

Figure 27 Lateral view, showing focal polymicrogyria (arrows) in a fetus with cytomegalovirus infection

pathological gliosis and mosaic pattern recently described in the germinal matrix of cases with long-standing perfusion pathology.

In the view of this author there is a close relationship between the distinctive macro- and microcirculation of the fetal and perinatal brain and the development of diffuse gliosis, as discussed elsewhere[2]. The hemodynamic and gas changes (O_2 and CO_2) can result in damage of endothelial cells with focal destruction of the blood–brain barrier and perivascular destruction of white matter (Figure 31), thus giving rise to pathological gliosis. These changes can only be demonstrated on histology, but might correspond to the diffuse transitory echodensities seen on ultrasound.

Pathological gliosis is an important tissue marker of hypoxic–ischemic events in the fetal

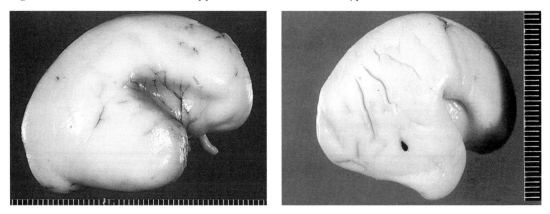

Figure 26 Lateral view at 20 weeks' gestation of normal brain (left) and brain showing focal abnormal cortication for the age (right). Intrauterine death with a congenital pneumonia associated with chorioamnionitis

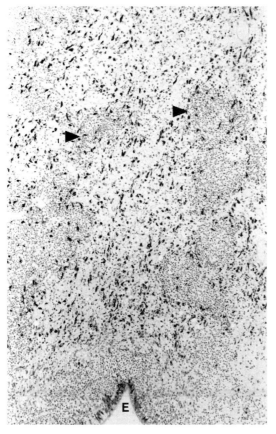

Figure 28 Staining of germinal matrix along the wall of the lateral ventricle (E) illustrates pathological gliosis (dark cells with fibrillary projections) and abnormal migration of neuroblasts (arrowheads). Termination of pregnancy at 22 weeks' gestation for HELLP syndrome. Glial fibrillary acidic protein, ×44

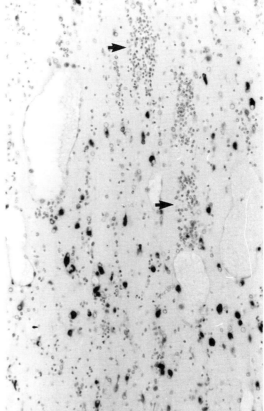

Figure 29 Pathological gliosis (dark cells with fibrillary projections) in white matter associated with foci of impaired migration of neuroblasts (arrows). Same case as Figure 28. Glial fibrillary acidic protein, ×135

brain. Its presence is a sign that one or several episodes of fetal stress were serious enough to give rise to brain damage.

FUNCTIONAL MORPHOLOGY AND BRAIN PATHOLOGY

Despite the ever-increasing capacity of neurosonography and its correlation with postmortem assessment, there is still a need for better definition of fetal brain damage and its clinical significance. In this context it is important to bear in mind that the presence of an organ anomaly and *dysfunction* confirms the pathological character of the condition. This dynamic rendering of the structural and

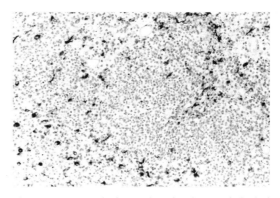

Figure 30 Germinal matrix, showing pathological gliosis (dark cells with fibrillary projections) and mosaic pattern. Same case as Figure 28. Glial fibrillary acidic protein, ×115

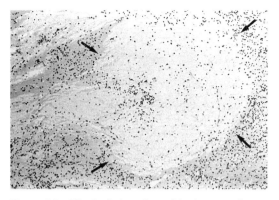

Figure 31 Histological section of brain parenchyma, showing focal congestion and rupture of microcirculation. Note perivascular necrosis of white matter (arrows). Same case as Figure 30. Hematoxylin–eosin, ×60

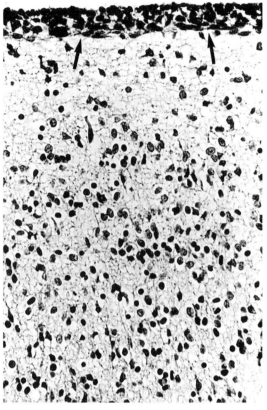

Figure 34 Higher magnification from Figure 32 showing a well-developed external granular layer (arrows). Hematoxylin–eosin, ×280. (From reference 2, with permission)

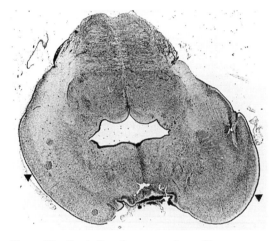

Figure 32 Cerebellum from control case. Note presence of the external granular layer (arrows). Hematoxylin–eosin, ×7. (From reference 2, with permission)

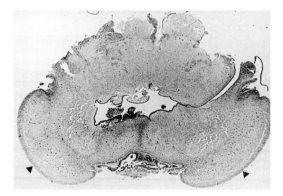

Figure 33 Shows absence of external granular layer in both cerebellar hemispheres (arrows). Hematoxylin–eosin, ×5. (From reference 2, with permission)

functional status was previously defined as functional morphology. In my view, this approach will result in major developments in the field of prenatal neurology that will help identify neurological abnormality in the fetus, its substratum and its clinical significance.

Real-time ultrasound has resulted in the establishment of the monitoring of fetal biophysical variables, which include, among other variables, fetal body movements, fetal breathing movements and fetal tone as a reflection of CNS function[28]. The quality and quantity of fetal movements and the development of behavioral states are probably the most sensitive parameters for the assessment of the function and integrity of the nervous system. Thus, the study of prenatal neurology has become a reality[29,30,31].

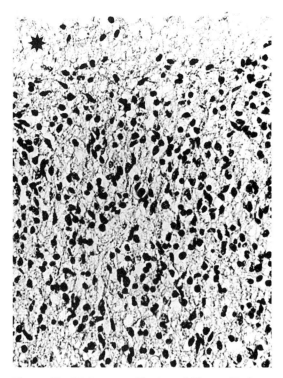

Figure 35 Higher magnification of Figure 33 shows absence of external granular layer (*) and an increased cellularity in the molecular layer as compared to control. Hematoxylin–eosin, ×280. (From reference 2, with permission)

A recently reported case illustrates the role of developmental neuropathology as an integral part of prenatal neurological examination[2]. A healthy 22-year-old nulliparous woman attended for genetic counselling because of a history of X-linked mental retardation in the family. Amniocentesis revealed a normal male karyotype and real-time ultrasound examination for fetal behavior was carried out which showed a hyperactive fetus with the onset of movements, and ongoing movements that were too abrupt[32]. The pattern of these movements showed a striking resemblance to the abnormal motility of anencephalic fetuses[33]. The postmortem revealed a complete absence of the superficial granular layer in both cerebellar hemispheres (Figures 33 and 35). The cerebella from two normal male fetuses (psychosocial interruptions) were used as controls (Figures 32 and 34).

The morphological findings in this case correspond to those described as primary degeneration of the granular layer of the cerebellum[34]. In view of the gestational age, only the absence of the external granular layer could be observed, without the presence of Purkinje cells, as has been described at a later stage in gestation[35].

This correlation between the findings of prenatal neurology and developmental neuropathology is not limited to fetal anomalies[32,33], but has also been observed with Fanconi's anemia[36].

CONCLUSION

Routine correlation between findings obtained by antenatal surveillance and morphological examination of postmortems, including the central nervous system, allow for a better understanding of fetal brain damage and its clinical relevance. Furthermore, this approach will gain importance when both prenatal neurological evaluations and neuropathological evaluations become a more established routine in antenatal care.

References

1. Visser, G.H.A. (1992). Antepartum events and subsequent handicap. In Fukuyama, Y., Suzuki, Y., Kamoshita, S. and Casaer, P. (eds.) *Fetal and Perinatal Neurology*, pp. 216–22.(Basel: Karger)
2. Laurini, R.N. (1994). Fetal brain pathology. In Kurjak, A. and Chervenak, F.A. (eds.) *The Fetus as a Patient*, pp. 89–106. (Carnforth, UK: Parthenon Publishing)
3. Pilu, G. (1994). Sonography of fetal ventriculomegaly: the never-ending story. *Ultrasound Obstet. Gynecol.*, **4**, 180–1
4. Holmes, L.B., Driscoll, S.G. and Atkins, L. (1976). Etiologic heterogeneity of neural-tube defects. *N. Engl. J. Med.*, **294**, 365–9
5. Harrod, M.J.E., Friedman, J.M., Santos-Ramos, R., Rutledge, J. and Weinberg, A. (1984). Etiologic heterogeneity of fetal hydrocephalus diagnosed by ultrasound. *Am. J. Obstet. Gynecol.*, **150**, 38–40
6. Laurini, R.N. (1986). *Aspects of Developmental Pathology*, pp. 11–33. (Groningen: Drukkerij van Denderen BV)
7. Goldstein, I., Reece, E.A. Pilu, G., Bovicelli, L. and Hobbins, J.C. (1987). Cerebellar measurements with ultrasonography in the evaluation of fetal growth

and development. *Am. J. Obstet. Gynecol.*, **156**, 1065–9

8. Birnholz, J.C. and Farrell, E.E. (1985). Towards an ultrasound characterisation of fetal brain development. In Jones, C.T. and Nathanielsz, P.W. (eds.) *The Physiological Development of the Fetus and Newborn*, pp. 617–20. (London: Academic Press)

9. Dorovin-Zis, K. and Dolman, C.L. (1977). Gestational development of the brain. *Arch. Pathol. Lab. Med.*, **101**, 192–5

10. Monteagudo, A., Timor-Tritsch, I.E. and Moomjy, M. (1994). In utero detection of ventriculomegaly during the second and third trimesters by transvaginal sonography. *Ultrasound Obstet. Gynecol.*, **4**, 193–8

11. Mintz, M.C., Grossman, R.I., Isaacson, G., Thickman, D.I., Kundel, H., Joseph, P. and DeSimone, D. (1987). MR imaging of fetal brain. *J. Comput. Assist. Tomogr.*, **11**, 120–3

12. Mirlesse, V., Werner, H., Jacquemard, F., Perotez, C., Daffos, F., Sonigo, P. and Brunelle, F. (1992). Magnetic resonance imaging in antenatal diagnosis of tuberous sclerosis. *Lancet*, **340**, 1163

13. Sonigo, P., Elmaleh, A., Fermont, L., Delezoide, A.L., Lallemand, D. and Brunelle, F. (1994). Apport de l'IRM cérébrale foetale dans le diagnostic prénatal de la sclérose tubéreuse de Bourneville. *Méd. Foetale Echogr. Gynécol.*, **19**, 13–16

14. Laurini, R.N. (1990). Abortion from a morphological viewpoint. In Huisjes, H.J. and Lind, T. (eds.) *Spontaneous Abortion*, pp. 79–113. (Edinburgh: Churchill Livingstone)

15. Marsal, K., Gunnarsson, G., Ley, D., Maesel, A. and Laurini, R.N. (1993). Cerebral circulation in the perinatal period. In Kurjak, A. and Chervenak, F. (eds.) *The Fetus as a Patient*, pp. 477–88. (Carnforth, UK: Parthenon Publishing)

16. Rizzo, G., Arduini, D. and Romanini, C. (1995). First-trimester fetal and uterine Doppler. In Copel, J.A. and Reed, K.L. (eds.) *Doppler Ultrasound in Obstetrics and Gynecology*, pp. 105–14. (New York: Raven Press)

17. Kurjak, A., Schulman, H., Predanic, A., Predanic, M., Kupesic, S. and Zalud, I. (1994). Fetal choroid plexus vascularization assessed by color flow ultrasonography. *J. Ultrasound Med.*, **13**, 841–4

18. Volpe, J.J. and Adams, R.D. (1972). Cerebrohepato-renal syndrome of Zellweger: an inherited disorder of neuronal migration. *Acta Neuropathol.*, **20**, 175–98

19. Melnick, M. (1979). Current concepts of the etiology of central nervous system malformations. *Birth Defects: Original Article Series*, **15**, 19–41. (New York: The National Foundation-March of Dimes)

20. Dobyns, W.B., Stratton, R.F., Parke, J.T., Greenberg, F., Nussbaum, R.L. and Ledbetter, D.H. (1983). Miller–Dieker syndrome and monosomy 17p. *J. Pediatr.*, **102**, 522–8

21. Jeret, J.S., Serur, D., Wisniewski, K.E. and Lubin, R.A. (1987). Clinicopathological findings associated with agenesis of the corpus callosum. *Brain Dev.*, **9**, 255–64

22. Bruyns, G.W. (1977). Agenesis septi pellucidi, cavum septi pellucidi and cavum vergae, and cavum veli interpositi. In Vinken, P.J. and Bruyns, G.W. (eds.) *Handbook of Clinical Neurology*, vol. 30, pp. 299–336. (Amsterdam: North-Holland)

23. Farhood, A.I., Morris, J.H. and Bieber, F.R. (1987). Transient cysts of the fetal choroid plexus: morphology and histogenesis. *Am. J. Med. Genet.*, **27**, 977–82

24. Furness, M.E. (1987). Choroid plexus cysts and trisomy 18. *Lancet*, **2**, 693

25. Gardner, E., O'Rahilly, R. and Prolo, D. (1975). The Dandy–Walker and Arnold Chiari malformation. Clinical, developmental and teratological considerations. *Arch. Neurol.*, **32**, 393–401

26. Monteagudo, A., Timor-Tritsch, I.E. and Moomjy, M. (1993). Nomograms of the fetal lateral ventricles using transvaginal sonography. *J. Ultrasound Med.*, **5**, 265–9

27. Pilu, G., Goldstein, I., Reece, E.A., Perolo, A., Foschini, M.P., Hobbins, J.C. and Bovicelli, L. (1992). Sonography of fetal Dandy–Walker malformation: a reappraisal. *Ultrasound Obstet. Gynecol.*, **2**, 151–7

28. Manning, F.A. (1985). Assessment of fetal condition and risk: analysis and combined biophysical variable monitoring. *Semin. Perinatol.*, **9**, 168–83

29. de Vries, J.I.P., Visser, G.H.A. and Prechtl, H.F.R. (1982). The emergence of fetal behaviour. I. Qualitative aspects. *Early Hum. Dev.*, **7**, 301–22

30. de Vries, J.I.P., Visser, G.H.A. and Prechtl, H.F.R. (1982). The emergence of fetal behaviour. II. Quantitative aspects. *Early Hum. Dev.*, **12**, 99–120

31. Nijhuis, J.G. (1986). Behavioural states: concomitants. Clinical implications and the assessment of the condition of the nervous system. *Eur. J. Obstet. Gynaecol. Reprod. Biol.*, **21**, 301–8

32. de Vries, J.I.P., Laurini, R.N. and Visser, G.H.A. (1989). Prenatal motor disorders in cases with abnormal cerebral development. In Versteegh, F.G., Ens-Dokkum, E.C.M., Kuypers, J.C., Pters, P.W.J. and van Velzen, D. (eds.) *1st International Congress in Paediatric Pathology* pp. 30. (Pijnacker, The Netherlands: Dutch Efficiency Bureau)

33. Visser, G.H.A., Laurini, R.N., de Vries, J.I.P., Bekedam, D.J. and Prechtl, H.F.R. (1985). Abnormal motor behaviour in anencephalic fetuses. *Early Hum. Dev.*, **12**, 173–82

34. Norman, R.M. (1940). Primary degeneration of the granular layer of the cerebellum: an unusual form of familial cerebellar atrophy occurring in early life. *Brain*, **63**, 365–79

35. Friede, R.L. (1989). *Developmental Neuropathology*, pp. 361–71. (Berlin: Springer-Verlag)

36. de Vries, J.I.P., Laurini, R.N. and Visser, G.H.A. (1994). Abnormal motor behaviour and developmental postmortem findings in a fetus with Fanconi anaemia. *Early Hum. Dev.*, **21**, 137–42

Transabdominal sonography of the fetal forebrain

3

C. H. Comstock and F. A. Chervenak

NORMAL ANATOMY

A thorough understanding of the normal anatomy of the cerebrum is essential in detecting any of the numerous possible abnormalities in this very complex area. Historically, transverse planes have been preferred for antenatal ultrasound over the coronal and sagittal planes used by neonatal ultrasonographers and pathologists, because the fetal head is most often in an occiput-transverse position (i.e. the side of the head lies parallel to the mother's abdominal wall). The membranous bones of the lateral fetal cranium can be penetrated by sound waves; they are more heavily calcified and rigid in postnatal life, when it becomes necessary to use the window provided by the fontanelles. Finally, a transverse plane produces a large cross-section of the brain, in which multiple landmarks may be visualized and quickly assessed at one time.

The ventricles

The lateral ventricles appear as paired echo-spared areas within the brain substance. The ventricle farthest from the ultrasound transducer is the most clearly visualized, since reverberation artifacts often obscure the anatomy of the proximal hemisphere. A prominent echogenic area is the choroid plexus within the lateral ventricle; it fills the width of the lateral ventricles (Figures 1 and 2).

In early fetal life, the ventricular system fills a large portion of the developing brain (Figure 3), and has the form of two smooth and parallel curved tubes joined to the central (and lower) third ventricle. The anterior portions are termed 'frontal horns' and the middle the 'bodies'; the wide point where the posterior horns join the body and temporal horns is known as the 'atrium'.

As gestation progresses, the ventricular system occupies a decreasing portion of the brain's volume. Sonographically, this change is manifested by a decrease in the proportion of the brain's cross-section occupied by the lateral ventricles. That is, as the biparietal diameter (BPD) increases, the actual side-to-side measurement of the ventricles remains the same. This evolution has been documented and nomograms generated that compare the width of the lateral ventricle to the width of the cerebral hemisphere at various gestational ages[1-3]. The width of the atrium of the lateral ventricle is well defined and should measure 1 cm or less at all gestational ages[4].

The axial or transverse plane

The most intensely studied transverse section of the fetus is at the level of the BPD. The two landmarks most consistently found are the paired, half-circular and non-echogenic thalami and two short anterior lines paralleling the midline, once thought to be the cavum septi pellucidi, but now known to be the medial walls of the lateral ventricles[5]. Other structures commonly observed in the same plane and near the midline are the third ventricle between the thalami and the frontal horns of the lateral ventricles (Figures 1 and 2).

In this plane, the BPD can be reproducibly measured as the distance from the proximal outer table to the distal inner table of the skull[6,7]. In addition, the head perimeter can be determined by direct measurement around the calvarium (excluding soft tissues). The ratio of BPD to occipitofrontal diameter (OFD) defines the cephalic index (normal values 75–85). A high value indicates brachycephaly and a low value dolichocephaly. Because the fetal head has such pliability, the BPD

43

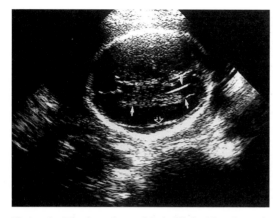

Figure 1 The lateral ventricle is filled with echogenic choroid plexus. The arrows mark the walls of the ventricle. Note that there is no space between the choroid and the medial wall of the lateral ventricle. The bright line (open arrow) paralleling the cranium should not be mistaken for the lateral ventricle wall: it is the surface of the brain

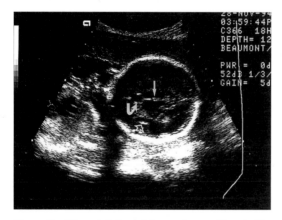

Figure 2 The axial view of the cerebrum. The slit-like third ventricle (arrow) lies between the half-circle-shaped thalami. The two parallel lines anterior to the thalami are the medial walls of the lateral ventricles (curved arrow). The insula (open arrow) is clearly seen

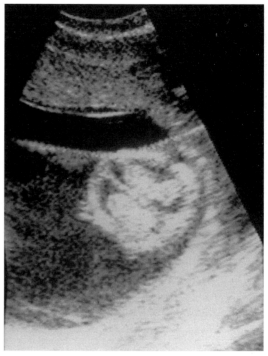

Figure 3 At 12 weeks, the choroid plexuses and ventricles are very large in comparison to the head itself

is often an inaccurate determinant of gestational age: the head circumference is, however, not affected by head shape.

There are several sonographic markers which have anatomic correlates that have been a source of confusion. During the second trimester and later, an echogenic line, once thought to be the sylvian fissure, is actually a reflection from the insular cortex with its associated middle cerebral artery[8]. Finally, parallel bright white lines are seen high in the vertex which have been mistaken for the lateral walls of the cerebral ventricles (Figure 4). Note, however, that they almost extend to the calvarium, both anteriorly and posteriorly; their actual source is unknown.

CRANIOSPINAL ANOMALIES

Anencephaly

Anencephaly is a congenital anomaly in which most of the brain is absent; what remains is not covered by the vault of the skull. Remnants of forebrain may be present and the medulla is generally well formed, but the cerebral hemispheres, and frequently the midbrain, are completely absent.

Etiology

Anencephaly is thought to be a result of a failure of closure of the rostral portion of the neural tube. This fusion normally begins in the region of the fourth somite and extends both rostrally and

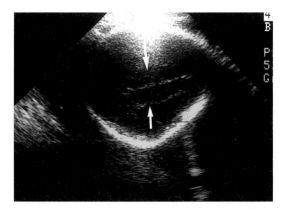

Figure 4 The high axial view demonstrates the midline falx and two parallel lines (arrows). The origin of these lines is not known, but they should not be mistaken for the walls of the ventricles

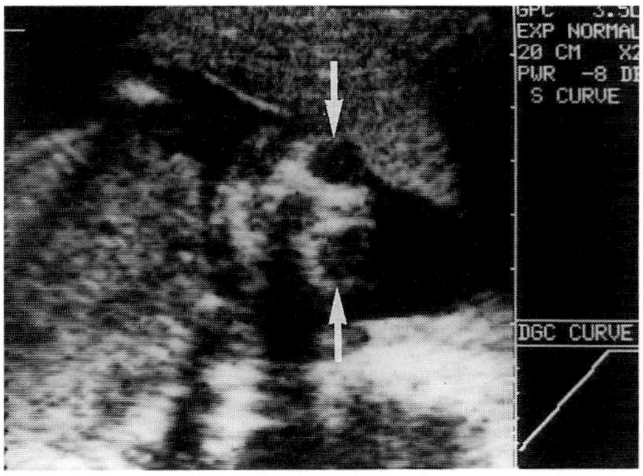

Figure 5 Anencephaly. Coronal plane with the top of the head to the right. The orbits (arrows) appear large when their upper border is absent

caudally. Closure in the region of the developing head is completed about 24 days after conception, and in the region of the sacrum at about 26 days. This common embryological origin may explain the concurrence of anencephaly with sacral spina bifida or complete non-closure of the neural tube. In place of the cerebral hemispheres, a mass of thin-walled vascular channels, known as the *area cerebrovasculosa*, may sometimes be seen protruding from the base of the skull. This mass, which may be a derivative of the choroid plexus, is usually covered by a membrane contiguous with the scalp. There is some evidence that anencephaly may also result from secondary degeneration of an already closed neural tube in which the skull did not form (acrania); brain tissue gradually decreases until the usual appearance of anencephaly is achieved[9,10].

Diagnosis

Anencephaly was the first fetal anomaly to be diagnosed by antenatal ultrasound. Ultrasound produces such a clear image of anencephaly that, as early as 1972, a pregnancy was terminated following an ultrasound diagnosis of anencephaly[11]. Anencephaly can now be reliably diagnosed during the second and third trimesters. However, caution is necessary when the diagnosis is made in the first trimester, because the normal immature brain may be difficult to differentiate from remnants of abnormal brain at this early stage[12].

The antenatal sonographic diagnosis of anencephaly is based upon the absence of the calvarium, the dome-like portion of the cranial vault (Figure 5). The orbits are clearly seen, but there is nothing above them. When the area cerebrovasculosa is prominent, an ill-defined mass of heterogeneous density may be seen by ultrasound. In addition, many of these pregnancies are complicated by hydramnios, presumably due to impaired fetal swallowing.

Although the diagnosis of anencephaly is usually straightforward, certain other entities should be considered. In severe microcephaly, the bones of the skull may be difficult to locate, but they are uniformly present. In the early amnion-rupture sequence, constricting bands may prevent the normal formation of the skull[10]. In this case, however, the malformation is usually asymmetrical and brain tissue is present. A large encephalocele might stimulate anencephaly until a brain-filled sac is localized. Lastly, anencephaly can be differentiated from *acrania*, because in the latter there is an outwardly normally formed brain, but absent skull. In actuality, although the brain in acrania appears normal on an ultrasound scan, it has many subtle abnormalities and outcome is poor.

Outcome/management

Anencephaly is a lethal anomaly. Most fetuses are either stillborn or, if liveborn, die shortly after birth. A single report describes an infant with anencephaly that survived for 5.5 months[13]. As anencephaly is diagnosable with a high degree of accuracy and is uniformly lethal, the authors believe that termination of pregnancy is an ethical option at any time in gestation[14]. If it is diagnosed during the third trimester and the parents elect termination, laminaria placement may facilitate induction of labor when the cervix is unripe.

Postmaturity is a common occurrence in anencephalic fetuses. Cesarean delivery is not recommended for fetal distress, but it may be necessary for maternal indication. If an anencephalic infant is liveborn, humane care should be provided until the time of its death. The use of anencephalic newborns as organ donors has been widely debated[15, 16].

The incidence of this disorder is highly variable, depending on an individual's geographic location, race and sex. Its incidence in the USA has been estimated at one in 1000 deliveries, but it is much more common in the UK, with an incidence as high as 6.7 in 1000 in Belfast. Anencephaly is more common in Whites than Blacks and Orientals, and approximately twice as common in female infants[17, 18].

The recurrence risk after the birth of an affected child for any open neural tube defect, including anencephaly, may be as low as 1.7% in the USA[19]. In populations in which anencephaly is more common, the risk may be greater. The rate of recurrence may be higher after the birth of two or more affected siblings, and a 25% recurrence risk exists in the rare instance in which anencephaly is part of the Meckel syndrome.

In future pregnancies, antenatal ultrasound examination should be performed in an attempt to make an anatomic diagnosis of an open neural tube defect and/or hydrocephalus.

Hydrocephalus

Hydrocephalus (ventriculomegaly) is an abnormal increase in the volume of the cerebral ventricles. It is almost always due to obstruction of the flow of cerebrospinal fluid (CSF) and the resulting increase in intracranial pressure. Very rarely, it may be due to an increase in CSF production or a relative decrease in the amount of brain tissue.

Hydrocephalus is said to be 'isolated' when there are no other anomalies that are not the direct result of the ventricular enlargment and intracranial pressure.

Etiology

The incidence of congenital hydrocephalus unassociated with neural tube defect is 5.8 in 10000 total births in the USA and 3.1 in 10000 total births in England and Wales[20]. There are many and varied causes of hydrocephalus. Some may be truly embryological (resulting from defects in primary morphogenesis) while others could be best described as defects acquired in utero. The first category includes hydrocephalus in a fetus with a chromosomal aberration, inherited following a Mendelian pattern, or in association with a malformation syndrome. Hydrocephalus may result from acquired defects in utero, as the result of infection with scarring and CSF obstruction, from intraventricular hemorrhage, arteriovenous malformations, or intracranial tumors. Unfortunately, many cases of hydrocephalus cannot be assigned to one or other of these categories.

A variety of fetal anomalies have been described in association with fetal hydrocephalus. The most frequent coincident anomaly is spina bifida which is thought to be due to the frequent association of spina bifida with the Arnold–Chiari malformation. In such cases, there is obstruction at the base of the fourth ventricle. The major causes of hydrocephalus are listed in Table 1.

In general there are four ways in which the ventricles grow to an abnormal size: (1) obstruction to outflow, usually at a point of narrowing in the system; (2) impaired resorption of CSF by the arachnoid granulations; (3) overproduction of CSF; and (4) underdevelopment or destruction of cortical tissue, with a relative increase in the size of the ventricles. Our experience and that of others suggests that obstructive causes are the most common in the fetal population, as is the case for the newborn[21–24].

Diagnosis

A variety of techniques have been advocated for the diagnosis of hydrocephalus. The traditional

Table 1 Etiology of hydrocephalus

Genetic causes
Aqueductal stenosis
Hydrocephalus with cerebellar agenesis
Achondroplasia
Osteogenesis imperfecta
With Dandy–Walker malformation
Triploidy
Trisomy 13
Trisomy 18
Trisomy 21
Balanced translocations

Other causes
Infection
Tumor
Subarachnoid cysts
Arteriovenous malformations
Hemorrhage
Spina bifida (Chiari malformation)

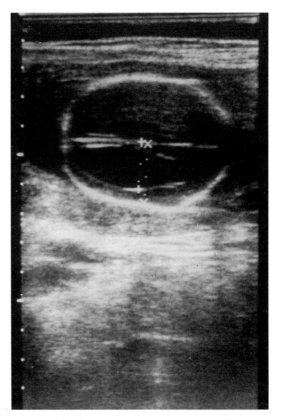

Figure 6 Hydrocephalus. The distance from the falx to the lateral wall of the lateral ventricle (+–+) is compared with the distance from the falx to the inner aspect of the calvarium (x–x). After 18 weeks, this ratio should be less than 1:2, but specific tables are available for each gestational age

method in the United States has been determination of the ratio of lateral ventricle to hemispheric width[1,2] (Figure 6). This method has several advantages. Measurements are taken in the largest part of the ventricular system that can be identified quickly and consistently. Further, these measurements do not depend on identification of the medial wall of the lateral ventricle, which was frequently difficult to visualize with earlier generation ultrasound machines and may still be a problem in difficult scanning situations.

Some have contended that the ratio of lateral ventricle to hemispheric width is insensitive to early hydrocephalus, as it ignores medial deviation of the medial wall of the lateral ventricle. Cardoza and colleagues[4] have presented strong evidence that a single measurement of the lateral ventricular atrium can accurately differentiate a normal ventricular system from one that is pathologically enlarged. Atrial measurements are obtained by placing calipers on the inner margins of the atrial walls, perpendicular to the long axis of the ventricle (and not to the midline axis) (Figure 7). Errors in measurement favor an increase in the size of the diameter, so that the smallest diameter is likely to be the most accurate[25]. In 100 normal fetuses, this measurement had a mean of 7.6 ± 0.6 mm (± SD) in the range of 14–38 weeks. All of 38 fetuses with hydrocephalus in this retrospective study had

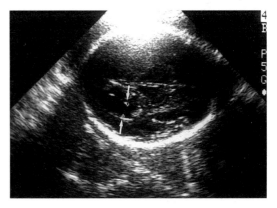

Figure 7 Measurement of the atrium of the lateral ventricle. The widest portion of the posterior pattern of the lateral ventricle is measured from inner surface to inner surface. The calipers (arrows) should be placed perpendicular to the axis of the ventricle, not to the axis of the falx

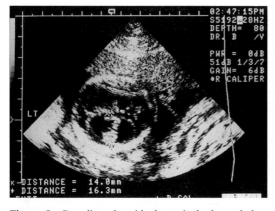

Figure 8 Dangling choroid plexus in hydrocephalus. The echogenic choroid is dangling at a right angle to the enlarged ventricle

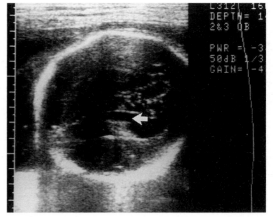

Figure 9 Hydrocephalus in fetus with heterozygous achondroplasia. There is a 4-mm separation (arrow) of the choroid plexus from the medial wall of the lateral ventricle

lateral ventricular atrial widths of ≥ 11 mm. Two recent studies of 500 fetuses[26] and 739 fetuses[27] confirm that almost all normal fetuses have atrial widths of < 10 mm. All fetuses from 12–17 weeks had ventricular measurments of ≤ 8 mm, and all but four out of 326 in the 17–25 week range also had diameters of < 8 mm[27].

There are other observations that may also be of value in the diagnosis of fetal hydrocephalus, of which evaluation of the choroid plexus may be one[28–31]. The choroid plexus usually fills the width of the lateral ventricles and appears symmetrical in both ventricles, regardless of the orientation of the fetal head to gravity. It is anchored anteriorly where it passes through the foramen of Munro, but is free posteriorly. In hydrocephalus, the posterior choroid plexus falls (or dangles) to the dependent side of the ventricles (Figure 8). Attempts have been made to quantify this dangling appearance by measuring a 'choroid angle' between the long axis of the choroid plexus in the dependent ventricle and the midline echo[30]. In addition, investigators have tried to define early hydrocephalus by an increased distance (> 3 mm) between the choroid plexus and the medial wall of the lateral ventricle at the level of the atrium[32] (Figure 9), or by evaluating changes in the shape of the frontal horn of the lateral ventricle[28]. If a ventricle is of normal width (< 10 mm) but the choroid plexus is separated from the medial walls of the ventricle by a fluid layer measuring more than 3 mm, hydrocephalus may still exist[33].

In cases of advanced hydrocephalus, any of these quantitative or qualitative assessments is bound to be accurate. In cases of mild ventricular enlargement or when hydrocephalus is studied in the early second trimester, it is the authors' opinion that a combination of these techniques in experienced hands is most likely to lead to accurate diagnosis. The crucial importance of serial examinations should be kept in mind in diagnosis or when fetal hydrocephalus is to be excluded. The absence of hydrocephalus at one point in gestation does not preclude its later development, and repeat examinations are indicated for a pregnancy at risk. Furthermore, and more importantly, when hydrocephalus is diagnosed as an isolated abnormality, serial scans should be performed, since hydrocephalus has been documented to regress *in utero*[34–36].

Communicating hydrocephalus, i.e. ventricular enlargement without obstruction within the ventricular system, has been diagnosed in a fetus with a choroid plexus papilloma. Dilatation of the ventricular system and of the subarachnoid space were documented sonographically[37].

When infection causes hydrocephalus, calcification of the periventricular or thalamic areas can sometimes be seen (Figure 10). These appear as brighter ventricular walls, rather than as discrete calcifications, and do not produce sound shadowing. There are often other findings, such as ascites, growth restriction and liver calcification[38].

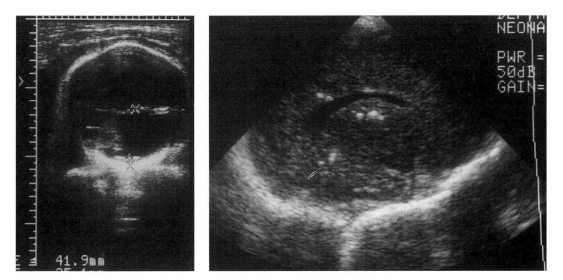

Figure 10 Hydrocephalus secondary to cytomegalovirus (left). Neonatal ultrasound in the sagittal plane (right) demonstrates tiny calcifications not seen in the antenatal scan

Certain pitfalls in the detection of early fetal hydrocephalus should be considered, to avoid false-positive diagnoses. Because artifactual echoes often obscure accurate measurement on the proximal side of the head, hydrocephalus is best assessed in the distal hemisphere. Another frequent source of confusion is a crescent-shaped, hypoechoic area, which is occasionally visualized in the distal hemisphere (Figure 1); the actual walls of the hemisphere must be identified[39].

Hydrocephalus may be distinguished from holoprosencephaly by the presence of midline structures and by separation of the ventricles. Even in lobar holoprosencephaly, the most mild form of holoprosencephaly, the anterior horns are fused. In hydranencephaly, there is no cortex whatsoever. Although head size is often normal in early hydrocephalus, it often increases disproportionately in later gestation. Since hydranencephaly is a replacement phenomenon rather than a result of pressure, the circumference of the head does not usually enlarge in hydranencephaly.

Outcome

Prior to the development of surgical shunting of the dilated ventricular system, the outlook for the infant with hydrocephalus was generally poor. Although even unoperated obstructive hydrocephalus can be slowly progressive or arrest spontaneously, massive head enlargement with blindness and mental retardation were far more common in the past and still exist in the Third World. In 1954, Feeny reported that, of 93 liveborn infants with hydrocephalus, only ten survived to leave the hospital[40]. In 1962, Laurence and Coates[41] reported that, among 182 patients with hydrocephalus for whom surgery was not performed, the newborns' chances of reaching adulthood were 20–23%. Of the survivors, only 38% had an IQ greater than 85. Furthermore, it should be appreciated that this was a selected group and even these figures are probably optimistic, when the prognosis for all newborn babies with hydrocephalus is considered.

The development of surgical shunting markedly improved the prognosis for the infant with hydrocephalus. This is illustrated by the experience in the early days of shunt therapy, when a prospective randomized trial comparing surgical shunting with conservative management in 30 infants was attempted by Lorber and Zachary[42]. The trial was terminated prematurely when 11 of the 13 infants in the control group needed surgery to arrest neurological deterioration or rapidly increasing head circumference. In another study, 200 consecutive infants with neonatal hydrocephalus at Children's Memorial Hospital in Chicago underwent shunt procedures[43]. Of these, only five died. Intellectual development in the survivors is related to the type of hydrocephalus, age at initial shunt placement and shunt function, but not to the severity of the hydrocephalus or to the number of shunt revisions. For Caucasians with isolated hydrocephalus, the mean IQ was 84 ± 25.8. Infants with other forms of hydrocephalus, such as those related to porencephaly or to Dandy–Walker cyst, had significantly lower mean IQs. In this series, those infants with congenital hydrocephalus were not clearly differentiated from those who developed hydrocephalus during the neonatal period. At the University of Washington School of Medicine, 16 of 19 infants with congenital hydrocephalus who were treated achieved IQs of at least 80[44]. A total of 32 of 37 infants with congenital hydrocephalus and microcephaly were managed at Georgetown University Medical Center; 17 had a normal IQ (above 80) and six had a borderline IQ (between 65 and 80)[45].

Others have confirmed the conclusion that well-treated infants *without associated congenital malformations* have an excellent chance to achieve normal intelligence, irrespective of the initial severity of their hydrocephalus. At the University of Pennsylvania, ten neonates were followed after computed tomography (CT) demonstrated virtual absence of the cerebral tissue[46]. Two well-defined clinical entities were distinguished. A total of five infants with hydranencephaly showed absence of cortical activity on electroencephalogram (EEG) and a CT picture of minimal occipital brain parenchyma. Although these infants received shunt therapy, no neurological or radiological improvement occurred with time. The remaining five infants had severe hydrocephalus, but retained minimal frontal cerebral mantle on CT and exhibited electrical activity on EEG. After shunting procedures, a remarkable increase in brain tissue was demonstrated in the latter group by serial CT scans, and neurological development was either normal or only slightly delayed. The probable reason for the retention of cerebral function with a markedly thinned cerebral cortex is that ventricular dilatation occurs at the expense of the white matter, whereas the gray matter on the convoluted surface of the cerebral cortex is unfolded and spread over a wider surface area, with no true damage to nerve cells[47]. This is supported by the normal appearance of the brain by CT following successful shunting in certain cases.

A total of 56 infants with severe congenital hydrocephalus (with 10 mm or less cortex remaining), treated with shunting have been followed over 8 years; 46 of the 56 infants survived[48]. Of these, five were of superior intelligence, 29 were of average-to-good intelligence, five were educably subnormal, and six were profoundly retarded. Intellectual outcome was better when the shunting procedure was performed prior to 6 months of age. Lorber concluded that 'Even the most extreme degrees of hydrocephalus are compatible with normal physical development and a normal-sized head and intelligence if operative treatment is not delayed'.

Several recent papers have focused on the outcome of hydrocephalus diagnosed during the fetal period. In each of these series, most of the fetuses (59–85%) had major structural and/or chromosomal anomalies in addition to hydrocephalus, and most died during the perinatal period[21–23,49–53]. The much higher death rate observed in these fetal studies as compared to studies of children with isolated hydrocephalus is at least partly attributable to the high frequency of associated anomalies.

Even if hydrocephalus is thought to be isolated, there may be undetected anomalies seen at birth[52]. In those fetuses who truly have isolated hydrocephalus, however, there is a possibility of developmental delay. A total of 28 fetuses with an atrial diameter of 11–15 mm and no other ultrasound findings have been followed to more than 1 year of life (mean follow-up period 30 months); 22 (79%) were developing normally and six (21%) were developmentally delayed. The nature of the delay was primarily that of speech and/or mild motor delay. One child had enough delay in cognitive development that special education was required[54].

Once fetal hydrocephalus is identified, a careful sonographic search for associated anomalies is indicated. Fetal echocardiography should be performed. Karyotype determination should be offered; at least a 10% incidence of chromosomal aberrations has been reported with fetal hydrocephalus[51]. Because so many cases of hydrocephalus are associated with meningomyelocele, it is important to exclude or identify such an association. Prognostic information is also provided in Chapter 14.

Management

The obstetric management of fetal hydrocephalus is dependent upon gestational age at the time of diagnosis and the association of other anomalies. Options include continuation of the pregnancy, termination prior to fetal viability, ventriculoamniotic shunt placement, or cephalocentesis prior to delivery.

The indications for and experience with ventriculoamniotic shunts is described elsewhere in this book. In order to minimize the potential ill effects of progressive ventricular enlargement, we recommend delivery of the fetus with hydrocephalus as soon as pulmonary maturity is demonstrated. At the present time, there is no clear guideline for preterm delivery when hydrocephalus worsens prior to fetal lung maturity. The risks of respiratory distress syndrome with resultant delay in ventriculoperitoneal shunt placement must be balanced against potential ill effects of progressive hydrocephalus. Serial sonography may be helpful in determining the management, arguing for early delivery if hydrocephalus is rapidly progressing. If delivery prior to fetal lung maturity is elected, then maternal corticosteroid administration is recommended to reduce the risk and severity of respiratory distress syndrome in the neonate.

In view of the potential for normal, and even superior, intelligence for those infants with hydrocephalus who are given optimum neonatal neurosurgical care, fetuses with isolated hydrocephalus and macrocephaly are best delivered by Cesarean section[51]. However, in those instances in which hydrocephalus is associated with anomalies that themselves carry a very poor prognosis (e.g. alobar holoprosencephaly or thanatophoric dysplasia with cloverleaf skull), cephalocentesis (with subsequent vaginal delivery) may be the most appropriate form of management. This procedure, which may avoid Cesarean section, is performed by passing a needle into a lateral cerebral ventricle, either transabdominally or transvaginally, and removing sufficient CSF to permit vaginal delivery. Simultaneous sonographic guidance facilitates cephalo-

centesis and the position of the needle tip should be followed throughout the procedure. After aspiration of CSF, overlapping of the cranial sutures can be observed with ultrasound. It is important to note that cephalocentesis is most often a destructive procedure; in one series, perinatal death occurred following 91% of the cephalocenteses. The sonographic visualization of intracranial bleeding during cephalocentesis, and the demonstration of this hemorrhage at autopsy, further emphasize the morbid nature of the procedure. Because fetal cortical mantle thickness correlates poorly with subsequent intelligence, the authors do not advocate cephalocentesis in cases of severe isolated hydrocephalus. If there is no demonstrable cortex, however, hydranencephaly is most probably present. Since this condition has a dismal prognosis, cephalocentesis may be appropriate[51].

The authors believe that Cesarean delivery may not be necessary for all cases if there is a normal progression of labor. Attempted vaginal delivery may be appropriate when the fetus, in a vertex presentation, has a normal-sized head (head biometry 2SD above the mean for gestational age), or has mild macrocephaly (e.g. BPD of 98 mm at 38 weeks of gestation). When fetal hydrocephalus is associated with a meningomyelocele, however, Cesarean delivery may be less traumatic than vaginal delivery[55,56].

Counselling

Although hydrocephalus has diverse causes, the identification of its source greatly aids in genetic counselling. Several heritable patterns have been identified. Sex-linked recessive aqueductal stenosis carries a 1 in 4 risk of recurrence for future pregnancies and a 1 in 2 risk for male fetuses[57]. Cerebellar agenesis with hydrocephalus is extremely rare, but also may be sex-linked and thus have a similar recurrence risk[58]. Several syndromes which manifest dominant inheritance are associated with hydrocephalus (e.g. achondroplasia and osteogenesis imperfecta)[59], but the occurrence is irregular and the risk of hydrocephalus in future pregnancies cannot be accurately predicted. The Dandy–Walker syndrome has been reported in siblings and may sometimes follow an autosomal recessive

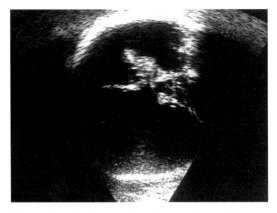

Figure 11 Hydranencephaly (coronal view). Note no cerebral cortex; however, the falx was still present. The echogenic mass to the right of the midline was blood

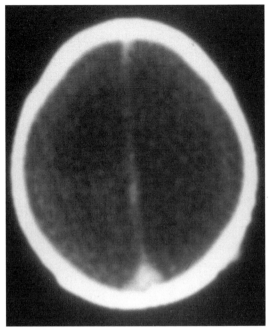

Figure 12 Hydranencephaly. Postnatal computed tomography demonstrated no cortical mantle

pattern with a recurrence risk of 1 in 4 for future pregnancies[60]. Several studies have suggested an increased risk of uncomplicated hydrocephalus in families with neural tube defects[61,62]. Lorber and De[63] studied uncomplicated congenital hydrocephalus and found an empiric risk of 4% for a central nervous system (CNS) malformation and of 2% for spina bifida or hydrocephalus in future pregnancies. Hydrocephalus may be associated with a variety of chromosomal abnormalities, including triploidy, trisomy 13, trisomy 18, trisomy 21 and certain balanced translocations. The risk of recurrence is low for sporadic chromosomal abnormalities, but may be much higher for balanced translocations[59].

Other causes of fetal hydrocephalus include prenatal infection, intracranial tumors and cysts, and vascular malformations. Such causes are unlikely to result in an increased risk of hydrocephalus in future pregnancies[59].

Hydranencephaly

Hydranencephaly is an intracranial anomaly characterized by replacement of the cerebral hemispheres with fluid. Only the basal ganglia and remnants of the mesencephalon remain within the normally formed skull above the tentorium cerebelli. The subtentorial structures are usually intact and the falx cerebri is frequently present. This anomaly is thought to arise by destruction of a normally forming brain some time during gestation. Bilateral occlusion of the internal carotid arteries has been proposed as one mechanism for this destruction.

The sonographic picture is of a normal cranial vault, filled with fluid and with a midline echo, but without cerebral cortex (Figures 11 and 12). The tentorium cerebelli and cerebellum are visible.

This disorder may be differentiated from hydrocephalus and severe porencephaly by the absence of any cerebral cortex. In holoprosencephaly, there is some cerebral cortex but no midline falx. In severe cases of hydrocephalus, a thin cortical mantle may be hard to detect by ultrasound, and intrauterine CT scanning or magnetic resonance imaging (MRI) may be useful modalities to generate a differential diagnosis[64,65].

Most infants with hydranencephaly die within the first year of life. Severe retardation is uniformly present among survivors. Sporadic familial recurrences have been reported, but these are most exceptional and, in general, the recurrence risk should be considered negligible.

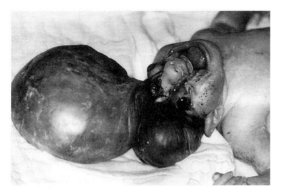

Figure 13 Encephalocele secondary to an amniotic band. Note the bilateral facial cleft

Cephalocele

A cephalocele is a protrusion of the meninges and, frequently, brain tissue through a defect in the cranium. The term includes both encephaloceles, which contain brain tissue, and cranial meningoceles, which do not. The incidence is approximately 1 in 2000 live births[20].

Etiology

Encephaloceles are thought to arise from a failure of closure of the rostral end of the neural tube during the fourth week of fetal life. This fusion begins in the region of the fourth somite and extends both rostrally and caudally. It has been suggested that either a primary overgrowth of neural tube tissue in the line of closure or a failure of induction by adjacent mesodermal tissues may interrupt this process. Since the majority of cephaloceles occur in the midline, this mechanism may explain their genesis. If disruption of neural tube fusion occurs in the caudal region at the same time, then spina bifida and a cephalocele may be present simultaneously. This helps to explain the observed concurrence of these two lesions in 7–15% of cephaloceles[66–68].

A cephalocele also may result from early disruption in the formation of the fetal skull. One clear example of this is the amnion rupture sequence. Rupture of the amnion early in gestation may produce bands of tissue capable of encircling any part of the fetus (Figure 13). Limb amputations, abdominal wall defects and malformations of the fetal skull are among the abnormalities that may result. In this disorder, cephaloceles do not have a single characteristic appearance or predictable location and often occur away from the midline[69].

A cephalocele may develop as an isolated lesion or as a part of various syndromes, several with high recurrence risks. The most important of these is Meckel's syndrome, which has an autosomal recessive pattern of inheritance, and is characterized by polycystic kidneys, cephalocele and polydactyly, as well as a variety of other defects[70]. A cephalocele may also occur as a part of Robert's, Chemke's, Knoblock's and cryptophthalmus syndromes and in dyssegmental dwarfism. These are all autosomal recessive disorders. In addition, cephaloceles have been reported with maternal warfarin ingestion[71].

Diagnosis

A cephalocele appears as a sac-like protrusion from the head, not covered by bone[72–75]. If only membranes have herniated, the sac is filled with fluid, but if the brain has herniated, the contents of the sac have a heterogeneous appearance. In the Western world, 75% of these lesions are occipital, but they also may be parietal, frontal or nasopharyngeal[76]. The incidence of anterior lesions appears to be considerably greater in the Orient[77]. The nasopharyngeal variety will be missed in most cases. Frequently, small frontal cephaloceles are missed, since they may not be in a standard scanning plane.

The diagnosis can be made with certainty only if a skull defect can be demonstrated (Figures 14 and 15). A diligent search with varying transducer angles is often necessary. If a defect in the skull is still not found, the differential possibilities include cystic hygroma, teratoma, cervical meningomyelocele (Figure 16) and hemangioma as well as cephalocele. It has been reported recently that fetal hair or a fetal ear[78] can mimic the sonographic appearance of a cephalocele. Again, the importance of finding a break in the skull is emphasized.

Once a cephalocele is diagnosed, a careful examination of fetal anatomy is indicated. Because hydrocephalus may be associated, intracranial anatomy should be evaluated. Since a second

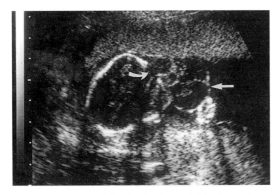

Figure 14 Encephalocele. Brain and falx (arrow) are visible outside the confines of the skull. There is a clear defect in the calvarium (curved arrow)

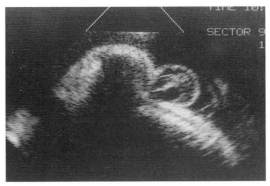

Figure 16 A cervical meningomyelocele can imitate an encephalocele. In this case the upper cervical spine was abnormal, and no defect could be seen in the cranium

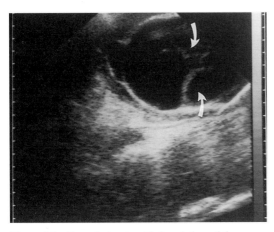

Figure 15 Encephalocele with herniation of the membranes only on the top of the head. This would be missed in many scans, because the head is not usually scanned in the coronal plane. Curved arrows, orbits

neural tube defect may be present, the spine should also be examined in detail. In addition, cephaloceles may be present in association with a variety of genetic syndromes, some features of which are currently detectable by ultrasound.

With cephaloceles, as with other open neural tube defects, levels of alpha-fetoprotein (AFP) may be elevated in both amniotic fluid and maternal serum. Thus, potential cases of cephalocele may be referred to the sonologist as a result of AFP screening. If the lesion is covered with skin, however, both maternal and amniotic fluid AFP levels may be normal[72]. Therefore, AFP is an unreliable adjunct to ultrasound diagnosis.

Outcome

Several investigators have attempted to determine the prognosis of children with cephaloceles[66–68,71,79]. The larger series have focused on occipital lesions, but certain principles appear constant for all locations. The presence of brain in the protruding sac is the most important discriminator[66–68,79]. Almost half of the infants with isolated meningoceles have normal development after surgery. In contrast, the outlook is dismal for those children with microcephaly secondary to brain herniation[68]. There are currently no good data regarding the significance of a small amount of brain in the sac. In one series, two infants in whom a small amount of brain tissue had herniated are currently alive with moderate developmental delays[72].

In the past, concurrent hydrocephalus was an adverse prognostic factor, but with modern shunt therapy, it has a lesser impact than the presence and amount of brain herniation. Frontal cephaloceles have a much better prognosis than those in other locations[66,71]. This may be because the defects are smaller, and, therefore, less brain herniates through them, or because the loss of frontal cortex produces fewer neurological deficits. If a cephalocele is present concomitantly with other defects, or as a part of certain severe genetic syndromes, the outlook is uniformly poor.

Management

If a cephalocele is diagnosed before fetal viability, many parents will elect termination of pregnancy.

After fetal viability has been reached, however, the mode of delivery at term becomes the critical issue. If a large amount of brain tissue is observed in the sac, and, especially, if one or more of the grave prognostic factors (i.e. microcephaly or associated anomalies) are also present, the parents should be counselled that the chance for a good outcome is remote, and Cesarean section is probably not advisable. In such cases, decompression of a large sac or associated hydrocephalus may be necessary to allow vaginal delivery[74].

There are, however, certain situations when Cesarean delivery should be considered:

(1) When a cephalocele is sufficiently large and solid enough to cause dystocia;

(2) When there is a viable, unaffected coincident twin with an indication for Cesarean delivery; or

(3) When an isolated cephalocele is sonographically identified and the parents accept the risks of significant developmental defects. In such cases, Cesarean delivery might minimize birth trauma and improve neonatal outcome.

The empiric risk for a cephalocele recurring in a subsequent pregnancy has been estimated at as high as 5%. If, however, those cases appearing as a part of genetic syndromes, especially the Meckel syndrome, are excluded, the recurrence risk for cephaloceles may be as low as 1.7%[19].

Holoprosencephaly

The term holoprosencephaly embraces a spectrum of cerebral abnormalities resulting from varying degrees of failure of division in the primitive prosencephalon, or forebrain. The incidence of holoprosencephaly has been reported to be between 1 in 5200 and 1 in 16000 live births[80, 81], but may affect as many as 0.4% of all conceptuses[82].

Holoprosencephaly is divided into alobar, semilobar and lobar categories, all based on the degree of separation of the cerebral hemispheres[83]. The alobar variety is the most severe, with no evidence of division of the cerebral cortex. The falx cerebri and interhemispheric fissure are absent. There is a single common ventricle and only a rudimentary corpus callosum, if one is present at all. The semilobar and lobar varieties represent a higher degree of brain development, with the semilobar having a partial separation of the hemispheres. There is much variability in the defects of the midline cerebral structures. Absent olfactory tracts and bulbs are usually associated with all of these conditions, hence the older term 'arhinencephaly'.

Etiology

In holoprosencephaly, perhaps more than any other malformation, an understanding of the embryology can lead directly to ultrasound diagnosis. Two intimately related abnormalities, namely hypotelorism and a single common ventricle, give rise to the sonographic markers of this abnormality: decreased intraorbital distance and absence of the midline echo.

A connective tissue mass between the oral cavity and the undersurface of the neural tube called the 'pre-chordal mesoderm' is thought to be the site of origin for both the development of the nasofrontal process and the division of the prosencephalon. The nasofrontal process gives rise to the ethmoid, nasal and pre-maxillary bones, the vomer and nasal septum. Failure of these structures to develop normally can result in the varying degrees of hypotelorism, cleft lip and palate, and nasal malformation seen in this disorder. The prosencephalon gives rise to the cerebral hemispheres, thalamus and hypothalamus. Failure of its sagittal division can result in a common ventricle, a fused thalamus, and cortex with neither lobes nor an interhemispheric fissure[83].

The etiology of holoprosencephaly is heterogeneous and often not known for an individual case. Chromosomal abnormalities including trisomies 13 and 18, triploidy, 13q–, and 18p have been associated[69]. Teratogenic agents, including ionizing radiation[84] and certain alkaloids[85] have produced this malformation in experimental animals. However, no such agent has been clearly identified in humans. A 200-fold increase in the incidence of holoprosencephaly has been reported in diabetic mothers[86]. Familial occurrence has been documented in several cases. Autosomal recessive inheritance with variable expression has been suggested

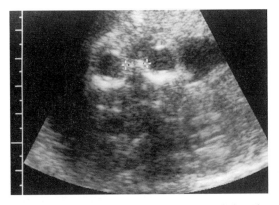

Figure 17 Hypotelorism in holoprosencephaly. The interorbital distance is small. If the orbits are very close together, there may be two globes, but only one opening

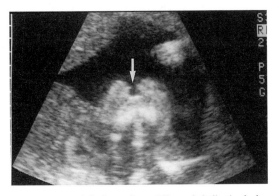

Figure 18 Axial view of a midline cleft lip in holoprosencephaly (arrow)

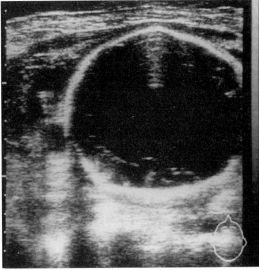

Figure 19 Holoprosencephaly. There is no division of the ventricles and, consequently, no falx. Note the anterior crescent of cortex, which is the most typical appearance

somal recessive inheritance. It is usually impossible to designate these families, although co-sanguinity or a previously affected child may be suggestive. Rarely, autosomal dominant inheritance could be present and predict a high recurrence. Close examination of both parents of the proband for minor signs of midline facial anomaly (e.g. hypotelorism) is mandatory, to seek evidence of this possibility.

Diagnosis

In holoprosencephaly, a spectrum of midline facial anomalies may be seen. Indeed, certain facies predict the presence of the alobar type. Cyclopia, the presence of a single median bony orbit with a fleshy proboscis above it, is the most severe of these malformations. Ethmocephaly, the least common, is characterized by two separate orbits with a proboscis in between. In cebocephaly, hypotelorism is associated with a normally placed nose with a single nostril. Hypotelorism with a midline facial cleft also predicts the presence of alobar holoprosencephaly (Figures 17 and 18). Holoprosencephaly also may be associated with milder forms of midline facial dysplasia or, occasionally, normal facies[83].

in some families, and autosomal dominant inheritance with both incomplete penetrance and variable expression in others. The recessively inherited Meckel's syndrome also may include holoprosencephaly.

The diagnosis of holoprosencephaly signals the need for a chromosomal determination to guide the management of future pregnancies. A chromosomal anomaly may predict either a low recurrence risk of less than 1%, if a trisomy is demonstrated, or a much higher risk, if the aneuploidy involves a translocation and one of the parents is a carrier of the translocation chromosomes.

In the absence of a chromosomal abnormality, an empirical recurrence risk of 6% has been calculated. However, some families may be faced with the 25% recurrence risk associated with auto-

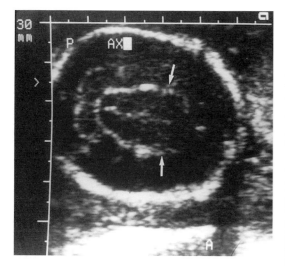

Figure 20 In holoprosencephaly, the thalami (arrows) appear large. The normal cerebellum lies to the left

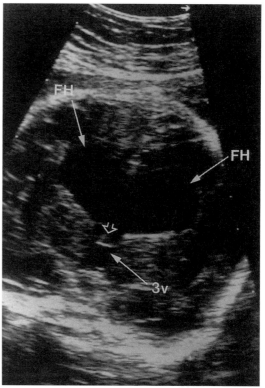

Figure 21 Lobar holoprosencephaly. Only the frontal horns (FH) are fused. The fused fornices (open arrow) in the third ventricle (3v) constitute a specific sign for lobar holoprosencephaly. (Printed with permission from reference 98)

The midline echo of the fetal head, seen sonographically, is generated in large part by the reflection of sound waves from acoustic interfaces at the interhemispheric fissure. This fissure is absent in alobar holoprosencephaly (Figure 19) and incomplete in the semilobar variety. The thalami are fused in the complete type (Figure 20). The hypotelorism frequently seen in holoprosencephaly may be detected antenatally, as the bony orbits can be visualized with ultrasound and interorbital distances can be compared with established nomograms[87,88]. In addition, the general appearance of the face, the position and configuration of the nose, and the integrity of the upper lip should be observed, as they may define a specific facies of holoprosencephaly. It is our observation that when the orbits are extremely closely approximated, although there may be two ocular globes, they often share one opening in the skin, giving the appearance of cyclops.

When hypotelorism and the absence of midline cerebral structures are observed, alobar holoprosencephaly is diagnosed with certainty[89–96]. Moreover, holoprosencephaly may be present with normal facies, or the face may be hidden from sonographic examination. Diagnosis is still possible if a common ventricle lacking in temporal and posterior horns is identified and prominence of the fused thalami observed[95]. Further support of the diagnosis is given if a dorsal cyst contiguous with the common ventricle in alobar holoprosencephaly is observed. It is not sufficient to see a central fluid collection in an abnormal brain, as this may also be present in hydranencephaly or a midline porencephalic cyst[96].

The degree of separation of the posterior cerebral hemispheres and the extent of thalamic fusion are best defined by postnatal studies. Such subtle differentiation of semilobar and lobar holoprosencephaly may not be possible before birth[95]. In lobar holoprosencephaly, only the frontal horns are fused; the remainder of the brain is differentiated into two parts. In the coronal view, the frontal horns will have a flat squared roof and the cavum septum pellucidum will be absent[97]. Additionally, the bright echo of the fused fornices may be seen in the third ventricle and is a sign specific to lobar holoprosencephaly (Figure 21). However, it is apparently not present in every case[98].

Outcome

The prognosis for alobar holoprosencephaly is uniformly poor. Most infants die shortly after birth, and the survivors have severe mental retardation[83,99]. Less is known about the prognosis in the lobar and semilobar varieties. Normal life span has been reported for some, but many are severely mentally retarded[82,83,100]. It is possible that individuals with subtle forms of lobar holoprosencephaly and very limited neurological abnormalities may exist.

Management

The obstetric management of holoprosencephaly is dependent upon gestational age at the time of diagnosis. If this condition is detected prior to 24 weeks of gestation, termination of pregnancy may be elected by the parents.

In the third trimester, macrocephaly may prevent spontaneous vaginal delivery. To avoid Cesarean delivery, cephalocentesis, the decompression of the distended fetal ventricular system using transabdominal needle placement under ultrasound guidance, should be considered[101]. The potentially destructive nature of this procedure must be explained to the parents. If parents, cognizant of the grave outlook in holoprosencephaly, elect to have a Cesarean delivery, attempts should be made to document fetal lung maturity.

Microcephaly

Strictly translated, microcephaly means 'small head'. However, the clinical importance of the entity is its association with microencephaly (small brain) and mental retardation. Estimates of the incidence of microcephaly based on observations made at birth vary from 1 in 6250 to 1 in 8500 births[102,103].

Etiology

As microcephaly is a heterogeneous entity, with many different morphological patterns, no simple

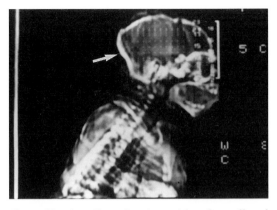

Figure 22 A small cranium (arrow) in a fetus affected by cytomegalovirus (lateral X-ray)

embryological aberration can lead to all the varied results. In general, a small head is the product of an underdeveloped brain; craniosynostosis (early fusion of the cranial sutures) appears to be a rare cause of microcephaly[104].

In some forms of microcephaly, a relative underdevelopment of the forebrain compared with the cerebellum has been observed. Studies have shown that the growth spurt in the cerebellum occurs later in gestation than that of the forebrain. Thus, a teratogenic insult of short duration might inhibit the growth of one structure and not the other[105].

The risk of recurrence of microcephaly is dependent upon the underlying etiology. A search for this etiology should include physical examination of the infant, maternal history of teratogenic exposure, careful family pedigree, chromosomal, microbiological and serological studies, and autopsy of stillborns and abortuses. It is increasingly recognized that fetal alcohol effects are a common cause of mental retardation, often with microcephaly. In general, if a chromosomal aberration or a defined genetic syndrome is identified, then that etiology defines the recurrence risk. Several patterns of inheritance have been described within the subgroup of microcephaly without associated anomalies, i.e. 'true' microcephaly. These include autosomal recessive, autosomal dominant with incomplete penetrance, and sporadic. If a teratogenic agent can be identified and removed, then the risk for future pregnancies should be no greater than that for the general population.

Table 2 Microcephaly – causes or associations

Genetic causes
Trisomies 13, 18, 21, 22
4p–, 5p–, 18p–, 18q–
Alpers' disease
Bloom syndrome
Börjeson–Forssman syndrome
Cockayne's syndrome
De Sanctis–Caccione syndrome
Dubowitz syndrome
Fanconi's pancytopenia
Focal dermal hypoplasia
Incontinentia pigmenti
Lissencephaly syndrome
Meckel–Gruber syndrome
Menkes' syndrome
Paine syndrome
Primary microcephaly
Robert's syndrome
Seckel bird-headed dwarfism
Smith–Lemli–Optiz syndrome
Williams syndrome

Environmental causes
Prenatal infections (rubella, cytomegalovirus, herpes,
    toxoplasmosis)
Fetal alcohol syndrome
Fetal hydantoin syndrome
Aminopterin syndrome

Unknown causes
Coffin–Siris syndrome
DeLange syndrome
Langer–Giedion syndrome
Rubenstein–Taybi syndrome

Infection with cytomegalovirus or toxoplasmosis can produce microcephaly (Figure 22). Suggestive additional signs would be hydrocephalus and periventricular or thalamic calcification. The major causes of microcephaly are listed in Table 2.

Diagnosis

The way to determine that a head is small is to measure it. This simplistic remark belies the difficulty in accurately determining when microcephaly is present and when it is clinically significant[106–109]. At the present time, there is no universally accepted anthropometric definition of microcephaly. When the standard of less than two standard deviations below the mean is used, the association with mental retardation is inconsistent. Three standard deviations below the mean for sex and age would appear to be a more reasonable criterion for the definition of microcephaly, as the correlation with mental retardation is stronger[102, 110–117].

Although the BPD has been used in attempts to diagnose and exclude microcephaly, a later series found that a BPD smaller than three standard deviations below the mean was normal in 44% of cases[107]. This large incidence of false-positive results was probably caused by normal variation in fetal head width, resulting from compressive forces within the uterus. Thus, in order to measure the size of a dolichocephalic head, it is necessary to consider the perimeter of the head, not just its width.

In some cases of microcephaly, there is a relative underdevelopment of the frontal lobes compared to the remainder of the brain. Nomograms documenting frontal lobe growth have been developed in an attempt to address this problem[109].

Since microcephaly can be a part of many malformation syndromes, a careful search for other associated anomalies is warranted. It should be noted that the cortical mass may be decreased in microcephaly, leading to ventriculomegaly in the absence of obstructive hydrocephalus.

Outcome

It is difficult to make definitive statements concerning the prognosis of an entity with an unclear definition and multiple etiologies. Several general remarks, however, can be made. (1) The majority of microcephalic infants are mentally retarded, many severely. (2) In general, the smaller the head, the worse the prognosis. (3) If microcephaly occurs as part of certain genetic syndromes (e.g. Meckel's syndrome) the outcome is uniformly poor. (4) Despite very decreased head size, a child may be born with normal intelligence. One child with a head perimeter 3.4 standard deviations below the mean has been reported to have an IQ above 90[102, 110–112, 116–118].

Management

Uncomplicated vaginal delivery of a microcephalic child is to be expected. There exists, however, the

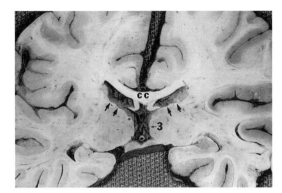

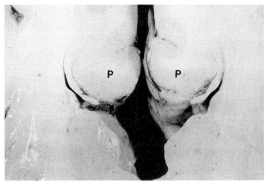

Figure 23 Normal brain in coronal section. The corpus callosum (cc) connects the two hemispheres. Note that it separates the interhemispheric fissure from the third ventricle (3). In its absence, these two structures connect. Note also the straight lower margin of the lateral ventricles (arrows). Published with permission. Comstock, C.H. (1992). *Female Patient*, **17**, 40

Figure 25 Agenesis of the corpus callosum. Gross specimen, coronal view. The bundles of Probst (P) indent the lateral ventricle, producing a 'batwing' or 'bell-horn' shape. Note that the interhemispheric fissure communicates directly with the third ventricle

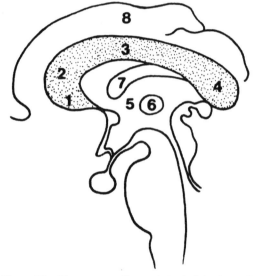

Figure 24 The corpus callosum (stippled) in the sagittal plane. 1, rostrum; 2, genu; 3, body; 4, splenium; 5, third ventricle; 6, massa intermedia; 7, fornix; 8, cingulate gyrus. Published with permission. Comstock, C.H. (1992). *Female Patient*, **17**, 40

possibility of shoulder dystocia, due to incomplete dilatation of the cervix by a small fetal head.

Agenesis of the corpus callosum

The corpus callosum is one of three bundles of fibers that connect the two cerebral hemispheres while forming the floor of the interhemispheric

fissure, and the roof of the third ventricle and the frontal horns (Figure 23). At 10–12 weeks, it begins to develop within the commissural plate, following the other two forebrain commissures (anterior and hippocampal) by 3 weeks. From anterior to posterior, the corpus callosum consists of four parts: the rostrum, genus, body and the bulb-shaped posterior portion known as the splenium (Figure 24). Although development begins at the genu and proceeds posteriorly, the last fibers are formed in the most anterior part or rostrum. Its outline is formed by 17 weeks, but it continues to thicken as the brain matures; completion of the occipital and temporal regions does not occur until the postnatal period. Myelination of the corpus begins at 4 months of neonatal life, starting in the splenium and proceeding to the genu; completion of thickening and myelination is achieved in the first year of neonatal age. Focal thinning at the junction of the body and splenium is found in 22% of persons and is considered to be a normal variation[119].

The entire corpus callosum can be absent (agenesis) or, more frequently, there may be overall thinning or absence of one or more parts (partial agenesis). Since the corpus callosum forms from genu to splenium and finally the rostrum, the posterior portions are the parts that are malformed or absent in partial agenesis (or part of the rostrum).

In complete agenesis of the corpus callosum (ACC) the fibers, instead of crossing the midline to

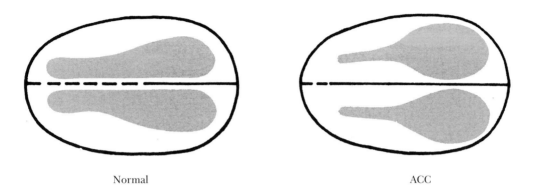

Normal   ACC

Figure 26 Axial plane. In agenesis of the corpus callosum (ACC), the medial wall of the lateral ventricle is displaced laterally toward the lateral wall. The ventricles are black in this drawing. Published with permission. Comstock, C.H. (1992). *Female Patient*, **17**, 40

the other hemisphere, run up to the interhemispheric fissure and then turn and run parallel to it, to form the longitudinal bundles of Probst. These bundles indent the medial borders of the lateral ventricles, giving them a characteristic shape in the coronal view (Figure 25). In the absence of the splenium, the occipital horns migrate superiorly into white matter, producing dilatation of the trigone, occipital horns and posterior temporal horns, or what is termed *colpocephaly*[120].

The frequency of ACC is difficult to determine, due to extreme ascertainment bias. However, Jellinger and associates[121] found an occurrence rate of 0.7% in pneumoencephalograms done for other reasons.

Diagnosis

MRI allows the best imaging of the corpus callosum and, therefore, has clarified the anatomy in this complex malformation. MRI allows sagittal cuts, which show the corpus callosum in its full length and depth without reconstruction. Additionally, the sagittal views obtainable with MRI best show the radiation of the sulci towards the third ventricle which occurs when the cingulate gyrus is absent and are the views of choice for visualization of the cerebellar tonsils (which can be abnormal). MRI has delineated clearly the typical abnormalities in both complete and incomplete dysgenesis of the corpus callosum. Atlas and co-workers[122] found that all the patients with complete ACC

examined with MRI had continuity of the third ventricle with the interhemispheric fissure, as did three out of four of the patients with partial ACC. All 11 had a high third ventricle and all but one had medially concave frontal horns. Only two of seven patients with complete ACC and none with incomplete ACC had an interhemispheric cyst. Six out of seven patients with complete ACC had colpocephaly, as did two out of four patients with partial ACC. Three out of seven of the patients with complete ACC had wide interhemispheric fissures, as did three out of four of the patients with incomplete ACC.

Malinger and Zakut have shown that the normal corpus callosum itself can be imaged and measured with vaginal ultrasound in the sagittal plane as early as 18 weeks, but that earlier than this it could not be differentiated from surrounding structures[123]. The body and genu could be measured as early as 18 weeks, but the splenium at that age is very attenuated. The genu enlarges from a thickness of 2 mm at 19 weeks to 4–5 mm at term. The body increases from 1mm at 18 weeks to 3mm near term and the length of the corpus increases in a linear manner from 17mm at 18–19 weeks to 44 mm at term. The cingulate gyri, which are absent in complete ACC, could not be visualized in the normal fetus until 28–29 weeks.

On the coronal scan, the corpus is a relatively hypoechoic area, the upper border of which is defined by the more hyperechogenic pericallosal cistern. However, the corpus callosum cannot be

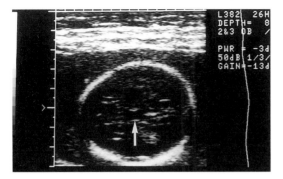

Figure 27 Axial view in agenesis of the corpus callosum. The third ventricle is high (arrow) and seen at the level of the lateral ventricles. The frontal horns produce parallel lines and the interhemispheric fissure is widened, so that the falx is surrounded by fluid and three midline lines are clearly seen

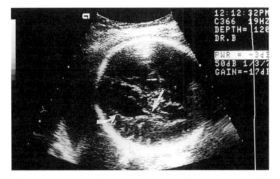

Figure 28 Agenesis of the corpus callosum. This axial view shows dilatation of the posterior lateral ventricle (colpocephaly) (curved arrow) and medial displacement of the anterior medial wall of the frontal horn (straight arrow), so that the entire ventricle has a tear-drop shape

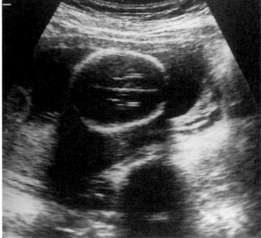

Figure 29 The displacement of the medial wall of the lateral ventricle away from the falx and toward the lateral wall appears as parallel lines, producing the pointed end of the tear drop or, alternatively, the 'railroad track' sign

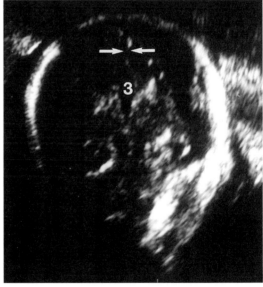

Figure 30 Coronal ultrasound in agenesis of the corpus callosum. The third ventricle (3) is higher than normal, and communicates directly with the interhemispheric fissure (arrows)

directly visualized on the axial scan obtained in screening ultrasound. Nevertheless, certain signs seen in this plane point to its malformation or absence. The findings reported in the fetus[124–129] are similar to the ultrasound appearance of complete ACC which has been well described in the neonate[130–133]: (1) lateral displacement of the medial walls of the frontal horns (Figure 26); (2) upward displacement of the third ventricle (Figure 27); (3) enlargement of the occipital horns and atria (Figure 28); and (4) increased fluid around the falx, due to widening of the interhemispheric fissure (Figure 27). Lateral displacement of the anterior horns and colpocephaly give a typical tear-drop shape to the lateral ventricles (Figure 28). The walls of the frontal horns are so close together, that they give a 'railroad track' appearance (Figure 29).

Confirmation can be made on the coronal view, in which the medial walls of the frontal horns are concave rather than convex, and the third ventricle is continuous with the hemispheric fissure, instead of being separated from it by the corpus callosum[134] (Figure 30). The cingulate gyrus, which should be visible by 28 weeks on the coronal scan, will be absent.

The ultrasound appearance in the fetus can be quite subtle. Since in many cases there is only partial absence of the corpus callosum, it may not be detectable at all, and many cases will go unrecognized. In fact, some cases in the literature appeared normal at 18 weeks and it was not until later that they appeared abnormal. It has been our experience that the ultrasound appearance may be normal at 18 weeks but quite abnormal just a few weeks later – probably due to continued formation of the corpus. Vergani and co-workers[129] found that although there may be ventriculomegaly at 18 weeks, the diagnosis could not be made with certainty before 20 weeks.

By prenatal ultrasound, it may be impossible to distinguish complete from incomplete agenesis, and it may not be important to distinguish them clinically, since some severe syndromes often have partial rather than complete agenesis. That is, prognosis may not be related to how much of the corpus is absent; there are individuals with complete absence who are outwardly normal and there are others with partial agenesis who are profoundly retarded[135]. In partial agenesis, the frontal horns become convex laterally instead of being concave, as they are when the genu is absent. Dilatation of the posterior horns and of the third ventricle have been reported in partial agenesis[125].

To date, MRI images do not appear to be as useful as a good ultrasound study. They have revealed the typical tear-drop-shaped ventricles and elevated third ventricle, but did not show the gyri or the actual corpus callosum[136]. The advantage of MRI is that it collects images in three dimensions, without the need for reconstruction, and may be useful when, due to technical factors, ultrasound images are suboptimal.

Outcome

All literature regarding ACC suffers from an ascertainment bias. Patients usually come to study because of some symptoms such as seizures or delayed development. Consequently, it is not possible to determine how many individuals have ACC with no apparent symptoms. Another problem is that most studies have used only ultrasound or CT as a 'gold standard' when in fact, it appears that only autopsy or MRI completely delineates all abnormalities. Curnes and associates[137] found that MRI is better than CT in diagnosing subtle abnormalities, such as lack of the normal configuration of the splenium.

Probably all individuals with ACC have at least subtle abnormalities of the CNS. The ability to distinguish two points on the skin of the thoracic region[138] and impaired rhyming ability are two such subtle defects. Those who have had MRI studies have all been found to have additional CNS malformations, not all of which are symptomatic in day-to-day life. For example, Atlas and co-workers[122] reported that all patients, whether with partial or complete ACC, had associated malformations of the limbic system (a combination of the parahippocampal and cingulate gyri and the hippocampus). All but one had absence of the cingulate gyrus and the anterior commissure. These limbic abnormalities are usually clinically undetectable. Parrish and associates[139] reviewed the 47 cases in the literature up to 1979 who had complete autopsies, 85% of which had CNS abnormalities and 62% other abnormalities. Gyral dysplasias, hypoplasia of the olfactory tracts or lobe, hypoplasia of the cerebellar vermis, meningomyelocele, and absent pyramidal tracts are very frequent. Other associated CNS anomalies include interhemispheric cysts, Dandy–Walker malformation, arachnoid cysts of the posterior fossa, Chiari II malformation, ethmoidal encephalocele and microphthalmia.

A very echogenic-appearing mass in the midline may be a lipoma of the corpus callosum. These may be associated with ACC and dysraphic conditions such as encephalocele, hypertelorism, medial cleft nose and myelomeningocele. Smaller ones may be located on the surface of the corpus callosum and may be asymptomatic[140, 141].

Miller–Diecker syndrome, in which the short arm of chromosome 17 is absent and there is lissencephaly, is commonly associated with ACC. Its primary manifestation is lissencephaly or smooth brain. These infants also have characteristic facies. Prognosis is dismal.

Of the many syndromes of which ACC is a part, acrocallosal syndrome and Aicardi's syndrome have been most thoroughly described. In the review of Thyen and colleagues[142], of all cases of acrocallosal syndrome described in the literature to early 1992 (27 cases), most had polydactyly (either pre- or post-axial). Five of 27 had congenital heart defects. Dandy–Walker malformation was also frequent. All had delayed development, which became more apparent as the child grew older; development proceeded in only a slightly delayed fashion at first, but the gap between expected and actual performance for age grew rapidly after the first year. This disorder is thought to be recessive, and reports of more than one individual in a family with this syndrome have been made.

The review of Donnenfeld and co-workers[143] of 18 cases of Aicardi's syndrome reveals that 72% had complete ACC and 28% partial ACC; 33% had unilateral microphthalmia, and 39% hemivertebrae. Aicardi's syndrome involves females only and appears to be sporadic, since no familial cases have been reported[144]. All new cases appear to be new mutations. The condition is thought to be X-linked, with early embryonic lethality in males[143]. Some degree of retardation and hypotonia is present in all cases, as are seizures. In their series, most did not develop beyond 12 months' developmental age, and only three ever walked.

ACC is present in 17% of individuals with Rubenstein–Taybi syndrome[145]. This is a syndrome also marked by mental and growth retardation, broad thumbs and toes, and a typical face characterized by frontal bossing. This is almost always sporadic.

ACC can also be found in Zellweger's syndrome, which is an autosomal recessive syndrome with extreme hypotonia, little mental development, renal cysts, and hepatic fibrosis. Multiple affected siblings have been reported. Cardiac defects and intra-uterine growth retardation are common. Although they have high bulging foreheads, to our knowledge this feature and none of others mentioned above have been identified in the antenatal period.

Although the background rate of occurrence is not known, sporadic reports have been made of association with 4–11 balanced location. Association with trisomies 8 and 18 has been reported. In trisomy 8, there is a prominent forehead, vertebral anomalies, mongoloid facies and mild hypertelorism.

ACC is heavily represented in children with metabolic diseases, such as non-ketetotic hyperglycemias[146, 147]. Diabetes insipidus was very common in a series of children with septo-optic dysplasia and/or ACC. It has been associated with teratogens in fetal alcohol syndrome[146] and possibly maternal ingestion of crack cocaine[148].

Septo-optic dysplasia is absence of the septum pellucidum and hypoplasia of the optic nerves – many cases include hypopituitary dwarfism, because affected individuals have either isolated growth hormone deficiency or pan-hypopituitarism. Actually, the septum pellucidum is absent in only half of affected individuals. The affected individuals are usually of normal intelligence, unless they also have holoprosencephaly. Either complete or partial ACC has been associated with this syndrome[137]. The syndrome is thought to be sporadic.

FG syndrome is characterized by sudden infant death, developmental delay, unusual facies, and abnormalities of the cardiac, gastrointestinal and central nervous systems[149].

There have been reports of familial cases which do not as yet fit a described syndrome. For example, Vici and colleagues[150] reported two brothers who had ACC, cutaneous hypopigmentation, cataracts, cleft lip and palate, and immunodeficiency. Both boys had psychomotor retardation, seizures and chronic candidiasis, and died of pneumonia at 2–3 years. Kang[151] reported a series of three Chinese brothers with frontal bossing, microcephaly, short broad hands and abnormal faces; the pattern of inheritance suggested that it was X-linked recessive. In that report, there is an excellent review of genetic syndromes associated with ACC.

Other case reports describe ACC in one individual with other anomalies. Kozlowski and Ouvrier[152] reported the case of a child with mental retardation, osseous lesions and wormian bones.

In the review of Parrish and colleagues[139] of the literature on ACC to 1979, the most common facial changes, whether syndromic or not, were ocular abnormalities, micrognathia, hypertelorism, and cleft lip or palate. In the musculoskeletal system, malformation of the digits and widespread skeletal dysplasia were most common. A list of non-CNS anomalies that have been associated with ACC and

Table 3 Potential ultrasound findings in syndromes with agenesis of the corpus callosum

	Potential ultrasound finding
Syndrome	
Aicardi	microphthalmia, hemivertebrae, female
Acrocallosal	polydactyly, (CHD) (DW)
Rubenstein–Taybi	frontal bossing, broad thumbs and toes
Zellweger's	renal cysts, IUGR, (CHD), bossing, vertebral anomalies, mild hypertelorism
Metabolic diseases	
Fetal alcohol	hypertelorism (CHD)
Septo-optic dysplasia	—
XXXXY	—
Andermann	—
FG	CHD

CHD, coronary heart disease; DW, Dandy–Walker; IUGR, intrauterine growth retardation

that are potentially detectable by antenatal ultrasound is given in Table 3.

The same warning applied to imaging applies to counselling regarding outcome – all literature suffers from an ascertainment bias. A very careful review of family history can reveal other affected individuals and help in counselling of the index patient. Specifically, most described syndromes to date have mental retardation as a hallmark. Careful questioning regarding relatives with mental retardation should be carried out. If there are such individuals, blindness, seizures, hydrocephalus and abnormalities of the skeletal system may point to patients with hereditary syndromes involving ACC. Note that although some syndromes (e.g. Aicardi's) are sporadic and have never been reported in more than one patient in a family, in others there can be multiple affected children.

If ultrasound has demonstrated that an affected fetus is female, Aicardi's syndrome must be mentioned, since no other abnormalities may be seen on scanning. It will be more frequent that subtle abnormalities of these myriad associated syndromes cannot be detected by ultrasound and therefore, the lack of demonstrated abnormalities does not help in establishing prognosis.

Many individuals will have no apparent functional abnormalities. Unlike patients who have had surgical resection of the corpus callosum, those with agenesis apparently can compensate in many ways through the other commissures. However, they do have subtle abnormalities of manual coordination and dexterity, which may be explained by the high frequency of pyramidal tract abnormalities[139].

When counselling a family with a previously affected child, ultrasound at 18 weeks, and then, if normal, at 20 weeks, should effectively exclude ACC in the hands of a physician experienced in its ultrasound diagnosis.

In summary, although a fetus may have no other detectable anomalies, either structural or chromosomal, and there is no family history that would suggest a hereditary pattern, it is impossible to predict outcome. Although many cases of ACC probably are undetectable without careful visual, sensory and speech testing, others may have metabolic diseases or have profound mental retardation. The abnormalities of facies and hands in many of these are not those that could be detected by ultrasound. All that can be offered are a thorough review of family history, amniocentesis and an attempt to find subtle ultrasound signs of a described syndrome.

Arteriovenous malformations

Most arteriovenous malformations of the brain have been thought to involve the vein of Galen, which is a midline vein located behind the third ventricle which drains into the straight sinus. However, an alternative explanation is that the aneurysm may actually result from persistence of the prosencephalic vein of Marhowski[153]. Whatever its origin, this malformation connects arteries directly to veins, with no intervening capillaries, resulting in (1) markedly increased blood flow to the brain; and (2) a round or cigar-shaped cyst behind the third ventricle. Blood supply is variable: the posterior cerebral, superior cerebellar, middle, and/or anterior cerebral arteries may supply arterial blood[154].

At least 14 vein of Galen aneurysms have been reported in the fetus[155–165] but never before 30 weeks, even in those with earlier scans[163].

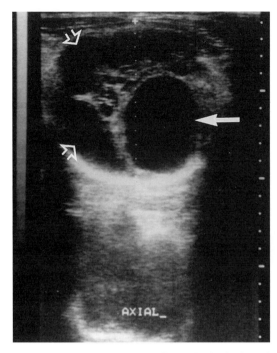

Figure 31 An arteriovenous malformation in the frontal lobe (arrow). Note the small circular areas around it, which are feeding vessels. There was also hydrocephalus (open arrows)

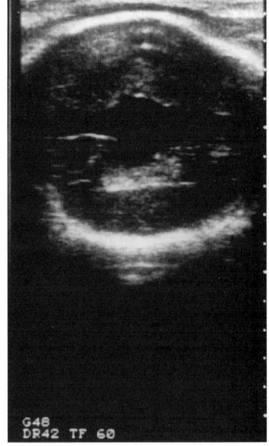

Malformations in vessels other than the vein of Galen are infrequent in fetuses and infants, but two have been reported in the fetus in the frontal region – one at 23.5 weeks and one at 34 weeks[163, 165] (Figure 31).

Figure 32 Typical appearance of a vein of Galen 'aneurysm'. Note the central location and cystic appearance

Diagnosis

The gray-scale appearance is that of a cystic area, sometimes surrounded by tubular structures (dilated blood vessels) (Figures 32 and 33). Color Doppler may show arterial jets within slower moving blood and dilated straight and sigmoid sinuses[163] (Color Plate A). Hydrocephalus is variable.

Resulting ascites and pleural effusion have produced hypoplastic lungs in one reported case[157]. Two fetuses with hydrops were shown to have retrograde circulation in the transverse aortic arch during both systole and diastole, such that blood travelling across the ductus was drawn up into the neck vessels rather than down the aorta[160]. Enlargement of the liver has been reported[157, 158].

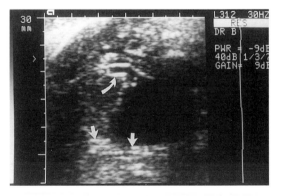

Figure 33 A close-up view of a vein of Galen aneurysm, demonstrating a feeding artery (curved arrow) and numerous other small vessels (arrows) surrounding the larger cystic area

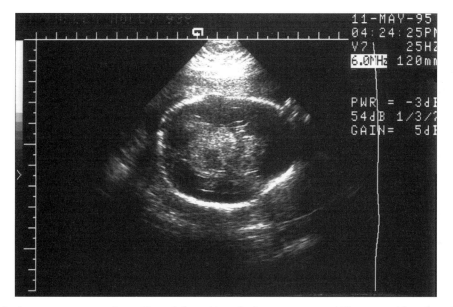

Figure 34 Immature teratoma in an 18-week fetus. Note the heterogeneous midline mass with an anterior cystic component (on the right). The mass was located in the interhemispheric fissure and grew rapidly over a 2-week period

Possible extra CNS signs include enlarged neck veins, cardiomegaly, hepatomegaly, ascites, pleural effusions and skin edema. The heart may be quite enlarged, so that the axis of the heart is rotated to the left[163]. Neck vessels may be enlarged, due to increased flow to the head. However, the heart should be evaluated well, since coarctation and transposition are thought to be more frequent in these infants[166].

Outcome

Many infants with arteriovenous malformations are born with high-output congestive heart failure. Recent therapy with a coil placed by catheterization or with embolization has been successful in closing off the arteriovenous malformation, often enabling surgical resection, and thus decreasing the cardiac load[167]. However, this will not correct any damage already done to the brain. Blood flow appears to be diverted from the normal brain to the arteriovenous malformation; the resultant anoxia can cause cerebral infarction or periventricular leukomalacia[168]. However, this is not invariable; just two of nine infants with arteriovenous malformations had demonstrable anoxic brain lesions in one series[169]. Thus, discussion of outcome must

include caution that despite successful embolization or surgery, there may still be persistent brain damage with spasticity.

Tumors

The vast majority of fetal brain tumors are teratomas (tumors that contain all three germ cell layers). However, there have been reports of a few other types of tumor which will be discussed later in less detail.

In the fetal and neonatal periods, teratomas are mature and behave as benign tumors – they invade locally as they grow rapidly but do not metastasize. Teratomas of the brain are thought to arise from the pineal gland and appear to involve the third ventricle at the beginning. Often hydrocephalus is noted, followed by a fast growing mass a few weeks later. Several cases have been reported in the antenatal period[170–174] (Figures 34 and 35). The mass distorts the normal architecture of the brain and usually appears primarily solid with some cystic components. Occasionally, they may be cystic with contained echogenic foci[170]. Although the mass itself may contain small cystic areas, most of the larger cystic areas reported in the literature

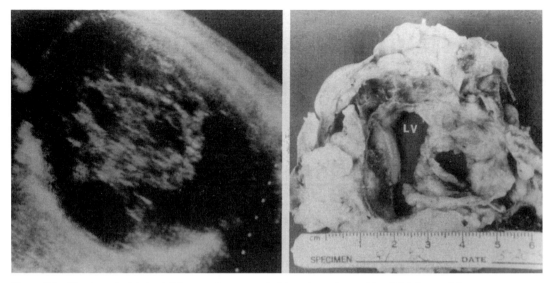

Figure 35   Teratoma (axial view). The mass is surrounded by enlarged ventricles. LV, left ventricle

have actually been distorted dilated ventricles. The tumor can grow through the base of the skull into the neck[170], midbrain[172] and orbits, but does not usually involve the posterior fossa (although one case has been reported of an extension into the posterior fossa[172]). Head size is always increased and the skull may be abnormally shaped in the area adjacent to the tumor[174]. Calcifications, when present, are more reliably detected in pathological specimens than on antenatal scans. Most fetal brain teratomas have been reported in the third trimester. The earliest reported teratoma was at 22 weeks[172], although, from the description of that case, it could probably have been seen at 20 weeks or earlier.

One case has been reported of antenatally seen skin edema over the skull and, in fact, at autopsy there was skin thickening over the body, an enlarged liver and a thickened placenta. Polyhydramnios is frequent, but not invariable. CT and MRI have not added additional information[175]. Maternal serum and amniotic AFP were increased in one case in which they were measured[175]. No familial inheritance has been shown, nor are there any commonly associated abnormalities.

Stillbirth is not uncommon. The prognosis is poor in those who survive to birth, with developmental delay even if surgery is successful. However, there is an occasional exception in which there is little residual brain damage[174]. Although teratomas are by far the most frequent type of tumor in the fetal brain, there are a few reports of other types: craniopharyngioma[176], neuroblastoma[177] and glioblastoma[178]. The appearance of these and teratomas are virtually indistinguishable and have similar outcomes. The appearance is also very similar to an intracranial bleed and even to advanced encephalomalacia[179].

Lipomas of the corpus callosum and of the pons have been reported[180]. These are very echogenic, without cystic areas. They are thought to arise from the leptomeninges and are usually midline, near the corpus callosum, third ventricle, pons and cerebellum. The outcome in reported antenatal cases has been variable with intrauterine demise in a fetus with a pontine lipoma[180], and ACC in those with lipomas near or in the corpus callosum. However, in the neonate, they have not produced abnormalities, unless they disturb function in a critical location or cause a mass effect and resulting hydrocephalus.

Choroid plexus cysts

The choroid plexus is located primarily in the lateral ventricles with a small amount in the roof of the third ventricle. It has a uniform echogenic appearance, which on closer inspection is actually

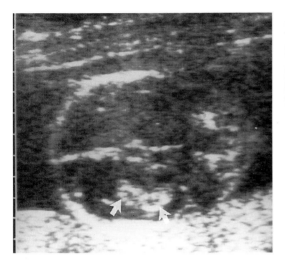

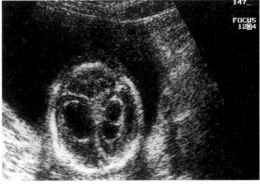

Figure 37 Large choroid plexus cysts, which occupy most of the ventricle and could be mistaken for hydrocephalus

Figure 36 Two small choroid plexus cysts (arrows)

finely heterogeneous. In about 1% of fetuses there may be cysts within the choroid plexus, usually in the lateral ventricles, but cysts of the third ventricle have also been reported[181]. Most of these disappear by 22–24 weeks[182–184], but a few will persist. Most are small (5mm), round and fluid-filled, with thin borders (Figure 36). However, they can be large and there can be multiple contiguous cysts[185] (Figure 37).

Choroid plexus cysts need to be distinguished from normal corpus striatum, which indents the lower portion of the lateral ventricles and can produce an appearance similar to that of a choroid cyst. When the transducer is tilted in an attempt to find a longer axis, however, they appear as rod- or cigar-shaped structures rather than remaining round. In the coronal plane, echolucent areas formed by the corpus striatum are always located at the bottom of the lateral ventricles. Choroid plexus cysts may be impossible to distinguish from subarachnoid cysts, which, unlike choroid cysts, persist past 24 weeks and may actually expand. Choroid cysts may be so large that they mimic hydrocephalus (Figure 37).

Choroid plexus cysts are usually of no consequence by themselves, unless located in a position in which they can obstruct CSF flow[184]. However, there is some suggestion that they may be associated with trisomies 18 and 21[185–189]. There has been conflicting information regarding whether or not larger choroid cysts more frequently indicate aneuploidy[186–189], but we and others have not found this to be true unless there are associated anomalies[190–196]. In any event, the question arises as to whether or not amniocentesis is advisable in all fetuses with choroid plexus cysts. Some individuals feel that most cases of trisomy 18 can be detected by meticulous scanning of the fetus, since in almost all cases of trisomy 18 there are anomalies of the hands (overlapping fingers, steerhorn fingers), and of the heart (ventriculoseptal defects are the most common). If the fetus has no ultrasound findings other than the choroid plexus cyst and there are no other factors, we and others feel that the risk of amniocentesis outweighs the risk of aneuploidy. However, if there are other risk factors (such as maternal age) or if a very thorough scan of the fetus by a physician experienced in detecting heart and hand abnormalities is not available, amniocentesis should be offered. The difficulty in arriving at a conclusion regarding management derives from the infrequent occurrence of trisomy 18 and the resulting statistical problems that then occur in accumulating the tens of thousands of screening scans needed to demonstrate a relationship or lack thereof.

Lissencephaly

Lissencephaly, or the absence of cerebral gyri, is also known as agyria. When the cells which normally

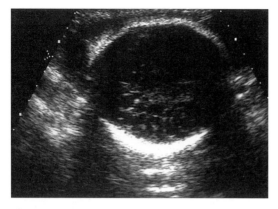

Figure 38 Normal gyri appear as curved echogenic lines along the brain surface. They are not clearly seen on a prenatal scan until the third trimester

form the gray matter of the brain fail to migrate outward from the primitive neural tube, the gyri are not formed, producing a smooth cerebral surface, hence the name, which means 'smooth brain'. There are two major types of lissencephaly: types I and II. In type I there are four, rather than six, layers of cortex, but the cortex is still thicker than usual. The normal myelinated white matter is very narrow, so that there is a ratio of 4 : 1 gray to white matter (normal is 1 : 10)[193]. Ventricular dilatation is present, particularly of the occipital horns (colpocephaly). There can be severe hypoplasia of the pyramidal tracts, thalami and brainstem[190]. There is usually ACC and slight microcephaly. Most patients with type I have either Miller–Diecker syndrome or isolated lissencephaly. In Miller–Diecker syndrome there is a characteristic facies and a higher incidence of extra-CNS anomalies: an up-turned nose, small mandible, prominent upper lip, dysphagia, failure to thrive and usually death at 3–4 months. ACC is frequent and midline calcification can be seen. Most have deletion of a part of the short arm of chromosome 17[191]. Since this cannot be detected by the usual karyotype, it is important to the geneticist to know that Miller–Diecker syndrome is being considered, so that special tests can be run to demonstrate this deletion.

Isolated lissencephaly is without facial abnormalities. The gyri are less often completely absent and instead show pachygyria – wide gyri with shallow sulci. This type can occasionally demonstrate

autosomal recessive inheritance[190]. Infrequently, a small part of the short arm of chromosome 17 is missing, but more frequently it is thought that the cause may be teratogens such as infection, disturbance in blood flow[190] or drugs.

In type II, there is always Dandy–Walker malformation and obstructive hydrocephalus. Occipital encephaloceles are common. Absence or hypoplasia of the optic nerve is often seen and thus microphthalmia is present.

Diagnosis

The gyri can usually be identified on the surface of the fetal brain by 28–30 weeks (Figure 38). With the transducer in the axial plane, a sweep should be made toward the vertex. Just before leaving the head, the gyri will be seen. However, the diagnosis of fetuses with lissencephaly have been made using signs of accompanying defects, such as ACC rather than gyral absence. Two patients with Miller–Diecker syndrome diagnosed *in utero* have been reported by Saltzman and associates[195]. In a fetus known to be at risk because of the birth of affected siblings, microcephaly and lack of gyral formation could be identified at 30 weeks. Polyhydramnios and decreased fetal movement were also noted. The polyhydramnios was presumed to be the antenatal manifestation of the postnatally observed dysphagia. In the second case, the diagnosis was suspected in a fetus in whom there were smooth gyri and slightly small head size. This fetus also had tetralogy of Fallot. In neither of these cases were additional findings mentioned, such as hydrocephalus or ACC, nor were the results of neonatal imaging mentioned. An additional case of Miller–Diecker syndrome, with severe hydrocephalus, was seen at 32 weeks by Holzgreve and colleagues[196]. No mention was made of MRI or other imaging modalities, so it is unknown whether ACC was present. One case of Walker–Warburg syndrome was also reported by Holzgreve and associates: hydrocephalus was the only antenatal finding, but at birth the child also had Dandy–Walker malformation and microphthalmos[196]. If, after 30–32 weeks, the diagnosis is suspected, MRI of the fetus should theoretically be helpful in diagnosis and thus management.

Outcome

Lissencephaly is almost always fatal in early infancy or childhood and is associated with severe mental retardation. One case of survival to 20 years has been reported, but is unique[190]. Since gyri cannot be demonstrated by ultrasound before 30 weeks, the diagnosis could not be made earlier, but could be suspected in a fetus at risk, if ACC, colpocephaly, hydrocephalus, or Dandy–Walker malformation are diagnosed. A fetus would be considered at risk if a previous sibling had had lissencephaly.

The possibility of type I lissencephaly must be included in counselling of parents of fetuses with either ACC or colpocephaly, whereas type II lissencephaly should be mentioned in counselling the parents of the fetus with Dandy–Walker malformation and hydrocephalus. In a series of 118 fetuses with hydrocephalus, lissencephaly was present in two cases, one each of Miller–Diecker syndrome and Walker–Warburg syndrome, so it is not a frequent cause of hydrocephalus[196].

Intracerebral hemorrhage

Hemorrhage can occur anywhere in the fetal brain: the ventricles, cortex, subarachnoid or subdural spaces, alone or in combination. In most fetuses, whatever the precipitating event, hemorrhage probably starts in the germinal matrix of the caudate nucleus in the frontal horn. It may progress into the ventricles or the remaining solid brain. Another starting place is the subdural area. The initial appearance of blood collections is an echogenic convex complex mass, which later may start to liquefy centrally, shrinking at its outer borders, so that they seem better defined[197,198]. Eventually, the mass may liquefy more, producing more echolucent areas and debris which, when in the ventricles, may produce a 'fluid level'[199].

Intraventricular hemorrhage

Blood in the fetal ventricles, either unilateral or bilateral, is initially seen as a dense and echogenic mass (Figure 39). Hydrocephalus, often asymmetric, may ensue. In fact, this is so frequent that,

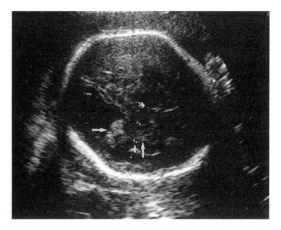

Figure 39 Intraventricular bleed. Echogenic irregular clot is identified by arrows. The cursor lies on the sylvian fissure, not on the lateral ventricular wall

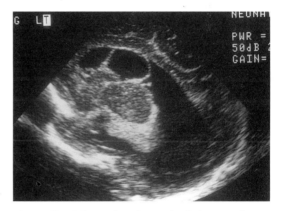

Figure 40 Subependymal cysts in their most characteristic location, in the head of the caudate nucleus. This is an immediately postnatal scan of a newborn who had had an intracerebral bleed identified by an antenatal scan

if asymmetric hydrocephalus is seen, it is wise to look for blood in the ventricles. A number of cases detected *in utero* have been reported[198,200–210]. Subependymal cysts are a common result (Figures 40 and 41).

Bleeding within the actual brain tissue is also thought to occur, although it is not clear from the literature whether these hemorrhagic areas connect with the ventricles, in which case they would be termed porencephalic cysts.

Porencephalic cysts, or cystic areas of brain degeneration, apparently form as they do in the

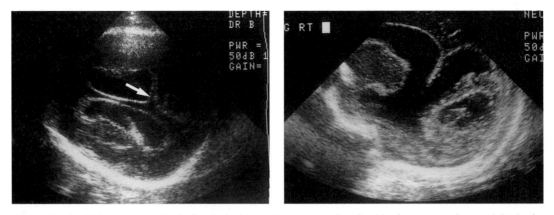

Figure 41 (Left) A cyst (arrow) in the head of a fetus with a presumed earlier bleed. A postnatal scan (right) in the coronal plane shows the cyst and attached clot

neonate but, unless large, they appear to be difficult to detect; there are numerous reports of detection immediately after birth in infants also scanned just before birth[200]. Encephalomalacia also appears to be difficult to detect in the antenatal period, but advanced cases at birth have been reported in neonates who had been scanned just before birth, when only interventricular hemorrhage was noted[200, 201]. Subarachnoid blood, which can be found over the surface of the brain in fetuses with interventricular hemorrhage, has not been reported antenatally[210]. Head size is often increased in relation to the abdomen, although abdominal size may also be increased if severe anemia has triggered hematopoiesis in the liver (with resulting hepatomegaly). Polyhydramnios occurs in some cases as well.

The cause of intracranial hemorrhage is occasionally clear, as in isoimmune thrombocytopenia. Severe maternal pancreatitis has been implicated in two cases, and warfarin in one. However, in most cases the cause is never known and the pregnancy has been uneventful. All cases in the literature have been reported in the mid- or late third trimester. The diffuse nature of the bleeding pattern in cases with no obvious cause suggests that many are due to subependymal hemorrhage characteristic of premature neonates. The described causes are listed in Table 4.

A marked decrease in movement has led to the scan in many instances. Outcome is difficult to predict by antenatal ultrasound, since it is apparently hard to see porencephalic cysts or

Table 4 Causes of intracerebral hemorrhage

Unknown
Trauma
Isoimmune thrombocytopenia
Anticoagulants
Maternal factor X deficiency
Pancreatitis?
Pre-eclampsia?
Maternal seizures
Cord thrombosis

encephalomalacia. In general, however, outcome has not been good, with intrauterine or neonatal death or frequent microcephaly, paresis and developmental delay. In some cases in which hemorrhage is fresh and in which the amount of bleeding is small, there has been good outcome.

Subdural hemorrhage

At least 30 cases of subdural hematomas have been reported in the antenatal period. A subdural hemorrhage may exist at the same time as interventricular hemorrhage, precede it, or occur by itself. The fluid collection clearly lies between the calvarium and the brain. It is initially very echogenic, but may gradually become echolucent with echogenic areas[211]. At this point, it must be distinguished from a subarachnoid cyst or subarachnoid hygroma.

Intraventricular hemorrhage may occur later[211]. In a case of subdural hemorrhage in the posterior

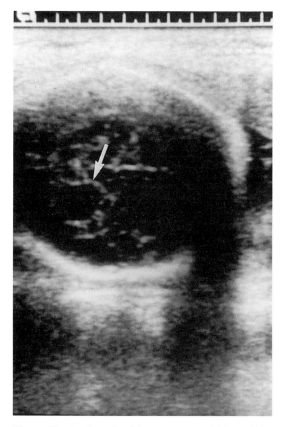

Figure 42 A subarachnoid cyst (arrow), which could be mistaken for a choroid plexus cyst. However, it did not decrease in size and appeared to compress the tissue around it. After birth, it continued to expand, and needed surgery

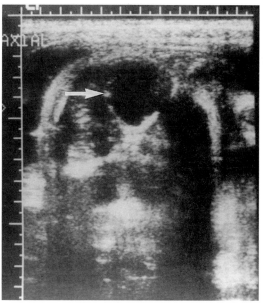

Figure 43 A subarachnoid cyst (arrow) at the base of the brain

fossa, there was reverse diastolic flow in the middle cerebral artery. If the nature of an echogenic intra-cerebral mass is not clear, magnetic resonance imaging may help determine whether it is clot or tumor, since blood has a characteristic MRI appearance.

Subdural hemorrhage usually results in fetal[212] or neonatal death, or delayed development and microcephaly[213], but a normal outcome has been

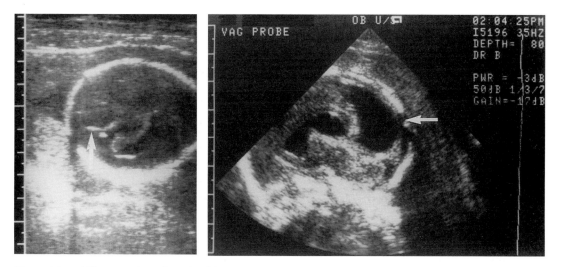

Figure 44 Midline posterior subarachnoid cyst (arrow). Left, axial view; right, vaginal probe, sagittal view

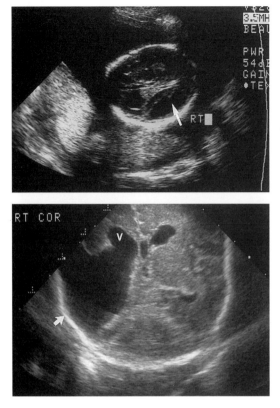

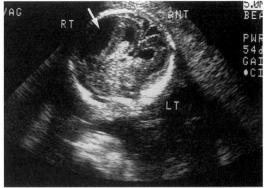

Figure 45 Unilateral schizencephaly. Axial view (top left) of the fetal head with a collection of fluid (arrow). Coronal view (top right), showing the collection of fluid (arrow). No definite connection to the atrial ventricle could be seen. Neonatal coronal scan (bottom), showing the collection (arrow) directly communicating with the lateral ventricle (V). Magnetic resonance imaging showed that the connecting channel was lined with gray matter

reported in a 30-week fetus with large bilateral subdurals[214].

Causes of subdural hemorrhage appear to be the same as interventricular hemorrhage, but in addition, maternal trauma is not uncommon. Gunn and colleagues[214] have reported a large number of cases in Pacific Islanders who apparently had healing by abdominal manipulation. Premature closure of the foramen ovale was thought to cause hydrops and hepatomegaly as well as subdurals in one fetus[214]. Subdural hemorrhages can be very large, resulting in severe fetal anemia[214].

Arachnoid cysts

Subarachnoid cysts can be located in the supra- or infratentorial parts of the brain (Figures 42–44). They are usually round, fluid-filled and surrounded by a thin wall. They can be located in the midline or asymmetrically and may or may not produce a mass effect. Occasionally, they can be difficult to distinguish from a choroid plexus cyst when they originate in a ventricle. The use of Doppler will differentiate them from arteriovenous malformations. Unlike porencephalic cysts, they do not connect with the lateral ventricles. A cystic neoplasm may be hard to differentiate, but usually contains some solid material and will enlarge rapidly. Although they may be ovoid, their borders are smooth and they do not contain any echogenic material.

Hydrocephalus can occur if the cyst blocks CSF circulation. In fact, an asymmetrically located subarachnoid cyst may be hard to distinguish from hydrocephalus, if the wall is hard to see. Growth can occur *in utero*. Sometimes, after evaluation in the neonatal period, surgery or shunting may be necessary, to relieve symptoms caused by expansion of the cyst or hydrocephalus. Outcome is usually good and has been good in prenatally diagnosed cases[215–218]. A very thorough review of the literature is given by Langer and co-workers[218].

Porencephaly

Porencephaly refers to a fluid-filled area within the brain substance that communicates with the ventricles. It is usually a result of destruction of the brain, with subsequent cavity formation, but there is a rare hereditary form in which there is probably a form of holoprosencephaly with a midline cyst. Since it is the result of destruction, it produces no mass effect. There can be numerous porencephalic cysts in cases of intracerebral bleeding. They are not always perfectly round, but may have irregular edges with some blood or debris attached to the wall. Outcome is related to size and location, but some neurological deficit is usual. These cysts, when present, are rarely detected in the antenatal period.

Schizencephaly

This term refers to fluid-filled bilateral clefts or passages from the lateral ventricles to the sub-arachnoid space under the calvarium. The cause is not known, but they occur in the blood supply area of the middle cerebral artery, suggesting that there may have been an early vascular accident or malformation of that vessel.

The clefts are lined with gray matter and are probably an infolding of the cortex. There are almost always other associated abnormalities of the brain, such as heterotopias and polymicrogyria.

Neurological disability seems to be related to the size of the cleft; if the cleft is narrow, fused in any part, or unilateral, the patient may be normal or have minimal developmental delay. If the clefts are large and bilateral, there is severe developmental delay. However, all patients have refractory seizures and motor dysfunction. Some may have septo-optic dysplasia.

Ultrasound will demonstrate clefts from the interior of the mid-calvarium into the bodies of the lateral ventricles. These may be small or large, unilateral (Figure 45) or bilateral. The anterior and posterior borders may be fused. The septum pellucidum is absent in all cases. It should be noted here that absence of the septum pellucidum may be difficult to diagnose. What has in the past been thought to be this structure is actually the medial walls of the lateral ventricles. The appearance in the fetus may change over a number of weeks; the initial appearance may be less worrisome than that 10–20 weeks later[219,220].

References

1. Jeanty, P., Dramaix-Wilmet, M., Delbeke, D., Rodesch, F. and Struyven, J. (1981). Ultrasonic evaluation of fetal ventricular growth. *Neuroradiology*, **21**, 127–31

2. Johnson, M.L., Dunne, M.G., Mack, L.A. and Rashbaum, C.L. (1980). Evaluation of fetal intracranial anatomy by static and realtime ultrasound. *J. Clin. Ultrasound*, **8**, 311–18

3. Pretorius, D.H., Drose, J.A and Manco-Johnson, M.L. (1986). Fetal lateral ventricular ratio determination during the second trimester. *J. Clin. Ultrasound*, **5**, 121

4. Cardoza, J.D., Goldstein, R.B. and Filly, R.A. (1988). Exclusion of fetal ventriculomegaly with a single measurement: the width of the lateral ventricular atrium. *Radiology*, **169**, 711–14

5. Thors, F. and Moogland, H.J. (1990). Ultrasonography of fetal brain: some remarks with respect to the interpretation of the 'caum sept. pellucid'. *J. Clin. Ultrasound*, **18**, 411–17

6. Shepard, M. and Filly, R.A. (1982). A standardized plane for biparietal diameter measurement. *J. Ultrasound Med.*, **1**, 145–50

7. Hadlock, F.P., Deter, R. L., Harrist, R.B. and Park, S.K. (1982). Fetal biparietal diameter: rational choice of plane of section for sonographic measurement. *Am. J. Roentgenol.*, **138**, 871–4

8. Jeanty, P., Chervenak, F.A., Romero, R., Michiels, M. and Hobbins, J.C. (1984). The Sylvian fissure: a commonly mislabeled cranial landmark. *J. Ultrasound Med.*, **3**, 15–18

9. Wilkins-Haug, L. and Freedman, W. (1991). Progression of exencephaly to anencephaly in the human fetus – an ultrasound perspective. *Prenat. Diagn.*, **11**, 227–33

10. Bronshtein, M. and Ornoy, A. (1991). Acrania: anencephaly resulting from secondary degeneration of a closed neural tube: two cases in the same family. *J. Clin. Ultrasound*, **19**, 230–4

11. Campbell, S., Johnstone, F.D., Hold, E.M. and May, P. (1972). Anencephaly: early ultrasonic diagnosis active management. *Lancet*, **2**, 1226–7

12. Goldstein, R.B., Filly, R.A. and Callen, P.W. (1989). Sonography of anencephaly: pitfalls in early diagnosis. *J. Clin. Ultrasound*, **17**, 397–402

13. Brackbill, Y. (1971). The role of the cortex in orienting: orienting reflex in an anencephalic infant. *Dev. Psychol.*, **5**, 195

14. Chervenak, F.A., Farley, M.A., Walters, L.E., Hobbins, J. C. and Mahoney, M.J. (1984). When is

termination of pregnancy during the third trimester morally justifiable? *N. Engl. J. Med.*, **310**, 501–4

15. Truog, R.D. and Fletcher, J.C. (1989). Anencephalic newborns. Can organs be transplanted before brain death? *N. Engl. J. Med.*, **321**, 388–91

16. Medearis, D.N. and Holmes, L.B. (1989). On the use of anencephalic infants as organ donors. *N. Engl. J. Med.*, **321**, 391–3

17. Lorber, J. and Ward, A.M. (1985). Spina bifida – a vanishing nightmare? *Arch. Dis. Child*, **60**, 1086–91

18. Warkany, J. (1971). *Congenital Malformations. Notes and Comments*, pp. 189–200. (Chicago: Year Book Medical Publishers)

19. Holmes, L.B., Driscoll, S.G. and Atkins, L. (1976). Etiologic heterogeneity of neural-tube defects. *N. Engl. J. Med.*, **294**, 365–9

20. International Clearing House for Birth Defects Monitoring System (1983). *Annual Report*, p. 13. (Washington, DC)

21. Nyberg, D.A., Mack, L.A., Hirsch, J., Pagon, R.O. and Shepard, T.H. (1987). Fetal hydrocephalus: sonographic detection and clinical significance of associated anomalies. *Radiology*, **163**, 187–91

22. Hudgins, R.J., Edwards, M.S.B., Goldstein, R., Callen, P.W., Harrison, M.R., Filly, R.A. and Golbus, M.S. (1988). Natural history of fetal ventriculomegaly. *Pediatrics*, **82**, 692–7

23. Drugan, A., Krause, B., Canady, A., Zador, I.E., Sacks, A.J. and Evans, M.I. (1989). The natural history of prenatally diagnosed cerebral ventriculomegaly. *J. Am. Med. Assoc.*, **261**, 1785–8

24. Chervenak, F.A., Berkowitz, R.L., Romero R., Tortora, M., Mayden, K., Duncan, C., Mahoney, M.J. and Hobbins, J.C. (1983). The diagnosis of fetal hydrocephalus. *Am. J. Obstet. Gynecol.*, **147**, 703–16

25. Heiserman, J., Filly, A.A. and Goldstein, R.B. (1991). The effect of measurement errors on the sonographic evaluation of ventriculomegaly. *J. Ultrasound Med.*, **10**, 121–4

26. Alagappan, R., Browning, P.D., Laorr, A. and McGahan, J.P., (1994). Distal lateral ventricular atrium: reevaluation of normal range. *Radiology*, **193**, 405–8

27. Farrell, T.A., Hertzberg, B.S., Kliewer, M.A., Harris, L. and Paine, S.S. (1994). Fetal lateral ventricles: reassessment of normal values for atrial diameter at US. *Radiology*, **193**, 409–11

28. Benacerraf, B.R. and Birnholz, J.C. (1987). The diagnosis of fetal hydrocephalus prior to 22 weeks. *J. Clin. Ultrasound*, **15**, 531–6

29. Benacerraf, B.R. (1988). Fetal hydrocephalous: diagnosis and significance. *Radiology*, **169**, 858–9

30. Cardoza, J.D., Filly, R.A. and Podarsky, A.E. (1988). The dangling choroid plexus: a sonographic observation of value in excluding ventriculomegaly. *Am. J. Radiol.*, **151**, 767–70

31. Chinn, D.C., Callen, P.W. and Filly, R.A. (1983).

The lateral cerebral ventricle in early second trimester. *Radiology*, **148**, 529–31

32. Mahony, B.S., Nyberg, D.A., Hirsch, J.H., Petty, C.N., Hendricks, S.K. and Mack, L.A. (1988). Mild idiopathic lateral cerebral ventricular dilatation *in utero*: sonographic evaluation. *Radiology*, **169**, 715–21

33. Hertzberg, B.S., Lile, R., Foosaner, D.E., Kliewer, M.A., Paine, S.S., Paulson, E.K., Carroll, B.A. and Bowie, J.D. (1994). Choroid plexus–ventricular wall separation in fetuses with normal-sized cerebral ventricles at sonography: postnatal outcome. *Am. J. Roentgenol.*, **163**, 405–10

34. Toi, A. (1987). Spontaneous resolution of fetal ventriculomegaly in a diabetic patient. *J. Ultrasound Med.*, **6**, 37–9

35. Chervenak, F.A., Hobbins, J.C., Wertheimer, I., O'Neal, J.P. and Mahoney, M.J. (1985). The natural history of ventriculomegaly in a fetus without obstructive hydrocephalus. *Am. J. Obstet. Gynecol.*, **152**, 574–5

36. Jorgensen, C., Ingemarsson, I., Svalenius, E., Montan, S. and Svenningsen, N.W. (1986). Ultrasound measurement of the fetal cerebral ventricles: a prospective consecutive study. *J. Clin. Ultrasound*, **14**, 185–90

37. Pilu, G., DePalma, L., Romero, R., Bovicelli, L. and Hobbins, J.C. (1986). The fetal subarachnoid cisterns: an ultrasound study with report of a case of congenital communicating hydrocephalus. *J. Ultrasound Med.*, **5**, 365–72

38. Drose, J.A., Dennis, M.A. and Thickman, D. (1991). Infection *in utero*: US findings in 19 cases. *Radiology*, **178**, 369–74

39. Reuter, K.L., D'Orsi, C.J., Raptopoulos, V.D., Barber, F.E. and Moss, L.J. (1982). Sonographic pseudoasymmetry of the prenatal cerebral hemispheres. *J. Ultrasound Med.*, **1**, 91–5

40. Feeney, J.K. and Barry, A.P. (1954). Hydrocephaly as a cause of maternal mortality and morbidity. *J. Obstet. Gynaecol. Br. Emp.*, **61**, 652–6

41. Laurence, K.M. and Coates, S. (1962). The natural history of hydrocephalus. *Arch. Dis. Child.*, **37**, 345–62

42. Lorber, J. and Zachary, R.B. (1968). Primary congenital hydrocephalus: long-term results of controlled therapeutic trial. *Arch. Dis. Child.*, **43**, 516–27

43. Raimondi, A.J. and Soare, P. (1974). Intellectual development in shunted hydrocephalic children. *Am. J. Dis. Child.*, **127**, 664–71

44. Shurtleff, D.B., Folz, E.L. and Loeser, J.D. (1973). Hydrocephalus: a definition of its progression and relationship to intellectual function, diagnosis, and complications. *Am. J. Dis. Child.*, **125**, 688–93

45. McCullough, D.C. and Balzer-Martin, L.A. (1982). Current prognosis in overt neonatal hydrocephalus. *J. Neurosurg.*, **57**, 378–83

46. Sutton, L.N., Bruce, D.A. and Schut, L. (1980).

Hydranencephaly versus maximal hydrocephalus: an important clinical distinction. *Neurosurgery*, **6**, 34–8

47. Rubin, R.C., Hochwald, G., Liwnicz, B., Tiell, M., Mizutani, H. and Shulman, K. (1972). The effect of severe hydrocephalus on size and number of brain cells. *Dev. Med. Child Neurol.*, **14**, 117–20

48. Lorber, J. (1968). The results of early treatment of extreme hydrocephalus. *Med. Child. Neurol.* (Suppl.), **16**, 21–9

49. Glick, P.L., Harrison, M.R., Nakayama, D.K., Edwards, M.S., Filly, R.A., Chinn, D.H., Callen, P.W., Wilson, S.L. and Golbus, M.S. (1984). Management of ventriculomegaly. *J. Pediatr.*, **105**, 97–105

50. Pretorius, D.H., Davis, K., Manco-Johnson, M.L., Manchester, D., Meier, P.R. and Clewell, W.H. (1985). Clinical course of fetal hydrocephalus: 40 cases. *Am. J. Roentgenol.*, **144**, 827–31

51. Chervenak, F.A., Berkowitz, R.L., Tortora, M. and Hobbins, J.C. (1985). The management of fetal hydrocephalus. *Am. J. Obstet. Gynecol.*, **151**, 933–42

52. Vintzileos, A.M., Campbell, W.A., Weinbaum, P.J. and Nochimson, P.J. (1987). Perinatal management and outcome of fetal ventriculomegaly. *Obstet. Gynecol.*, **69**, 5–12

53. Bromley, B., Frigoletto, F.D. and Benacerraf, B.R. (1991). Mild fetal lateral cerebral ventriculomegaly: clinical course and outcome. *Am. J. Obstet. Gynecol.*, **164**, 863–7

54. Patel, M.D., Filly, A.L., Hersh, D.R. and Goldstein, R.B. (1994). Isolated mild fetal cerebral ventriculomegaly: clinical course and outcome. *Radiology*, **192**, 759–64

55. Luthy, D.A., Wardinsky, T., Shurtleff, D.B., Hollenbach, K.A., Hickok, D.E., Nyberg, D.A. and Benedetti, T.J. (1991). Cesarean section before the onset of labor and subsequent motor function in infants with meningomyelocele diagnosed antenatally. *N. Engl. J. Med.*, **324**, 662–6

56. Chervenak, F.A., Duncan, C., Ment, L.R., Tortora, M., McClure, M. and Hobbins, J.C. (1984). Perinatal management of meningomyelocele. *Obstet. Gynecol.*, **63**, 376–80

57. Edwards, J.H. (1961). The syndrome of sex-linked hydrocephalus. *Arch. Dis. Child.*, **36**, 486–93

58. Riccardi, V.M. and Marcus, E.S. (1978). Congenital hydrocephalus and cerebellar agenesis. *Clin. Genet.*, **13**, 443–7

59. Smith, D.W. (1982). *Recognizable Patterns of Human Malformation*, 3rd edn, pp. 298, 436. (Philadelphia: W.B. Saunders)

60. Wynne-Davis, R. (1973). Disorders in Orthopedic Practice, pp. 156–62. (Oxford: Blackwell Scientific Publications)

61. Lorber, J. (1984). The family history of uncomplicated congenital hydrocephalus: an epidemiological study based on 270 probands. *Brit. Med. J.*, **289**, 281–4

62. Adams, C., Johnston, W.P. and Nevin, N.C. (1982).

Family study of congenital hydrocephalus. *Dev. Med. Child Neurol.*, **24**, 493–8

63. Lorber, J. and De, N.C. (1970). Family history of congenital hydrocephalus. *Dev. Med. Child Neurol.* (Suppl.), **22**, 94

64. Coady, D.J., Snyder, J.R., Lustig-Gillman, I., Suidan, J., Hori, S. and Young, B.K. (1985). Hydranencephaly: prenatal and neonatal ultrasonographic appearance. *Am. J. Perinatal*, **2**, 228–30

65. Greene, M.F., Benacerraf, B. and Crawford, J.M. (1985). Hydranencephaly: ultrasound appearance during *in utero* evolution. *Radiology*, **156**, 779–80

66. Mealey, J., Ozenitis, A.J. and Hockley, A.A. (1970). The prognosis of encephaloceles. *J. Neurosurg.*, **32**, 209–18

67. Field, B. (1974). The child with an encephalocele. *Med. J. Aust.*, **1**, 700

68. Lorber, J. and Schofield, J.K. (1979). The prognosis of occipital encephalocele. Z. Kinderchirurg. *Grenzgeb.*, **28**, 347–51

69. Cohen, M.M. and Lemire, R.J. (1982). Syndromes with cephaloceles. *Teratology*, **25**, 161–72

70. Mecke, S. and Passarge, E. (1971). Encephalocele, polycystic kidneys, and polydactyly as an autosomal recessive trait simulating certain other disorders. The Meckel syndrome. *Ann. Genet.*, **14**, 97–103

71. Chervenak, F.A., Isaacson, G., Mahoney, M.J., Berkowitz, R.L., Tortora, M. and Hobbins, J.C. (1984). Diagnosis and management of fetal cephalocele. *Obstet. Gynecol.*, **64**, 86–90

72. Sabbagha, R.E., Tamura, R.K., Dal Campo, S., Elias, S., Salvino, C., Shkolnik, A. and Gerbie, A.B. (1980). Fetal cranial and carniocervical masses: ultrasound characteristics and differential diagnosis. *Am. J. Obstet. Gynecol.*, **138**, 511–17

73. Graham, D., Johnson, T.R.B. Jr, Winn, K. and Sanders, R.C. (1982). The role of sonography in the prenatal diagnosis and management of encephalocele. *J. Ultrasound Med.*, **1**, 111–15

74. Fiske, C.E. and Filly, R.A. (1982). Ultrasound evaluation of the normal and abnormal fetal neural axis. *Radiol. Clin. N. Am.*, **20**, 285–96

75. Chervenak, F.A., Isaacson, G., Rosenberg, J.C. and Kardon, N.B. (1986). Antenatal diagnosis of frontal cephalocele in a fetus with atelosteogenesis. *J. Ultrasound Med.*, **5**, 111–13

76. Ingraham, F.D. and Swan, H. (1943). Spina bifida and cranium bifidum. I. A survey of five hundred and forty six cases. *N. Engl. J. Med.*, **228**, 559

77. Suwanwela, C. and Suwanwels, N. (1972). A morphological classification of sincipital encephalomeningoceles. *J. Neurosurg.*, **36**, 201–11

78. Fink, I.J., Chinn, D.H. and Callen, P.W. (1983). A potential pitfall in the ultrasonographic diagnosis of fetal encephalocele. *J. Ultrasound Med.*, **2**, 313–14

79. Mclaurin, R.L. (1964). Parietal encephaloceles. *Neurology*, **14**, 764–72

80. Saunders, E.S., Shortland, D. and Dunn, P.M. (1984). What is the incidence of holoprosencephaly? *J. Med. Genet.*, **21**, 21–6

81. Roach, E., DeMyer, W., Conneally, P.M., Palmer, C. and Marrit, A.D. (1975). Holoprosencephaly: birth data, genetic and demographic analyses of 30 families. Birth defects. *Orig. Article Serv.*, **11**, 294–313

82. Matsunaga, E. and Shiota, K. (1977). Holoprosencephaly in human embryos: epidemiologic studies of 150 cases. *Teratology*, **16**, 261–72

83. DeMyer, W. and Seman, W. (1963). Alobar holoprosencephaly (arrhinencephaly) with median cleft lip and palate. *Confin. Neurol.*, **23**, 1

84. Dekaban, A. (1969). Effects of X-radiation on mouse fetus during gestation: emphasis on distribution of cerebral lesions. Part 2. *J. Nucl. Med.*, **10**, 68–77

85. Keeler, R.F. (1970). Teratogenic compounds of veratrum californium (Durand) X. Cyclopia in rabbits produced by cyclonamine. *Teratology*, **3**, 175–80

86. Barr, M., Hanson, J.W., Currey, K., Sharp, S., Toriello, H., Schmickel, R.D. and Wilson, G.N. (1983). Holoprosencephaly in infants of diabetic mothers. J. Pediatr., 102, 565–8

87. Mayden, K.L., Tortora, M. and Berkowitz, R.L. (1982). Orbital diameters: a new parameter for prenatal diagnosis and dating. *Am. J. Obstet. Gynecol.*, **144**, 289–97

88. Jeanty, P., Dramaix-Wilmet, M., Van Gansbeke, D., van Regemorler, N. and Rodesch, F. (1982). Fetal ocular biometry by ultrasound. *Radiology*, **143**, 513–16

89. Blackwell, D.E., Spinnato, J.A., Hirsch, G., Giles, H.R. and Sackler, J. (1982). Antenatal ultrasound diagnosis of holoprosencephaly: a case report. *Am. J. Obstet. Gynecol.*, **143**, 848–9

90. Hill, L.M., Breckle, R. and Bonebrake, C.R. (1982). Ultrasonic findings with holoprosencephaly. *J. Reprod. Med.*, **27**, 172

91. Mok, P.M. and Douglas-Jones, A.G. (1983). Prenatal diagnosis of holoprosencephaly by sonography. *Aust. Radiol.*, **27**, 5–7

92. Filly, R.A., Chinn, D.H. and Callen, P.W. (1984). Alobar holoprosencephaly: ultrasonic prenatal diagnosis. *Radiology*, **151**, 455–9

93. Chervenak, F.A., Isaacson, G., Mahoney, M.J., Tortora, M., Mesologites, T. and Hobbins, J.C. (1984). The obstetric significance of holoprosencephaly. *Obstet. Gynecol.*, **63**, 115–21

94. Chervenak, F.A., Isaacson, G., Hobbins, J.C., Chitkara, U., Tortora, M. and Berkowitz, R.L. (1985). Diagnosis and management of fetal holoprosencephaly. *Obstet. Gynecol.*, **66**, 322–6

95. Nyberg, D.A., Mack, L.A., Bronstein, A., Hirsch, J. and Pagon, R.A. (1987). Holoprosencephaly: prenatal sonographic diagnosis. *Am. J. Roentgenol.*, **149**, 1051–8

96. Pilu, G., Romero, R., Rizzo, N., Jeanty, P. Bovicelli, L. and Hobbins, J.C. (1987). Criteria for the prenatal diagnosis of holoprosencephaly. *Am. J. Perinat.*, **4**, 41–9

97. Pilu, G., Sandri, F., Perolo, A., Giangaspero, F., Cocchi, G., Savlioli, G. P. and Bouicelli, L. (1992). Prenatal diagnosis of labor holoprosencephaly. *Ultrasound Obstet. Gynecol.*, **2**, 88–94

98. Pilu, G., Ambrosetto, P., Sandri, F., Tani, G., Perolo, A., Grisolia, G. and Ancora, G. (1994). Intraventricular fused fornices: a specific sign of fetal lobar holoprosencephaly. *Ultrasound Obstet. Gynecol.*, **4**, 65–7

99. DeMyer, W. (1977). Holoprosencephaly. In Vinken, P.J. and Bruyn, G.W. (eds.) *Handbook of Clinical Neurology*, vol. 30, pp. 431–78. (New York: Elsevier Biomedical)

100. Manelfe, C. and Sevely, A. (1982). Neuroradiological study of holoprosencephalies. *J. Neuroradiol.*, **9**, 15–45

101. Chervenak, F.A. and Romero, R. (1984). Is there a role for fetal cephalocentesis in modern obstetrics? *Am. J. Perinatol.*, **1**, 170–3

102. Book, J.A., Schut, J.W. and Reed, S.C. (1953). A clinical and genetical study of microcephaly. *Am. J. Ment. Defic.*, **57**, 637–60

103. Koch, G. (1969). Genetics of microcephaly in man. *Acta Genet. Med. Gemellol. (Roma)*, **8**, 75–86

104. Hsia, Y.E., Bratu, M. and Herberdt, A. (1971). Genetics of the Meckel syndrome (dysencephalia splanchnocystica). *Pediatrics*, **48**, 237–47

105. Dobbing, J. and Sands, J. (1973). Quantitative growth and development of the human brain. *Arch. Dis. Child*, **48**, 757–67

106. Kurtz, A.B., Wapner, R.J., Rubin, C.S., Cole-Beuglet, C., Ross, R.D. and Goldberg, B.B. (1980). Ultrasound criteria for *in utero* diagnosis of microcephaly. *J. Clin. Ultrasound*, **8**, 11–16

107. Chervenak, F.A., Jeanty, P., Cantraine, F., Chitkara, U., Venus, I., Berkowitz, R.L. and Hobbins, J.C. (1984). The diagnosis of fetal microcephaly. *Am. J. Obstet. Gynecol.*, **149**, 512–17

108. Chervenak, F.A., Rosenberg, J., Brightman, R.C., Chitkaru, U. and Jeanty, P. (1987). A prospective study of the accuracy of ultrasound in predicting fetal microcephaly. *Obstet. Gynecol.*, **69**, 908–10

109. Goldstein, I., Reece, E.A., Pilu, G., O'Connor, T.Z., Lockwood, C.J. and Hobbins, J.C. (1988). Sonographic assessment of the fetal frontal lobe: a potential tool for prenatal diagnosis of microcephaly. *Am. J. Obstet. Gynecol.*, **158**, 1057–62

110. Avery, G.B., Menesses, L. and Lodge, A. (1972). The clinical significance of 'measurement microcephaly.' *Am. J. Dis. Child.*, **123**, 214–17

111. Martin, H.P. (1970). Microcephaly and mental retardation. *Am. J. Dis. Child.*, **119**, 128–31

112. Sells, C.J. (1977). Microcephaly in a normal school population. *Pediatrics*, **59**, 262–5

113. Bell, W.E. (1977). Abnormalities in size and shape of the head. In Shaffuer, A.J. and Avery, M.E. (eds.)

Diseases of the Newborn, 4th edn, pp. 717–19. (Philadelphia: W.B. Saunders)

114. Warkany, J. (1971). *Microcephaly, Congenital Malformations*, pp. 237–244. (Chicago: Year Book Medical Publishers)

115. Ross, J.J. and Frias, J.L. (1977). Microcephaly. In Vinken, P.J. and Bruyn, G.W. (eds.) *Handbook of Clinical Neurology*, pp. 507–24. (New York: North-Holland)

116. Brandon, M.W.G., Kirman, B.H. and Williams, C.E. (1959). *Microcephaly. J. Ment. Sci.*, **105**, 721–47

117. Davies, H. and Kirman, B.H. (1962). Microcephaly. *Arch. Dis. Child.*, **37**, 623–7

118. Hecht, F. and Kelly, J.V. (1979). Little heads: inheritance and early detection. *J. Pediatr.*, **95**, 731–2

119. Macleod, N.A., William, J.P., Muchen, B. and Lum, G.B. (1987). Normal and abnormal morphology of the corpus callosum. *Neurology*, **37**, 1240–2

120. Georgy, B.A., Hesselink, J.R. and Jernigan, T.L. (1993). MR imaging of the corpus callosum. *Am. J. Roentgenol.*, **160**, 949–55

121. Jellinger, F., Gross, H. and Kaltenback, E. (1981). Holoprosencephaly and agenesis of the corpus callosum frequency of associated malformations. *Acta. Neurol. Pathol.*, **55**, 1–10

122. Atlas, S.W., Zimmerman, R.A., Bilaniuk, L.T., Rorke, L., Hackney, D.B., Goldberg, H.I. and Grossman, R.I. (1986). Corpus callosum and limbic system: neuroanatomic MR evaluation of developmental anomalies. *Neuroradiology*, **160**, 355–62

123. Malinger, G. and Zakut, H. (1993). The corpus callosum: normal fetal development as shown by transvaginal sonography. *Am. J. Roentgenol.*, **161**, 1041–3

124. Comstock, C.H., Culp, D., Gonzales, J. and Boal, D.B. (1985). Agenesis of the corpus callosum in the fetus: its evolution and significance. *J. Ultrasound Med.*, **4**, 613–16

125. Bertino, R.E., Nyberg, D.A., Cyr, D.R. and Mack, L.A. (1988). Prenatal diagnosis of agenesis of the corpus callosum. *J. Ultrasound Med.*, **7**, 251–60

126. Lockwood, C.J., Ghidini, A., Aggarwal, R. and Hobbins, J.C. (1988). Antenatal diagnosis of partial agenesis of the corpus callosum: a benign cause of ventirculomegaly. *Am. J. Obstet. Gynecol.*, **159**, 184–6

127. Meizner, I., Barki, Y. and Hertzanu, Y. (1987). Prenatal sonographic diagnosis of agenesis of corpus callosum. *J. Clin. Ultrasound*, **15**, 262–4

128. Mulligan, G. and Meier, P. (1989). Lipoma and agenesis of the corpus callosum with associated choroid plexus lipomas: *in utero* diagnosis. *J. Ultrasound Med.*, **8**, 583–8

129. Vergani, P., Ghidini, A., Strobelt, N., Locatelli, A., Mariani, S., Bertalero, C. and Cavallone, M. (1993). Prognostic indicators in the prenatal diagnosis of agenesis of corpus callosum. *Am. J. Obstet. Gynecol.*, **170**, 753–8

130. Skeffington, F.S. (1982). Agenesis of the corpus callosum: neonatal ultrasound appearances. *Arch. Dis. Child.*, **57**, 713–14

131. Gabarski, S.S., Gebarski, K.S., Bowerman, R.A. and Silver, T.M. (1984). Agenesis of the corpus callosum: sonographic features. *Radiology*, **151**, 443–8

132. Babcock, D.S. (1984). The normal, absent, and abnormal corpus callosum: sonographic findings. *Radiology*, **151**, 449–53

133. Atlas, S.W., Shkoinik, A. and Naidick, T.P. (1985). Sonographic recognition of agenesis of the corpus callosum. *Am. J. Roentgenol.*, **145**, 167–73

134. Sarwar, M., Virapongse, C., Bhimani, S. and Freilich, M. (1984). Interhemispheric fissure sign of dysgenesis of the corpus callosum. *J. Comput. Assist. Tomogr.*, **8**, 637–44

135. Lacey, D.J. (1985). Agenesis of the corpus callosum. *Am. J. Dis. Child.*, **139**, 953–5

136. Resta, M., Greco, P., D'Addario, V., Florio, C., Dardes, N., Caruso, G., Spagnolo, P., Clement, R., Vimercati, A. and Selvaggi, L. (1994). Magnetic resonance imaging in pregnancy: study of fetal cerebral malformations. *Ultrasound Obstet. Gynecol.*, **4**, 7–20

137. Curnes, J.T., Laster, D.W., Koubek, T.D., Moody, D.M., Ball, M.R. and Witcofski, R.L. (1986). MRI of corpus callosal syndromes. *Am. J. Neuroradiol.*, **7**, 617–22

138. Schiavetto, A., Lepore, F. and Lassonde, M. (1993). Somesthetic discrimination thresholds in the absence of the corpus callosum. *Neuropsychologia*, **31**, 695–707

139. Parrish, M.L., Roessman, V. and Levinsohn, M.W. (1979). Agenesis of the corpus callosum: a study of the frequency of associated malformations. *Ann. Neurol.*, **6**, 349–54

140. Boechat, M.I., Kangarloo, H., Diament, M.J. and Krauthamer, R. (1983). Lipoma of the corpus callosum: sonographic appearance. *J. Clin. Ultrasound*, **11**, 447–8

141. Christensen, R.A., Pinckney, L.E., Higgins, S. and Miller, K.E. (1987). Sonographic diagnosis of lipoma of the corpus callosum. *J. Ultasound Med.*, **6**, 449–51

142. Thyen, U., Aksu, F., Bartsch, O. and Herb, E. (1992). Acrocallosal syndrome: association with cystic malformation of the brain and neurodevelopmental aspects. *Neuropediatrics*, **23**, 292–6

143. Donnenfeld, A.E., Packer, R.J., Zackai, E.H., Chee, C.M., Sellinger, B. and Emanuel, B.S. (1989). Clinical, cytogenetic, and pedigree findings in 18 cases of Aicardi syndrome. *Am. J. Med. Genet.*, **32**, 461–7

144. Erenberg, G. (1983). Aicardi's syndrome: report of an autopsied case and review of the literature. *Cleve. Clin. Q.*, **50**, 341–5

145. Guion-Almeida, M.L. and Richieri-Costa, A. (1992). Callosal agenesis, iris coloboma, megacolon

in a Brazilian boy with Rubinstein–Taybi syndrome. *Am. J. Med. Genet.*, **43**, 929–31

146. Dobyns, W.B. (1989). Agenesis of the corpus callosum and gyral malformations are frequent manifestations of nonketotic hyperglycemia. *Neurology*, **39**, 817–20

147. Bamforth, F., Bamforth, S., Poskett, K., Applegarth, D. and Hall, J. (1988). Abnormalities of corpus callosum in patients with inherited metabolic diseases. *Lancet*, **2**, 451–2

148. Dominguez, R., Vila-Coro, A.A., Slopis, J.M. and Bohan, T.P. (1991). Brain and ocular abnormalities in infants with *in utero* exposure to cocaine and other street drugs. *Am. J. Dis. Child.*, **145**, 688–95

149. McCurdle, P. and Wilson, B. (1993). Language and development in FG syndrome with callosal agenesis. *J. Commun. Disord.*, **26**, 83–100

150. Vici, C.D., Sabetta, G., Gambarara, M., Vigevano, F., Bertini, E., Boldrini, R., Parisi, S.G., Quinti, I., Aiuti, F. and Fiorilli, M. (1988). Agenesis of the corpus callosum, combined immunodeficiency, bilateral cataract, and hypopigmentation in two brothers. *Am. J. Med. Genet.*, **29**, 1–8

151. Kang, W.M., Huang, C.C. and Lin, S.J. (1992). X-linked recessive inheritance of dysgenesis of corpus callosum in a Chinese family. *Am. J. Med. Genet.*, **41**, 419–23

152. Kozlowski, K. and Ouvrier, R.A. (1993). Agenesis of the corpus callosum with mental retardation and osseous lesions. *Am. J. Med. Genet.* (*Neuropsychiatr. Genet.*), **48**, 6–9

153. Raybaud, C.A., Strother, C.M. and Hald, J.K. (1989). Aneurysms of the vein of Galen: embryologic considerations and anatomical features relating to the pathogenesis of the malformation. *Neuroradiology*, **31**, 109–28

154. Gold, A.P., Ransohoff, J. and Carter, S. (1964). Vein of Galen malformation. *Acta Neurol. Scand.* (Suppl. 11), **4**, 1–31

155. Hirsch, J.H., Cyr, D., Eberhardt, H. and Zunkel, D. (1983). Ultrasonographic diagnosis of an aneurysm of the vein of Galen *in utero* by duplex scanning. *J. Ultrasound Med.*, **2**, 231–3

156. Mao, K. and Adams, J. (1983). Antenatal diagnosis of intracranial arteriovenous fistula by ultrasonography. Case report. *Br. J. Obstet. Gynaecol.*, **90**, 872–3

157. Vintzileos, A.M., Eisenfeld, L.I., Campbell, W.A., Herson, V.C., DiLeo, P.E. and Chameides, L. (1986). Prenatal ultrasonic diagnosis of arteriovenous malformation of the vein of Galen. *Am. J. Perinatol.*, **3**, 209–11

158. Reiter, A.A., Huhta, J.C., Carpenter, R.J. Jr, Segall, G.K. and Hawkins, E.P. (1986). Prenatal diagnosis of arteriovenous malformation of the vein of Galen. *J. Clin. Ultrasound*, **14**, 623–8

159. Rizzo, G., Arduini, D., Colosimo, C., Boccolini, M.R. and Mancuso, S. (1987). Abnormal fetal cerebral blood flow velocity waveforms as a sign of an aneurysm of the vein of Galen. *Fetal Ther.*, **2**, 75–9

160. Johnson, W., Berry, J.M. Jr, Einzig, S. and Bass, J.L. (1988). Doppler findings in nonimmune hydrops fetalis and cerebral arteriovenous malformation. *Am. Heart J.*, **115**, 1138–40

161. Mendelsohn, D.B., Mertzaner, T. and Butterworth, A. (1984). *In utero* diagnosis of a vein of Galen aneurysm by ultrasound. *Neuroradiology*, **26**, 417–18

162. Jeanty, P., Kepple, D., Roussis, P. and Shah, D. (1990). *In utero* detection of cardiac failure from an aneurysm of the vein of Galen. *Am. J. Obstet. Gynecol.*, **163**, 50–1

163. Comstock, C.H. and Kirk, J.S. (1991). Arteriovenous malformations: locations and evolution in the fetal brain. *J. Ultrasound Med.*, **10**, 361–5

164. Dan, U., Shaley, E., Greif, M. and Weiner, E. (1992). Prenatal diagnosis of fetal brain arteriovenous malformation: the use of color Doppler imaging. *J. Clin. Ultrasound*, **20**, 149–51

165. Lee, W., Kirk, J.S., Pryde, P., Romero, R. and Qureski, F. (1994). Atypical presentation of fetal arteriovenous malformation. *J. Ultrasound Med.*, **13**, 645–7

166. Watson, D.G., Smith, R.R. and Brann, A.W. (1976). Arteriovenous malformation of the vein of Galen. *Am. J. Dis. Child.*, **130**, 520–5

167. Fox, A.J., Pelz, D.M. and Lee, D.H. (1990). Arteriovenous malformations of the brain: recent results of endovascular therapy. *Radiology*, **177**, 51–7

168. Norman, M.G. and Becker, L.E. (1974). Cerebral damage in neonates resulting from arteriovenous malformation of the vein of Galen. *J. Neurol. Neurosurg. Psychiatry*, **37**, 252–8

169. Westra, S.J., Curran, J.G., Duckwiler, G.R., Zaninovic, A.C., Hall, T.R., Martin, N.A., Boechat, M.I. and Vinuela, F. (1993). Pediatric intracranial vascular malformations: evaluation of treatment results with color Doppler US. *Radiology*, **186**, 775–83

170. Hoff, N.R. and Mackay, I.M. (1980). Prenatal ultrasound diagnosis of intracranial teratoma. *J. Clin. Ultrasound*, **8**, 247–9

171. Crade, M. (1982). Ultrasonic demonstration *in utero* of an intracranial teratoma. *J. Am. Med. Assoc.*, **247**, 1173

172. Lipman, S.P., Pretorius, D.H., Rumack, C.M. and Manco-Johnson, M.L. (1985). Fetal intracranial teratoma: US diagnosis of three cases and a review of the literature. *Radiology*, **157**, 491–4

173. Sherer, D.M., Abramowicz, J.S., Eggers, P.C., Metlay, L.A., Sinkin, R.A. and Woods, J.R. Jr (1993). Prenatal ultrasonographic diagnosis of intracranial teratoma and massive craniomegaly with associated high-output cardiac failure. *Am. J. Obstet. Gynecol.*, **168**, 97–9

174. Ulreich, S., Hanieh, A. and Furness, M.E. (1993). Positive outcome of fetal intracranial teratoma. *J. Ultrasound Med.*, **3**, 163–5

175. Oi, S., Tamaki, N., Kondo, T., Nakamura, H., Kudo, H., Suzuki, H., Sasaki, M., Matsumoto, S., Ueda, Y., Katayama, K. and Mochizuki, M. (1990).

Massive congenital intracranial teratoma diagnosed *in utero*. *Child's Nerv. Syst.*, **6**, 459–61

176. Snyder, J.R., Lustig-Gillman, I., Milio, L., Morris, M., Pardes, J.G. and Young, B.K. (1986). Antenatal ultrasound diagnosis of an intracranial neoplasm (craniopharyngioma). *J. Clin. Ultrasound*, **14**, 304–6

177. Suresh, S., Indrani, S., Vijayalakshmi, S., Nirmala, J. and Meera, G. (1993). Prenatal diagnosis of cerebral neuroblastoma by fetal brain biopsy. *J. Ultrasound Med.*, **5**, 303–6

178. Riboni, G., De Simoni, M., Leopardi, O. and Molla, R. (1985). Ultrasound appearance of a glioblastoma in a 33-week fetus *in utero*. *J. Clin. Ultrasound*, **13**, 345–6

179. Belfar, H.L., Kuller, J.A., Hill, L.M. and Kislak, S. (1991). Evolving fetal hydranencephaly mimicking intracranial neoplasm. *J. Ultrasound Med.*, **10**, 231–3

180. Winter, T.C. III., Laing, F.C., Mack, L.A. and Born, D.E. (1992). Prenatal sonographic diagnosis of a Pontine lipoma. *J. Ultrasound Med.*, **11**, 559–61

181. Lam, A.H. and Villanueva, A.C. (1992). Symptomatic third ventricular choroid plexus cysts. *Pediatr. Radiol.*, **22**, 413–16

182. Chudleigh, P., Pearce, J.M. and Campbell, S. (1984). The prenatal diagnosis of transient cysts of the fetal choroid plexus. *Prenat. Diagn.*, **4**, 135–7

183. DeRoo, T.R., Harris, R.D., Sargent, S.K., Denholm, T.A. and Crow, H.C. (1988). Fetal choroid plexus cysts: prevalance, clinical significance, and sonographic appearance. *Am. J. Roentgenol.*, **151**, 1179–81

184. Fakhry, J., Schechter, A., Tenner, M.S. and Reale, M. (1985). Cysts of the choroid plexus neonates: documentation and review of the literature. *J. Ultrasound Med.*, **4**, 561–3

185. Hertzberg, B.S., Kay, H.H. and Bowie, J.D. (1989). Fetal choroid plexus lesions: relationship of antenatal sonographic appearance to clinical outcome. *J. Ultrasound Med.*, **8**, 77–82

186. Nicolaides, K.H., Rodeck, C.H. and Gosden, C.M. (1986). Rapid karyotyping in non-lethal fetal malformations. *Lancet*, **1**, 283–7

187. Ostlere, S.J., Irving, H.C. and Lilford, R.J. (1990). Fetal choroid plexus cysts: a report of 100 cases. *Radiology*, **175**, 753–5

188. Porto, M., Murata, Y., Warneke, L.A. and Keegan, K.A. Jr (1993). Fetal choroid plexus cysts: an independent risk factor for chromosomal anomalies. *J. Clin. Ultrasound*, **21**, 103–8

189. Fitzsimmons, J., Wilson, D., Pascoe-Mason, J., Shaw, C.M., Cyr, D.R. and Mack, L.A. (1989). Choroid plexus cysts in fetuses with trisomy 18. *Obstet. Gynecol.*, **73**, 257–60

190. Nadel, A.S., Bromley, B.S., Frigoletto, F.D. Jr, Estroff, J.A. and Benacerraf, B.R. (1992). Isolated choroid plexus cysts in the second-trimester fetus: is amniocentesis really indicated? *Radiology*, **185**, 545–8

191. Twining, P., Zuccollo, J., Clewes, J. and Swallos, J. (1991). Fetal choroid plexus cysts: a prospective study and review of the literature. *Br. J. Radiol.*, **64**, 98–102

192. Gabrielli, S., Reece, E.A., Pilu, G., Perolo, A., Rizzo, N., Bovicelli, L. and Hobbins, J.C. (1989). The clinical significance of prenatally diagnosed choroid plexus cysts. *Am. J. Obstet. Gynecol.*, **160**, 1207–10

193. Kuchelmeister, K., Bergmann, M., Gullotta, F. (1993). Neuropathology of lissencephalies. *Child's Nerv. Syst.*, **9**, 394–9

194. Dobyns, W.B., Stratton, R.F., Parke, J.T., Greenberg, F., Nussbaum, R.L. and Ledbetter, D.H. (1983). Miller–Dieker syndrome: lissencephaly and monosomy. *J. Pediatr.*, **102**, 552–8

195. Saltzman, D.H., Krauss, C.M., Goldman, J.M. and Benacerraf, B.R. (1991). Prenatal diagnosis of lissencephaly. *Prenat. Diagn.*, **11**, 139–43

196. Holzgreve, W., Feil, R., Louwen, F. and Minz, P. (1993). Prenatal diagnosis and management of fetal hydrocephaly and lissencephaly. *Child's Nerv. Syst.*, **9**, 408–12

197. Jackson, J.C. and Blumhagen, J.D. (1983). Congenital hydrocephalus due to prenatal intracranial hemorrhage. *Pediatrics*, **72**, 344–6

198. Mintz, M.C., Arger, P.H. and Coleman, B.G. (1985). *In utero* sonographic diagnosis of intracerebral hemorrhage. *J. Ultrasound Med.*, **4**, 375–6

199. Chinn, D.H. and Filly, R.A. (1983). Extensive intracranial hemorrhage *in utero*. *J. Ultrasound Med.*, **2**, 285–7

200. Kim, M. and Elyaderani, M.K. (1982). Sonographic diagnosis of cerebroventricular hemorrhage *in utero*. *Radiology*, **142**, 479–80

201. Donn, S.M., Barr, M. Jr and McLeary, R.D. (1984). Massive intracerebral hemorrhage *in utero*: sonographic appearance and pathologic correlation. *Obstet. Gynecol.*, **63**, 28S–30S

202. Bondurant, S., Boehm, F.H., Fleischer, A.C. and Machin, J.E. (1984). Antepartum diagnosis of fetal intracranial hemorrhage by ultrasound. *Obstet. Gynecol.*, **63**, 25S–27S

203. McGahan, J.P., Haesslein, H.C., Meyers, M. and Ford, K.B. (1984). Sonographic recognition of *in utero* intraventricular hemorrhage. *Am. J. Roentgenol.*, **142**, 171–3

204. Minkoff, H., Schaffer, R.M., Delke, I. and Grunebaum, A.N. (1985). Diagnosis of intracranial hemorrhage *in utero* after a maternal seizure. *Obstet. Gynecol.*, **65**, 22S–24S

205. Morales, W.J. and Stroup, M. (1985). Intracranial hemorrhage *in utero* due to isoimmune neo-natal thrombocytopenia. *Obstet. Gynecol.*, **65**, 20S–21S

206. Pretorius, D.H., Singh, S., Manco-Johnson, M.L. and Rumack, C.M. (1986). *In utero* diagnosis of intracranial hemorrhage resulting in fetal hydrocephalus. *J. Reprod. Med.*, **31**, 136–8

207. Herman, J.H., Jumbelic, M.I., Ancona, R.J. and

Kickler, T.S. (1986). *In utero* cerebral hemorrhage in alloimmune thrombocytopenia. *Am. J. Pediatr. Hematol. Oncol.*, **8**, 321–17

208. Fogarty, K., Cohen, H.L. and Haller, J.O. (1989). Sonography of fetal intracranial hemorrhage: unusual causes and a review of the literature. *J. Clin. Ultrasound*, **17**, 366–70

209. DeVore, G.R., (1991). In-utero cerebral vascular accident prior to external cephalic version. *J. Clin. Ultrasound*, **19**, 227–9

210. Lustig-Gillman, I., Young, B.K., Silverman, F., Raghavendra, B.N., Wan, L., Reitz, M.E., Aleksic, S., Greco, A. and Snyder, J.R. (1983). Fetal intraventricular hemorrhage: sonographic diagnosis and clinical implications. *J. Clin. Ultrasound*, **11**, 277–80

211. Rotmensch, S., Grannum, P.A., Nores, J.A., Hall, C., Keller, M.S., McCarthy, S. and Hobbins, J.C. (1991). *In utero* diagnosis and management of fetal subdural hematoma. *Am. J. Obstet. Gynecol.*, **164**, 1246–8

212. Kawabata, I., Imai, A. and Tamaya, T. (1993). Antenatal subdural hemorrhage causing fetal death before labor. *Int. J. Gynecol. Obstet.*, **43**, 57–60

213. Nogueira, G.J. (1992). Chronic subdural hematoma *in utero*. Report of a case with survival after treatment. *Child's Nerv. Syst.*, **8**, 462–4

214. Gunn, T.R., Pui, H. and Becroft, D.M. (1985). Subdural hemorrhage *in utero*. *Pediatrics*, **76**, 605–10

215. Hanigan, W.C., All, M.B., Cusack, T.J., Miller, T.C. and Shah, J.J. (1985). Diagnosis of subdural hemorrhage *in utero*. *J. Neurosurg.*, **63**, 977–9

216. Diakowmakis, E.E., Weinberg, B. and Mollin, J. (1986). Prenatal sonographic diagnosis of suprasellar arachnoid cyst. *J. Ultrasound Med.*, **5**, 529–30

217. Meizner, I., Barki, Y., Tadmor, R. and Katz, M. (1988). *In utero* ultrasonic detection of fetal arachnoid cyst. *J. Clin. Ultrasound*, **16**, 506–9

218. Langer, B., Haddad, J., Favre, R., Frigue, V. and Schlaeder, G. (1994). Fetal arachnoid cyst: report of two cases. *Ultrasound Obstet. Gynecol.*, **4**, 68–72

219. Barkovich, A.J. and Norman, D. (1988). MR imaging of schizencephaly. *Am. J. Roentgenol.*, **150**, 1391–6

220. Klingensmith, W.C. and Cioffi-Ragan, D.T. (1986). Schizencephaly: diagnosis and progression *in utero*. *Radiology*, **159**, 617–18

The fetal posterior fossa

4

C. H. Comstock

NORMAL ANATOMY

Cerebellum

The fetal cerebellum is much smaller in relation to the cerebrum than is that of adults. Starting to form at 6 weeks, the final configuration consists of two lobes, or hemispheres, covered with foglia (gyri). Lying between the cerebellar hemispheres is the vermis, an echogenic midline structure that parallels the midbrain and covers the roof of the fourth ventricle. The cerebellum occupies most of the posterior fossa; it is bounded inferiorly and posteriorly by the cisterna magna, superiorly by the tentorium and quadrigeminal cisterns, and anteriorly by the roof of the fourth ventricle, the pons and the medulla (Figures 1 and 2).

Measurements of the lateral width of the cerebellum (Table 1) may be used to determine age in normally grown fetuses[1,2]. An axial plane, with the usual midplane landmarks of the septum pellucidum and thalamus, is obtained and the transducer is then angled slightly to bring the cerebellum into view (Figure 3). If an axial-view measurement cannot be obtained, one in the coronal plane can be used[3,4]. It is possible to measure the cerebellar diameter accurately as early as 12–14 weeks with a vaginal transducer[5]. The ratio of cerebellar diameter to abdominal circumference is 13.7% and has been shown to be independent of gestational age in normally grown fetuses[6].

The area of the vermis (in the sagittal plane) has also been found to correlate closely with gestational age[7,8], as have vermian circumference and maximum vertical length[8]. In fact, Co and colleagues found that vermian area and circumference correlated with age better than did transverse cerebellar width. Although these vermian measurements were obtained in the newborn from gestational ages 25 weeks and up, they could theoretically be used for the fetus if an appropriate sagittal plane could be obtained.

Although cerebellar width correlates well with age in a normally grown fetus, it may not be as useful in symmetric intrauterine growth retardation (IUGR). When placental insufficiency is long-standing or severe enough to decrease the head circumference, there is probably some effect on the cerebellum. This has, in fact, been shown in animals such as sheep and monkeys, and in neonates, as summarized by Hill and associates[9]. All of these studies have shown a reduction in cerebellar weight, which explains why measurement of cerebellar diameter alone does not always demonstrate a decrease in size. Although Reece and co-workers[10] found no difference in the cerebellar diameters of growth retarded vs. normal weight fetuses, no distinction was made between symmetric IUGR (head-affected) and asymmetric IUGR (head-spared), and the degree and duration of growth retardation was not mentioned. Hill and colleagues however, in their larger study, found the transverse cerebellar diameter to be 2SD or more below the mean in 59% of growth retarded fetuses, with symmetrically and asymmetrically growth retarded fetuses equally affected[9]. Lee and associates[11] found the transverse cerebellar diameter to be a good predictor of gestational age in asymmetric IUGR but reduced and, therefore, not as useful in symmetric IUGR[11]. However, cerebellar diameter was still a more accurate predictor of gestational age than was head circumference, abdominal circumference or femur length. Perhaps a measurement of cerebellar *area* or *volume* would reflect changes in IUGR to a greater degree than does diameter alone. Birnholz measured vermian *area* and demonstrated a clear reduction in neonates with IUGR[7]. As might be expected, cerebellar

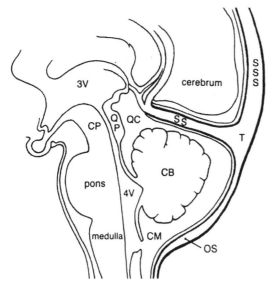

Figure 1 Sagittal drawing of the posterior fossa. CB, cerebellum; CM, cisterna magna; CP, cerebral peduncle; QC, quadrigeminal cistern; QP, quadrigeminal plate; 3V, third ventricle; 4V, fourth ventricle; T, torcula; SS, straight sinus; SSS, superior sagittal sinus; OS, occipital sinus. From reference 20, with permission

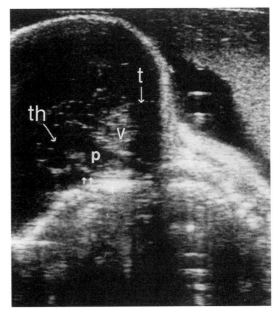

Figure 2 Sagittal scan through the posterior fossa in the exact midline. th, thalamus; V, vermis; p and small arrows, pons; t, tentorium. From reference 20, with permission

diameters are an accurate predictor of gestational age in fetuses that are large for gestational age[12].

Fourth ventricle

The axis of the fourth ventricle lies parallel to the midbrain (Figure 1) with the vermis forming its roof. It can be visualized in most fetuses, optimally in the mid- to late-second trimester. It is so small that visualization can be difficult before 17 weeks[13]. On the fourth-ventricle view (a slight caudad rotation from the usual transcerebellar view) (Figure 4) the shape can be triangular, round, or like a boomerang. The normal anterior–posterior diameter and width gradually increase with gestational age[13]. The fourth ventricle should be smaller than usual in aqueductal stenosis or Chiarri II malformation.

Cisterna magna

The cisterna magna surrounds the cerebellum laterally and inferiorly and fills the V-shaped space between the cerebellar hemispheres (Figures 1–3).

It is increasingly difficult to see the cisterna magna in the axial view as pregnancy progresses, due to shadowing from the posterior cranium, but it can almost always be visualized in the coronal plane.

Standard measurements of the sagittal height of the cisterna magna in newborns have been published[14] and, presumably, would apply in near-term fetuses as well, since no measurements of the fetal cisterna magna in this sagittal plane have yet been published. However, measurements of the depth of the normal fetal cisterna magna in the modified axial plane are available[15,16] (the distance between the interior wall of the posterior cranium and the vermis) (Figure 3). Between 15 and 36 weeks, the size of the cisterna does not change; the mean is 5 mm (SD 3mm) with a range of 1–10 mm. The largest cisterna magna in a normal fetus measured 10 mm in this plane. If the angle of the transducer was increased in relation to the true axial plane, the cisterna magna measured to a maximum of 13mm. The cisterna was visualized in such a manner in 94% of fetuses of 15–28 weeks in one study[15] and 97% of fetuses of 15–25 weeks in another[17].

Table 1 Relationship between cerebellar diameter, biparietal diameter and gestational age (data from reference 1)

Cerebellar diameter (mm)	Biparietal diameter (mm)			Gestational age (weeks)	Cerebellar diameter (mm)	Biparietal diameter (mm)			Gestational age (weeks)
	Mean	+SE	−SE			Mean	+SE	−SE	
15	34.7	38.0	31.5	17.0	35	74.4	78.2	70.7	30.0
16	37.2	40.6	34.0	17.5	36	75.8	79.5	72.1	31.0
17	39.8	43.2	36.4	18.5	37	77.1	80.8	73.4	31.5
18	42.2	45.7	38.8	19.0	38	78.3	82.0	74.7	32.0
19	44.6	48.1	41.1	20.0	39	79.5	83.1	75.9	32.7
20	46.9	50.5	43.4	20.5	40	80.6	84.2	77.0	33.0
21	49.2	52.8	45.6	21.0	41	81.7	85.2	78.1	33.5
22	51.4	55.0	47.8	22.0	42	82.6	86.2	79.1	33.7
23	53.5	57.2	49.9	23.0	43	83.6	87.1	80.1	34.0
24	55.6	59.3	51.9	23.5	44	84.4	87.9	81.0	34.0
25	57.6	61.3	53.9	24.2	45	85.3	88.6	81.9	34.5
26	59.6	63.3	55.8	25.0	46	86.0	89.3	82.7	35.0
27	61.5	65.2	57.7	25.5	47	86.7	89.9	83.5	35.5
28	63.3	67.1	59.5	26.5	48	87.3	90.5	84.2	35.5
29	65.1	68.8	61.3	27.0	49	87.9	91.0	84.8	36.0
30	66.8	70.6	63.0	27.5	50	88.4	91.4	85.4	36.0
31	68.4	72.2	64.7	27.7	51	88.8	91.8	85.9	36.5
32	70.0	73.8	66.3	28.5	52	89.2	92.1	86.4	36.5
33	71.6	75.3	67.8	29.0	53	89.6	92.3	86.8	37.0
34	73.0	76.8	69.3	29.5	54	89.8	92.5	87.2	37.0

SE, standard error. If the biparietal diameter cannot be used because of changes in shape or hydrocephalus, it should be estimated from the gestational age of the fetus

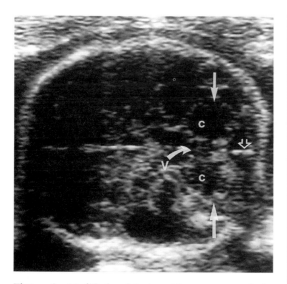

Figure 3 Modified axial view. Measurement of the width of the cerebellum is taken from the outer margin of one cerebellar hemisphere (c) to the other (solid arrows). The vermis (V) lies between the hemispheres. Hollow arrow, dural fold traversing the cisterna magna

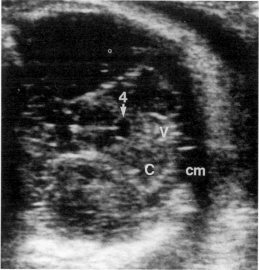

Figure 4 Fourth-ventricle view showing an ellipsoid shape of the fourth ventricle (4). C, cerebellar hemispheres; V, vermis; cm, cisterna magna. Note the two dural folds traversing the cisterna magna

In most fetuses, an echogenic line or lines or circle can be seen in the cisterna just posterior to the vermis (Figure 3). This has been previously described as the straight or occipital sinus, but has recently been shown actually to be an arachnoid septum or dural folds [18, 19].

Quadrigeminal cistern

The quadrigeminal cistern lies slightly superior to the anterior cerebellum (Figure 1). Subarachnoid cysts have occasionally been seen in this cistern [20–22]. They are located directly posterior to the third ventricle (in the midline) and anterior to the cerebellum.

Tentorium

The tentorium is an infolding of the dura that separates the contents of the posterior fossa from the rest of the cranial vault. The transverse sinuses run between its leaves, where it attaches laterally and posteriorly to the cranium. Anterolaterally, it is attached to the superior border of the petrous portion of the temporal bone and posterior clinoid processes of the sphenoid bones. Anteriorly, the midbrain passes through the incisura, the U-shaped medial–anterior border of the tentorium. It slopes upward to the midline and is continuous with the falx cerebi (Figure 5). The tentorium is elevated in many cases of Dandy–Walker malformation; such elevation is considered to be part of the classic malformation, but has not yet been visualized and described in an antenatal scan.

ABNORMALITIES OF THE POSTERIOR FOSSA

Dandy–Walker malformation

Abnormalities in the formation of the vermis include Dandy–Walker syndrome and variant, Joubert's syndrome, tecto-cerebellar dysraphia, and rhombencephalosynapsis. Because the vermis may not be completely formed in fetuses less than 17½ weeks of gestation, the diagnosis of

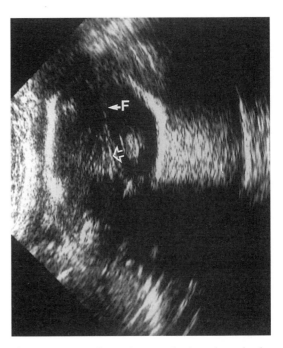

Figure 5 Tentorium. A coronal view through the posterior cranium shows the tent-shaped tentorium (hollow arrow) continuous with the midline falx (F)

hypoplasia of the vermis should not be firmly made before that time [23].

The Dandy–Walker complex encompasses a continuum of abnormalities, all of which have in common varying degrees of vermian hypoplasia. At one end of the spectrum is the Dandy–Walker malformation and at the other is the Dandy–Walker variant.

If, on the true axial view, the cisterna magna is enlarged and there is no visible vermis, the diagnosis is Dandy–Walker malformation (Figures 6 and 7). The absence of the vermis allows the fourth ventricle to enlarge, so that it fills the entire cisterna magna. Despite the fact that the cerebellar hemispheres are mildly or severely hypoplastic, the transcerebellar diameter may be normal or only slightly increased, due to wide separation as the fourth ventricle balloons into the area normally occupied by the cisterna magna [24]. There is almost always hydrocephalus, or at least enlargement of the atria [24]. In Dandy–Walker malformation, the torcula is very high, resulting in an actual marked enlargement of the entire posterior fossa. This widens the angle between the sagittal and

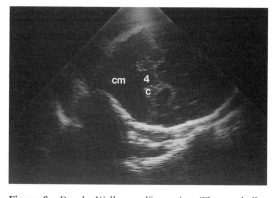

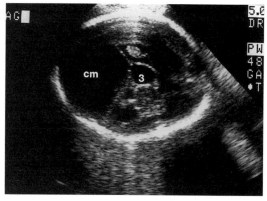

Figure 6 Dandy–Walker malformation. The cerebellar (c) hemispheres are very small. Note no intervening vermis. The fourth ventricle (4) is box-shaped. The cisterna magna (cm) is much enlarged. From reference 20, with permission

Figure 7 Dandy–Walker malformation. Note the huge cisterna magna (cm). The cerebellar hemispheres are barely visible. There was moderate hydrocephalus. 3, dilated third ventricle

straight sinuses (in the leaves of the tentorium) from a normal of 55–75° to 80° or greater[25]. This abnormality has not been used for diagnoses in the fetus, but with color Doppler the sinuses could theoretically be visualized in the sagittal plane.

The back of the skull should be evaluated; Hirsch found a 17.5% incidence of encephaloceles. Agenesis of the corpus callosum (ACC) varies from 7.5 to 17.5%[26,27] and consequently the position of the medial walls of the lateral ventricles should be evaluated, even in the presence of hydrocephalus. Although ACC by itself may be benign, the combination of Dandy–Walker malformation and ACC indicates a major disturbance in embryology and implies that there are probably other abnormalities of the brain that cannot be seen.

Even in cases with a normal karyotype, facial and cardiac anomalies and polydactyly are more frequent than usual[28]. Facial hemangiomas have been reported in as many as 10% of patients[25,27,29].

Familial Dandy–Walker with port-wine nevi[30] and Aicardi's syndrome are associated with Dandy–Walker in some cases. Lissencephaly and Dandy–Walker malformation are essential parts of Walker–Warburg syndrome. In this recessive syndrome, Dandy–Walker malformation may be the only abnormal finding until 30 weeks. Retinal malformation, microphthalmos, cleft lip and occipital encephaloceles are common. Profound mental retardation and hypotonia are usual. A more extensive list of associated syndromes is outlined by Romero and colleagues[31].

In most instances, Dandy–Walker malformation is sporadic, but the absence of hydrocephalus or the presence of other anomalies is associated with a high incidence of chromosomal anomalies[29,32]. However, it is probably wise to obtain a karyotype in all cases of Dandy–Walker malformation, since some anomalies characteristic of trisomies 13 and 18 are difficult to detect by antenatal ultrasound examination.

Prognosis in Dandy–Walker malformation varies widely. Low IQ to normal development has been reported, even in cases with agenesis of the corpus callosum[33]. However, the range of IQ of 16 surviving children in Sawaya's series was 83 or more in four, 69–82 in five, 52–68 in one, 36–51 in three, and 20–35 in one[26]. The two children in that series with agenesis of the corpus callosum had IQ scores of 50 and 75. Similar findings have been reported by Tal and associates[34]. Most patients with Dandy–Walker malformation do not have specific signs characteristic of cerebellar dysfunction, such as ataxia or gait disturbance, but this is variable[34].

Dandy–Walker variant

The vermis normally contains nine lobules, numbered 1–9 from superior to inferior. It forms by

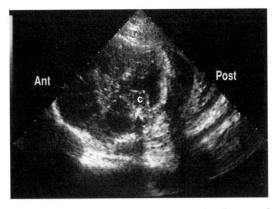

Figure 8 Dandy–Walker variant. Note the absence of the lower vermis between the cerebellar hemispheres (c)

the superior to inferior fusion of the cerebellar hemispheres from 9 to 15 weeks. Until it is completely formed, the fourth ventricle and cisterna may be seen to communicate in the 'fourth-ventricle view' of the cerebellum. In fact, Estroff and colleagues all found that this communication could be seen until 17½ weeks[23]. In Dandy–Walker variant, the lower part of the vermis alone is absent or hypoplastic. If part of the vermis is missing, it is always the inferior portion, but degree of hypoplasia has been extremely difficult to determine antenatally. Theoretically, vermian area measurements developed by Co for neonates could be used in similarly aged fetuses[8]. If the cisterna is continuous with the fourth ventricle, it is presumed that

there is some degree of hypoplasia, even if the vermis can be seen. The connection may be very wide in cases of marked hypoplasia, or narrow in cases in which the inferior vermis only is missing (Figure 8). It is important to evaluate the cerebellum from cephalad to caudal, because in partial agenesis the upper cerebellum may appear normal, whereas at a lower level there will be the typical keyhole deformity (Figure 9). When evaluating the posterior fossa, care should be taken to turn the transducer only slightly from the axial plane. If the plane is exaggerated such that the cervical spine or thick nuchal tissues are seen, the vallecula (anterior extension of the cisterna) is elongated and gives a false impression of Dandy–Walker or Dandy–Walker variant (Figure 10)[35]. However, the cleft in the variant is key-hole shaped rather than V-shaped.

Keeping these points in mind, differentiation between Dandy–Walker variant and a normal posterior fossa can be very difficult (Table 2). If the posterior fossa, cerebellar hemispheres and fourth ventricle are normal-sized, but the cisterna communicates with the fourth ventricle, this is termed Dandy–Walker variant. The cisterna is usually enlarged. Pilu and associates[36] discussed 12 cases in which the cerebellum was normal in the trans-cerebellar view, but on what they termed the 'fourth ventricle (lower) view', a U-shaped prolongation of the cisterna connected with the fourth ventricle. In nine of those 12 patients, atrial width was increased[36].

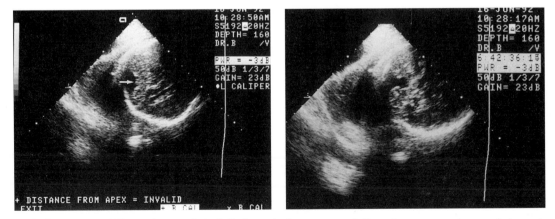

Figure 9 Dandy–Walker variant. A plane (left) through the upper cerebellum demonstrates the vermis (arrow); a lower plane (right) shows absence of the vermis with a keyhole deformity

Table 2 Differentiation between Dandy–Walker malformation and Dandy–Walker variant

	Dandy–Walker malformation	*Dandy–Walker variant*
Cisterna enlarged	+++	+
Cerebellum hypoplastic	+, ++, +++	no
Atria enlarged	no, +, +++	no, +
Vermis on axial view	no	yes
Vermis on fourth-ventricle view	no	no
Fourth ventricle enlarged	yes	no

Although no outcome was given for that series, eight of the 17 cases described by Estroff and co-workers[37] had concurrent anomalies of systems other than the CNS. Five had abnormal karyotypes, of which two also had agenesis of the corpus callosum (one: trisomy 21; two: trisomy 18; one: trisomy, 13-translocation; one: partial trisomy, 11q+). Those fetuses with normal karyotypes and no other findings did well.

After birth, confirmation of absence of the inferior vermis can only be made confidently by magnetic resonance imaging and computerized tomography; neonatal ultrasound scanning may not show the vermis well. If ultrasound is the only modality available, examination through locations other than the anterior fontanelle should be attempted.

Meckel–Gruber syndrome (encephalocele and cystic kidneys) has been associated in some fetuses (two out of six) with vermian hypoplasia[38]. Familial aplasia of the cerebellar vermis has also been reported in four families with a dominantly inherited ataxia associated with hypoplasia of the cerebellar vermis. Twelve of 14 cases have involved females with normal intelligence and truncal ataxia[39]. The COACH syndrome (cerebellar vermis hypoplasia, oligophrenia, congenital ataxia, coloboma, hepatic fibrocirrhosis) appears to be autosomal recessive[40]. Reduced size of the vermis is a common finding in autism (lobules VI and VII)[41].

Joubert's syndrome

This is a syndrome which has a very typical clinical presentation characterized by global developmental delay and usually (but not always) by episodic apnea interspersed with hyperpnea, abnormal eye movements, rhythmic protrusion of the tongue and ataxia[42]. Facial asymmetry, occipital encephalocele, polydactyly and sacral dermoids have also been reported. Agenesis of the corpus callosum is more than occasional[43]. These associated anatomical findings are summarized in Table 3. The vermis is segmented in an unusual way, or it has a deep groove from top to bottom, or it is severely hypoplastic or absent. The brainstem is hypoplastic. Hydrocephalus is not a part of Joubert's syndrome.

It is thought to be autosomal recessive. If there has been no family history, it would be difficult to distinguish this entity from Dandy–Walker variant, since the diagnosis truly rests on the clinical presentation, which results from a combination of pontine and vermian hypoplasia. Cases of Joubert's syndrome have been identified antenatally, but always in fetuses at risk[44].

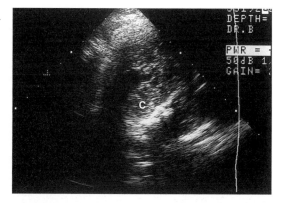

Figure 10 False impression of Dandy–Walker variant. This is a very low plane, below the vermis, showing the extension of the cisterna under the cerebellum (c) – compare with the right-hand scan of Figure 9

Table 3 Ultrasound findings in Joubert's syndrome

Dysgenesis of the vermis – partial/complete
No hydrocephalus
Occipital encephalocele*
Agenesis of the corpus callosum*
Polydactyly*
Asymmetry of the face*
Polycystic kidneys*

*Variable

Table 4 Most frequent causes of the finding of enlarged cisterna magna

Dandy–Walker malformation
Dandy–Walker variant
Trisomy 18
Hydrocephalus
Normal variation
Measurement error (sharp angulation)

Rhombencephalosynapsis

If the cerebellar hemispheres are fused in the midline and there is no intervening vermis, rhombencephalosynapsis may be present. In this anomaly, the cerebellar hemispheres are small. There may be hydrocephalus. A fetus with this disorder has been described[45], as have some children[46,47].

Tecto-cerebellar dysraphia

This syndrome, to our knowledge, has not been seen by ultrasound of the fetus to date. However, the combination of an encephalocele and vermian hypoplasia or aplasia (but with normal kidneys) should suggest it. This is a disorder which affects all midline structures of the brain: the maxillary bodies and corpus callosum may be absent and the cerebral hemispheres are often disproportionate with occipital lobe fusion and polygyria. The thalami are often fused[48]. Differential diagnosis would include Meckel–Gruber with abnormal kidneys, an encephalocele, and sometimes absence of the vermis (Dandy–Walker) or Joubert's syndrome which can also be associated with anencephalocele. Outcome of tecto-cerebellar dysraphia is poor, probably due to the cerebral anomalies rather than those of the cerebellum.

The enlarged cisterna magna

An enlarged cisterna magna can be a normal finding in adults. It can also be associated with communicating hydrocephalus (in which all spaces containing cerebrospinal fluid are larger than normal). However, in the fetus and newborn, in the absence of hydrocephalus or Dandy–Walker malformation, an enlarged cisterna magna should suggest the possibility of cerebellar hypoplasia, a finding suggestive of trisomy 18 (Figure 11)[29,49,50]. The most frequent causes of an enlarged cisterna are listed in Table 4.

The differential diagnosis of an enlarged cisterna magna includes not only Dandy–Walker malformation and cerebellar hypoplasia (discussed below), but also an extra-axial or subarachnoid cyst. These collections of fluid accumulate between layers of arachnoid and usually do not communicate with the cisterns or ventricles. They may lie in the midline or to the side[51]. Even postnatally it may be difficult to distinguish a Dandy–Walker malformation from a post-axial cyst. If a normal vermis and a fourth ventricle can be seen and no connection can be demonstrated between the cisterna and the fourth ventricle by cisternography, the diagnosis is probably that of an extra-axial cyst. Hydrocephalus

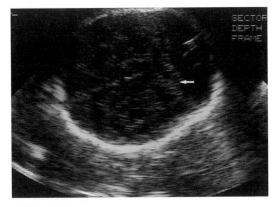

Figure 11 An enlarged cisterna magna in trisomy 18. The cerebellum (arrow) is small, but the vermis is intact

Table 5   Most frequent causes of small cerebellum

Growth retardation (symmetric)
Spina bifida
Incorrect dates
Trisomy 18
Normal variation

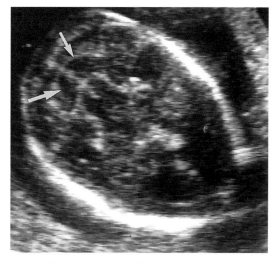

Figure 12   Banana sign. The cerebellum (arrows) has lost its bilobate appearance. The cisterna magna is smaller than normal

may accompany both Dandy–Walker malformation and a post-axial cyst and will not help to distinguish between them. Agenesis of the corpus callosum (with an accompanying high, dilated third ventricle, and laterally displaced lateral ventricles) is much more common in Dandy–Walker malformation.

Cerebellar hypoplasia

Cerebellar *weight* has been shown to be decreased in trisomies 13, 18 and 21[52,53]. The cerebellar diameter can be measurably small in trisomy 18[29,49,50,54,55]. Hill and colleagues[56] found that the cerebellar diameter was small in two out of seven fetuses with trisomy 18 under 21 weeks vs. nine out of 12 above 21 weeks. This suggests that the normal growth spurt seen in the cerebellum after 21 weeks may not take place in these fetuses. Cerebellar hypoplasia in trisomy 18 may be manifested by an enlarged cisterna magna (i.e. over 10 mm in depth) (Figure 11)[29,49,50]. In trisomy 21, however, the cerebellar transverse diameter is not decreased sufficiently to separate these fetuses from those with normal karyotypes[56].

The cerebellar diameter is decreased in fetuses with spina bifida, in addition to other posterior fossa changes discussed below[57,58]. Other causes of cerebellar hypoplasia include viral infection[59], inherited hypoplasia[60], teratogens[61] and necrosis of the fetal brainstem[62]. The most frequent causes of cerebellar hypoplasia are listed in Table 5.

Asymmetry has been reported in a case of Moebius' syndrome (cranial nerve palsies, reductive limb defects)[63]. It appears that asymmetry of the cerebellar hemispheres may occasionally be seen in neurologically normal infants[49]. Actual agenesis of both hemispheres is rarely seen[64].

Cerebellar atrophy can be distinguished from hypoplasia in the postnatal period by enlargement of the sulci or fissures separating the cerebellar foglia. This distinction probably cannot be made antenatally.

The cerebellum in spina bifida

The weight of the cerebellum is decreased in newborns with meningomyeloceles compared to that of normal newborns[65]. Presumably the same is true of the fetus. Not only is the cerebellar diameter decreased in spina bifida, but, in almost all cases of open spina bifida, the cerebellum is displaced downward into the foramen magnum. This is known as the Arnold–Chiari or Chiari Type II malformation. Campbell and associates[57] could not visualize the cerebellum in nine (of 26) fetuses with spina bifida. In 16 of the remaining 17 in which the cerebellum could be seen, it was abnormally shaped; the indentation at the level of the vermis was obliterated, giving the cerebellum the appearance of a banana (Figure 12). In 13 of these 17, the cerebellar diameter was more than 2SD below the mean. Nicolaides' group found this 'banana' sign in 72% of fetuses with spina bifida before 24 weeks[66]. Benacerraf and colleagues[67] found it to be even more reliable (22 out of 23) in fetuses of 16–27 weeks. A more reliable sign of spina bifida in all studies has been obliteration of the cisterna magna (see below).

The small cisterna magna

Obliteration or a decrease in size to less than 4 mm (Figure 12) is a more reliable sign of open spina bifida than the 'banana' or 'lemon' signs (anterior scalloping of the skull). In all 19 cases of spina bifida examined by Pilu and co-workers[58], the cisterna could not be visualized. In seven of these, the cerebellum also could not be seen, but in the remaining 12, a small cerebellum was present with no visible cisterna. (The spinal defects involved three or more vertebrae.) Goldstein and associates[68] found the cisterna obliterated (18) or small

(one) in 19 open defects. Interestingly, in two reported *closed* defects (one a lipomeningocele), the cisterna was not obliterated or small. Unfortunately, a small or obliterated cisterna is not specific for spina bifida, since Goldstein found it in 38% of fetuses with hydrocephalus from other causes.

Cerebellar hemorrhage

Cerebellar hemorrhage appears as a dense mass in the posterior fossa[69,70]. It can occur without any obvious reason[70]. In the case reported by Hadi and co-workers[70], decreased fetal movement was noted before the scan. There was accompanying interventricular hemorrhage. At birth, blood gases were normal, as were all hematological indices other than hematocrit.

References

1. McLeary, R.D., Kuhns, L.R. and Barr, M. (1984). Ultrasonography of the fetal cerebellum. *Radiology*, **151**, 439–42

2. Goldstein, I., Reece, E.A., Pilu, G., Bovicelli, L. and Hobbins, J.C. (1987). Cerebellar measurements with ultrasonography in the evaluation of fetal growth and development. *Am. J. Obstet. Gynecol.*, **156**, 1065–9

3. Kofinas, A.D., Simon, N.V., King, K., Clay, D. and Deardorf, J. (1992). Comparison of fetal cerebellar measurements by two different techniques. *J. Ultrasound Med.*, **11**, 257–9

4. Sarno, A.P., Rose, G.S. and Harrington, R.A. (1992). Coronal transcerebellar diameter: an alternate view. *Ultrasound Obstet. Gynecol.*, **2**, 158–61

5. Kushnir, U., Shalev, J., Bronstein, M., Bider, D., Lipitz, S., Nebel, L., Mashiach, S. and Ben-Rafael, Z. (1989). Fetal intracranial anatomy in the first trimester of pregnancy: transvaginal ultrasonographic evaluation. *Neuroradiology*, **31**, 222–5

6. Campbell, W.A., Nardi, D., Vintzileos, A.M., Rodis, J.F., Turner, G.W. and Egan, J.F.X. (1991). Transverse cerebellar diameter/abdominal circumference ratio throughout pregnancy: a gestational age-independent method to assess fetal growth. *Obstet.Gynecol.*, **77**, 893–6

7. Birnholz, J. (1982). Newborn cerebellar size. *Pediatrics*, **70**, 284–7

8. Co, E., Raju, T.N.K. and Aldana, O. (1991). Cerebellar dimensions in assessment of gestational age in neonates. *Radiology*, **181**, 581–5

9. Hill, L.M., Guzick, D., Rivello, D., Hixson, J. and Peterson, C. (1990). The transverse cerebellar diameter cannot be used to assess gestational age in the small for gestational age fetus. *Obstet. Gynecol.*, **75**, 329–33

10. Reece, E.A., Goldstein, I., Pilu, G. and Hobbins, J.C. (1987). Fetal cerebellar growth unaffected by intrauterine growth retardation: a new parameter for prenatal diagnosis. *Am. J. Obstet. Gynecol.*, **157**, 632–8

11. Lee, W., Barton, S., Comstock, C., Bajorek, S., Batton, D. and Kirk, J.S. (1991). Transverse cerebellar diameter: a useful predictor of gestational age for fetuses with asymmetric growth retardation. *Am. J. Obstet. Gynecol.*, **165**, 1044–50

12. Hill, L.M., Guzick, D., Fries, J., Hixson, J. and Rivello, D. (1990). The transverse cerebellar diameter in estimating gestational age in the large for gestational age fetus. *Obstet. Gynecol.*, **75**, 981–5

13. Baumeister, L.A., Hertzberg, B.S., McNally, P.J., Kliewer, M.A. and Bowie, J.D. (1994). Fetal fourth ventricle: US appearance and frequency of depiction. *Radiology*, **192**, 333–6

14. Goodwin, L. and Quisling, R.G. (1983). The

neonatal cisterna magna: ultrasonic evaluation. *Radiology*, **149**, 691–5

15. Mahony, B.S., Callen, P.W., Filly, R.A. and Hoddick, W.K. (1984). The fetal cisterna magna. *Radiology*, **153**, 773–6

16. Watson, W.J., Katz, V.L., Chescheir, N.C., Miller, R.C., Menard, K. and Hansen, W.F. (1992). The cisterna magna in second-trimester fetuses with abnormal karyotypes. *Obstet. Gynecol.*, **79**, 723–5

17. Filly, R.A., Cardoza, J.D., Goldstein, R.B. and Barkovich, A.J. (1989). Detection of fetal CNS anomalies: a practical level of effort for a 'routine' sonogram. *Radiology*, **172**, 403–8

18. Knutzon, R.K., McGahan, J.P., Salamat, M.S. and Brant, W.E. (1991). Fetal cisterna magna septa: a normal anatomic finding. *Radiology*, **180**, 799–801

19. Pretorius, D.H., Kallman, C.E., Grafe, M.R., Budorick, N.E. and Stamm, E.R. (1992). Linear echoes in the fetal cisterna magna. *J. Ultrasound Med.*, **11**, 125–8

20. Comstock, C.H. (1994). The fetal posterior fossa. In Sabbagha, R. (ed.) *Diagnostic Ultrasound Applied to Obstetrics and Gynecology*, 3rd edn., pp. 417–29. (Chicago: J.B. Lippincott)

21. Rumack, C.M. and Johnson, M.L. (1984) Intracranial neoplasms, cysts, and vascular malformations. *Perinatal and Infant Brain Imaging*, pp. 175–96. (Chicago: Year Book Medical Publishers)

22. Kwon, T. and Jeanty, P. (1991). Supratentorial arachnoid cyst. *Fetus*, **1**, 1–5

23. Bromley, B., Wade, I.A., Packer, S., Estroff, J. and Benacerraf, B.R. (1994). Closure of the cerebellar vermis: evaluation with second trimester ultrasound. *Radiology*, **193**, 761–3

24. Pilu, G., Romero, R., De Palma, L., Rizzo, N., Jeanty, P., Copel, J.A., Bovicelli, L. and Hobbins, J.C. (1986). Antenatal diagnosis and obstetric management of Dandy–Walker syndrome. *J. Reprod. Med.*, **31**, 1017–22

25. Barkovich, A.J., Kjos, B.O., Norman, D. and Edwards, M. (1989). Revised classification of posterior fossa cysts and cystlike malformations based on the results of multiplanar MR imaging. *Am. J. Neuroradiol.*, **10**, 977–88; *Am. J. Roentgenol.*, **153**, 1289–300

26. Sawaya, R. and McLaurin, R.L. (1981). Dandy–Walker syndrome: clinical analysis of 23 cases. *J. Neurosurg.*, **55**, 89–98

27. Hirsch, J., Pierre-Kahn, A., Renier, D., Sainte-Rose, C. and Hoppe-Hirsch, E. (1984). The Dandy–Walker malformation: a review of 40 cases. *J. Neurosurg.*, **61**, 515–22

28. Nyberg, D.A., Cyr, D.R., Mack, L.A., Fitzsimmons, J., Hickok, D. and Mahony, B.S. (1988). The Dandy–Walker malformation prenatal sonographic diagnosis and its clinical significance. *J. Ultrasound Med.*, **7**, 65–71

29. Nyberg, D.A., Mahony, B.S., Hegge, F.N., Hickok, D., Luthy, D.A. and Kapur, R. (1991). Enlarged cisterna magna and the Dandy–Walker malformation: factors associated with chromosome abnormalities. *Obstet. Gynecol.*, **77**, 436–42

30. Nova, H.R. (1979). Familial communicating hydrocephalus, posterior cerebellar agenesis, mega cisterna magna, and port-wine nevi. *J. Neurosurg.*, **51**, 862–5

31. Romero, R., Pilu, G., Jeanty, P., Ghidini, A. and Hobbins, J.C. (1988). *Prenatal Diagnosis of Congenital Anomalies*. (Norwalk, CT: Appleton & Lange)

32. Russ, P.D., Pretorius, D.H. and Johnson, M.J. (1989). Dandy–Walker syndrome: a review of fifteen cases evaluated by prenatal sonography. *Am. J. Obstet. Gynecol.*, **161**, 401–6

33. Gardner, E., O'Rahilly, R. and Prolo, D. (1975). The Dandy–Walker and Arnold–Chiari malformations. *Arch. Neurol.*, **32**, 393–407

34. Tal, Y., Freigang, B., Dunn, H.G., Durity, F.A. and Moyes, P.D. (1980). Dandy–Walker syndrome: analysis of 21 cases. *Dev. Med. Child Neurol.*, **22**, 189–201

35. Laing, F.C., Frates, M.C., Brown, D.L., Benson, C.B., DiSalvo, D.N. and Doubilet, P.M. (1994). Sonography of the fetal posterior fossa: false appearance of mega-cisterna magna and Dandy–Walker variant. *Radiology*, **192**, 247–51

36. Pilu, G., Goldstein, I., Reece, E.A., Perolo, A., Foschini, M.P., Hobbins, J.C. and Bovicelli, L. (1992). Sonography of fetal Dandy–Walker malformation: a reappraisal. *Ultrasound Obstet. Gynecol.*, **2**, 151–7

37. Estroff, J.A., Scott, M.R. and Benacerraf, B.R. (1992). Dandy-Walker variant: prenatal sonographic features and clinical outcome. *Radiology*, **185**, 755–8

38. Nyberg, D.A., Hallesy, D., Mahony, B.S., Hirsch, J.H., Luthy, D.A. and Hickok, D. (1990). Meckel–Gruber syndrome: importance of prenatal diagnosis. *J. Ultrasound Med.*, **9**, 691–6

39. Fenichel, G.M. and Phillips, J.A. (1989). Familial aplasia or the cerebellar vermis. *Arch. Neurol.*, **46**, 582–3

40. Verloes, A. and Lambotte, C. (1989). Further delineation of a syndrome of cerebellar vermis hypo/aplasia, oligophrenia, congenital ataxia, coloboma and hepatic fibrosis. *Am. J. Med. Genet.*, **32**, 227–32

41. Murakami, J.W., Courchesne, E., Press, G.A., Yeung-Courchesne, R. and Hesselink, M.R. (1989). Reduced cerebellar hemisphere size and its relationship to vermal hypoplasia in autism. *Arch. Neurol.*, **46**, 689–94

42. Joubert, M., Eisenring, J., Robb, J.P. and Andermann, F. (1969). Familial agenesis of the cerebellar vermis. *Neurology*, **19**, 813–25

43. Cantani, A., Lucenti, P., Ronzani, G.A. and Santoro, C. (1990). Joubert syndrome review of the fifty-three cases so far published. *Ann. Genet.*, **33**, 96–8

44. Campbell, S., Tsannatos, C. and Pearce, J.M. (1984). The prenatal diagnosis of Joubert's syndrome of familial agenesis of the cerebellar vermis. *Prenat. Diagn.*, **4**, 391–5

45. Litherland, J., Ludlam, A. and Thomas, W. (1993). Antenatal ultrasound diagnosis of a cerebellar vermian agenesis in a case of rhombencephalosynapsis. *J. Clin. Ultrasound*, **21**, 636–8

46. Truwit, C.L., Barkovich, A.J., Shanaken, R. and Maroido, T.V. (1991). MR imaging of rhombencephalosynapsis: report of three cases and review of the literature. *Am. J. Neuroradiol.*, **12**, 957–65

47. Simmons, G., Damiano, T.R. and Truwit, C.L. (1993). MRI and clinical findings in rhombencephalosynapsis. *J. Comput. Assist. Tomogr.*, **17**, 211–14

48. Friede, R.L. (1978). Uncommon syndromes of cerebellar vermis aplasia. II. Tecto-cerebellar dysraphia with occipital encephalocele. *Develop. Med. Child. Neurol.*, **20**, 764–72

49. Comstock, C.H. and Boal, D.B. (1985). Enlarged fetal cisterna magna: appearance and significance. *Obstet. Gynecol.*, **66**, 25–8S

50. Thurmond, A.S., Nelson, D.W., Lowensohn, R.I., Young, W.P. and Davis, L. (1989). Enlarged cisterna magna in trisomy 18: prenatal ultrasonographic diagnosis. *Am. J. Obstet. Gynecol.*, **161**, 83–5

51. Locatelli, D., Bonfanti, N., Sfogliarini, R., Gagno, T.M. and Pezzotta, S. (1987). Arachnoid cysts: diagnosis and treatment. *Childs Nerv. Syst.*, **3**, 121–4

52. Warkany, J., Passarge, E. and Smith, C.C. (1966). Congenital malformations in autosomal trisomy syndromes. *Am. J. Dis. Child.*, **112**, 502–17

53. Norman, R.M. (1966). Neuropathological findings in trisomies 13–15 and 17–18 with special reference to the cerebellum. *Dev. Med. Child Neurol.*, **8**, 170–7

54. Hill, L.M., Martin, J.G., Fries, J. and Hixson, J. (1991). The role of the transcerebellar view in the detection of fetal central nervous system anomaly. *Am. J. Obstet. Gynecol.*, **164**, 1220–4

55. Nakamura, Y., Hashimoto, T. and Sabaguri, Y. (1986). Brain anomalies found in 18 trisomy: CT scanning, morphologic and morphometric study. *Clin. Neuropathol.*, **5**, 47–52

56. Hill, L.M., Rivello, D., Peterson, C. and Marchese, S. (1991). The transverse cerebellar diameter in the second trimester is unaffected by Down syndrome. *Am. J. Obstet. Gynecol.*, **164**, 101–3

57. Campbell, J., Gilbert, W.M., Nicolaides, K.H. and Campbell, S. (1987). Ultrasound screening for spina bifida: cranial and cerebellar signs in a high-risk population. *Obstet. Gynecol.*, **70**, 247–50

58. Pilu, G., Romero, R., Reece, E.A., Goldstein, I., Hobbins, J.C. and Bovicelli, L. (1988). Subnormal cerebellum in fetuses with spina bifida. *Am. J. Obstet. Gynecol.*, **158**, 1052–6

59. Ceballos, R., Ch'ien, L.T., Whitley, R.J. and Brans, Y.W. (1976). Cerebellar hypoplasia in an infant with congenital cytomegalovirus infection. *Pediatrics*, **57**, 155–7

60. Wichman, A., Frank, L.M. and Kelly, T.E. (1985). Autosomal recessive congenital cerebellar hypoplasia. *Clin. Genet.*, **27**, 733–82

61. Fischer, D.S. and Jonas, H.M. (1965). Cerebellar hypoplasia resulting from cytosine arabinoside treatment in the neonatal hamster. *Clin. Res.*, **13**, 540

62. Gessaga, E.C., Herrick, M.K. and Urich, H. (1986). Necrosis of the fetal brain stem with cerebellar hypoplasia. *Acta Neuropathol.*, **7**, 1077–8

63. Harbord, M.G., Finn, J.B., Hall-Craggs, M.A., Brett, E.M. and Baraitser, M. (1989). Moebius syndrome with unilateral cerebellar hypoplasia. *J. Med. Genet.*, **26**, 579–82

64. Macchi, G. and Bentivoglio, M. (1977). Agenesis or hypoplasia of cerebellar structures. In Vinken, P.J. and Bruyn, G.W. (eds.) *Congenital Malformations of the Brain and Skull. Handbook of Clinical Neurology*, pp. 367–93. (Amsterdam: North Holland Publishing)

65. Variend, S. and Emery, J.L. (1973). The weight of the cerebellum in children with myelomeningocele. *Dev. Med. Child Neurol.*, **15**, 17–83

66. Van den Hof, M.C., Nicolaides, K.H., Campbell, J. and Campbell, S. (1990). Evaluation of the lemon and banana signs in one hundred thirty fetuses with open spina bifida. *Am. J. Obstet. Gynecol.*, **162**, 322–7

67. Benacerraf, B.R., Stryker, J. and Frigoletto, F.D. (1989). Abnormal US appearance of the cerebellum (banana sign): indirect sign of spina bifida. *Radiology*, **171**, 151–3

68. Goldstein, R.B., Podrasky, A.E., Filly, R.A. and Callen, P.W. (1989). Effacement of the fetal cisterna magna in association with myelomeningocele. *Radiology*, **172**, 409–13

69. Jennett, R.J., Daily, W.J.R., Tarby, T.J. and Manwaring, K.H. (1990). Prenatal diagnosis of intracerebellar hemorrhage: case report. *Am. J. Obstet. Gynecol.*, **162**, 1472–5

70. Hadi, H.A., Finley, J., Mallette, J.Q. and Strickland, D. (1994). Prenatal diagnosis of cerebellar hemorrhage: medicolegal implications. *Am. J. Obstet. Gynecol.*, **170**, 1392–5

Transvaginal fetal neurosonography: the first trimester of pregnancy

5

R. Achiron and A. Achiron

INTRODUCTION

Until quite recently, reviews describing the imaging of the fetal central nervous system (CNS) began with the description of brain development from the 12th menstrual week[1]. However, the introduction of advanced, high-resolution transvaginal equipment has allowed detailed study of the first-trimester fetus, opening a new era in evaluating the fetal brain during the early stages of gestation[2].

The major contributions of high-frequency transvaginal transducers are: the capability to evaluate normal embryological changes occurring during the first trimester; early detection of fetal brain malformations, and evaluation of these malformations in relation to gestational age and other system abnormalities. Extensive knowledge of normal fetal CNS development is therefore a prerequisite for those who perform first-trimester transvaginal examinations. This chapter describes the normal development of fetal brain anatomy as shown by transvaginal ultrasonography (TVS) during the first trimester of pregnancy, and outlines the feasibility of diagnosis of fetal brain anomalies with this new mode of imaging.

Technique and terminology

Transvaginal examination is performed on the patient with an empty bladder, and in the lithotomy position. With the transvaginal approach, the full bladder does not act as a spacer between the area of interest and the transducer, therefore the distance between the developing fetus and transducer element is shortened, allowing the use of higher-frequency transducers (6.5–7.5 MHz). The advantage of higher-frequency transducers, particularly of 7.5 MHz, is their ability, due to a greater axial and lateral resolution, to clear the image, making small details better distinguishable. For vaginal insertion, the probe is covered with coupling gel and introduced into one of the digits of a sterile surgical rubber glove, which is also lubricated with the gel.

Throughout this chapter, the postmenstrual (gestational) age is given in weeks in correlation with the crown–rump length (CRL). Table 1 indicates the relationship between CRL, embryo age and milestone appearance of the fetal brain structures. Ultrasonographic examinations are described according to the classical imaging planes: transverse–axial, longitudinal–sagittal and frontal–coronal.

IMAGING OF THE NORMAL BRAIN IN RELATION TO EMBRYOLOGICAL DEVELOPMENT

Embryonic CNS development begins with the 'neurulation' period, which is defined as the time interval between 32 days from menstruation (gestational age) to 41 days or six weeks' gestation[3]. During this period, ectoderm that lies on the dorsal portion of the embryo, along with the underlying notochord and chordal mesoderm, induces formation of the neural plate. The lateral edges of the plate soon become elevated, forming the neural folds; the depressed region between the folds is known as the neural groove. With further development, the neural folds become more elevated, approach each other in the midline and finally fuse, resulting in the formation of the neural tube. When the embryo has reached 5 weeks, the cephalic end of the neural tube differentiates into three primary brain vesicles:

Table 1 Milestones of embryological and fetal development of the central nervous system: relationship between ultrasound, menstrual age, crown–rump length and biparietal diameter

Developmental stage*	Menstrual age (weeks)	Crown–rump length (mm)	Biparietal diameter (mm)	Ultrasound findings		
				Prosencephalon (forebrain)	Mesencephalon (midbrain)	Rhombencephalon (hindbrain)
Neurulation	6	2–6	—	echogenic embryonic pole; no clear central nervous system is detected		
Secondary canalization	7	9–14	2–4	three primary brain vesicles		
Retrogressive differentiation	8	15–22	5–8	Y-shaped telencephalon – small hemispheres diencephalon – large third ventricle, communicating through foraminas of Monro with lateral ventricles	large cerebral cavity	diamond-shaped posterior cavity
Five secondary brain vesicles	9	23–32	9–12	telencephalon – large lateral ventricles filled with choroid plexus diencephalon – hypoechoic thalamus, slit-like third ventricle	thickening forms cerebral peduncles with large cerebral aqueduct (Sylvius)	metencephalon – ventrally pons; dorsally cerebellum myelencephalon – not visible
Fetal period	10	33–42	13–16	telencephalon – butterfly shape of echogenic choroid plexus diencephalon – hypoechoic thalami	echogenic lamina tecti	echogenic cerebellar tentorium; heart-shaped pons; hypoechoic cerebellum
	11	43–51	7–19	midline cavum verge basal ganglia in the floor of the lateral ventricles	distinguished cerebral peduncle	measurable cerebellum and cisterna magna

* From reference 4

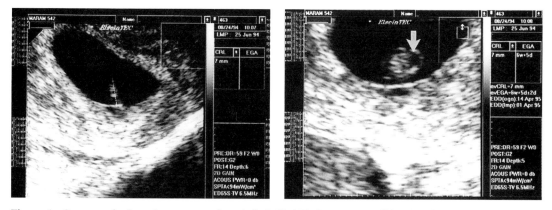

Figure 1 Seven weeks from last menstrual period: (left) CRL 7 mm compatible with 47 days' embryo; (right) magnification of the embryonic pole reveals posterior hypoechoic vesicle (arrow) representing the rhombencephalon

the prosencephalon (forebrain), mesencephalon (midbrain) and rhombencephalon (hindbrain)[4]. Between 6 and 8 weeks from the last menstruation, a secondary canalization period occurs, in which development of the brain progresses considerably. During this period, five components of the secondary brain vesicles can be distinguished – the prosencephalon differentiates into the telencephalon and diencephalon, the mesencephalon undergoes little change, and the rhombencephalon divides into the metencephalon and myelencephalon[3].

Transvaginal sonography at 6 weeks' gestation demonstrates the embryonic pole as an echogenic structure of about 5 mm, with acting heart beats. The neural system cannot be delineated. Towards the end of the 6th week, and during the 7th week (embryonic CRL 7–14 mm), the cephalic pole becomes clearly distinguishable from the embryonic torso, mainly due to the appearance of hypoechoic vesicles below the calvarial roof (Figure 1). At the 8th week, for a 16 mm CRL embryo, a retrogressive differentiation period begins, and brain structures assume a considerable size, amenable to detailed TVS. The transverse diameter of the head (biparietal diameter (BPD)) is about 5–6 mm, and its longitudinal occipitofrontal diameter (OFD) is 10 mm: in this plane, a posterior prominent hypoechoic region is equivalent to the rhombencephalon, while an anterior Y-shaped cavity corresponds to the prosencephalon (Figure 2, left). A delicate echogenic line that

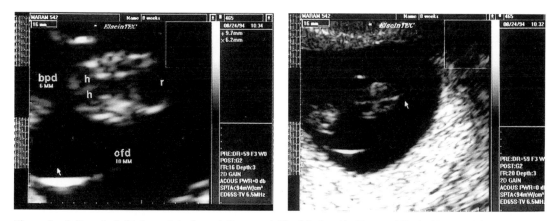

Figure 2 At 8 weeks (left) the occipitofrontal diameter (ofd) of the head is 10 mm while the biparietal diameter (bpd) is 6 mm; note the developing hypoechoic hemispheres (h) and prominent rhombencephalon (r); (right) an echogenic line representing the future falx cerebi can be delineated (arrow)

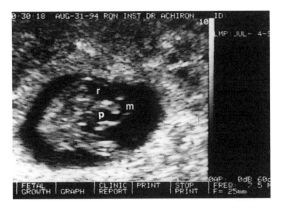

Figure 3 Sagittal section at 8 weeks and 5 days; magnification of the embryonic head demonstrates the three brain vesicles. The large cavity of the rhomben-cephalon (r) lies at the top; the cavity of the mesen-cephalon (m) lies anteriorly, communicating with the large third ventricle of the prosencephalon (p)

forms the future falx cerebri can be identified by a lower axial scan (Figure 2, right).

An oblique sagittal image at this age reveals the three primary brain vesicles: the posterior and the longest represents the rhombencephalon, the central represents the mesencephalon, and the anterior rostral represents the prosencephalon (Figure 3). A posterior coronal section during the 8th week of gestation clearly identifies the prominent hypoechoic rhombencephalon (Figure 4, left). Moving the transducer to the mid-coronal section, the two components of the prosen-cephalon, the diencephalon and the telence-

phalon, are visualized as Y-shaped (Figure 4, right). The diencephalon, which gives rise to the future third ventricle, appears as a large central cavity, interposed between the two developing hypoechoic hemispheres (telencephalon). The wide foraminas of Monro can already be recognized at this age.

Before the 8th week, the hemispheres can be measured in only 17% of cases, while after the 8th week, the hemispheres can be evaluated quantitatively in 79% of cases. At 7 weeks and 4 days, the mean length, width and height of the hemispheres are 1.7 mm (0.6–3.4 mm), 1 mm (0.42–2.1 mm) and 1.8 mm (0.8–3.2 mm), respectively, and their growth is found to be curvilinear.

The mean length of the diencephalon at 7 weeks and 3 days is 2.1 mm (0.8–3.4 mm) and the mean height is 1.1 mm (0.3–1.8 mm), both measurements showing a linear growth pattern during the embryonic period. The width of the diencephalon cavity is about 1.2 mm (0.7–1.7 mm) at this stage, and decreases with further brain development, due to the rapid growth of the thalamus that gradually projects into the lumen of the diencephalon[5]. The most prominent structure seen at this stage of gestation is the rhomben-cephalon, which lies on the top of the embryo and stretches posteriorly. This huge, hypoechoic region was previously misinterpreted as an abnormal CNS cystic structure[6]. With further development of the brain, the rhombencephalon complex is reduced in size to its normally

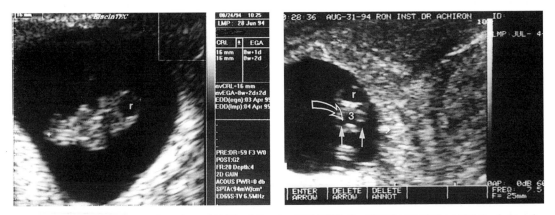

Figure 4 Coronal section at the 8th week (CRL 16 mm) reveals (left) the rhombencephalon (r) lying below the calvarial roof, moving the transducer anteriorly into the mid-coronal plain; (right) the Y-shape of the prosencephalon becomes evident; note the large third ventricle (3) communicating through the foramina of Monro (curved arrow) with the hemispheres (straight arrows)

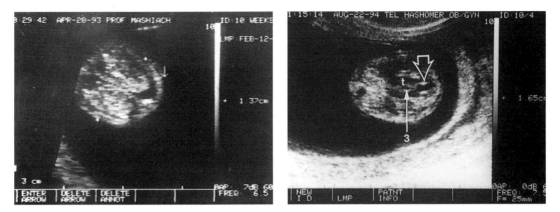

Figure 5 High axial scan of 10-week fetus: (left) biparietal diameter of 13 mm with spongy appearance of the choroid plexus within the lateral ventricle; (right) caudal scan to that on the left, demonstrating the hypoechoic thalami (t) surrounding a narrow, slit-like third ventricle (3-arrow); note the still-large cavity of the mesencephalon (open arrow)

proportioned posterior fossa. An early anatomical study in 1921 by Jenkins[7] compared the relative sizes of the embryonic and fetal brain compartments: the rhombencephalon that accounted for 54% of the fetal brain at the secondary canalization stage (7th gestational week) had changed to 36% at the retrogressive stage (9th gestational week).

During the 9 weeks, growth of the prosencephalon is faster than that of the mesencephalon or rhombencephalon. The telencephalon forms the cerebral hemisphere and the lateral ventricles with the choroid plexus, and the diencephalon gives rise to the thalamus and third ventricle. The head begins to assume its round shape and the BPD measures between 9 and 12 mm.

At high axial scan, the hemispheres are occupied by lateral ventricles where the echogenic choroid plexus can be observed. The mean length, width and height of the choroid plexus are 2.8 mm (1.2–5.1 mm), 1.3 mm (0.5–2.4 mm) and 1.8 mm (0.9–3.0 mm), respectively[5]. Caudally to the BPD plane, an axial scan reveals the cavity of the mesencephalon that develops to form the lumen of the cerebral aqueduct (of Sylvius), connected between the third and fourth ventricles. The growth of the cerebral peduncles, which are the thickening of the mesencephalon, eventually reduce the lumen of the cerebral aqueduct. Blood flow in the mid-cerebral artery can be demonstrated by pulsed Doppler mounted on the TVS transducer anteriorly to the brainstem. A sagittal

scan during the 9 weeks shows the hemisphere with the echogenic choroid plexus within the lateral ventricle, the central echogenic thickening of the mesencephalon and the reduced size of the posterior cavity of the rhombencephalon. Changes occurring in the rhombencephalon can be detected by posterior coronal section. At the beginning of the 9th week, the dorsal part of the rhombencephalon, mainly the metancephalon, starts its thickening that forms the future cerebellum.

At the beginning of the 10th week, the embryonic period is over, and the fetal period begins. A transverse anatomic section of the head is optimal for evaluation of the fetal brain at this gestational age. When this plane has been established, the transducer ascends and descends to obtain details of the various anatomic levels. The most prominent intrahemispheric structures seen on a high horizontal scan through the fetal head are the lateral ventricles. These are identified by the echogenic choroid plexus, which almost completely fills the bodies of the lateral ventricles, forming the typical butterfly appearance that is surrounded by a thin hypoechoic rim of brain parenchyma. The BPD during the 10th week is 13–16 mm (Figure 5, left). Caudally, a hypoechoic thalamus, the dominant portion of the developing diencephalon, can be visualized. As a result of rapid growth, the thalamus gradually projects into the lumen of the diencephalon, i.e. the third

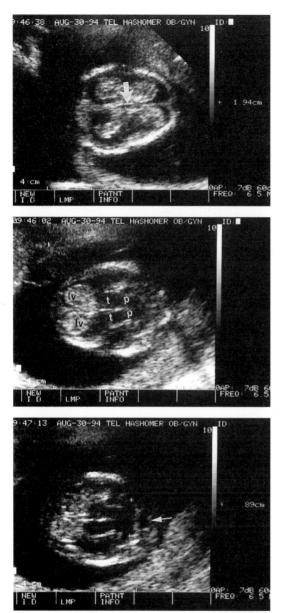

Figure 6 Series of axial scans of an 11-week fetus at various levels: (top) high plane demonstrating the lateral ventricles with the typical filling of the choroid plexus (biparietal diameter 19 mm), cavum verge is located between the ventricles (arrow); (middle) oblique scan to that above, showing only partial view of the lateral ventricles (lv), the floor occupied by the thalami (t) with slit-like third ventricle; posteriorly, the echodense cerebral peduncles (p) are visible; (bottom) further oblique scan reveals the characteristic appearance of the posterior fossa: the cerebellar diameter is 8.9 mm (between calipers) and the cisterna magna is observed as a hypoechoic region lying below the cerebellum (arrow)

ventricle, reducing its lumen to a narrow cleft with a slit-like appearance. The mesencephalon, which is morphologically the most primitive of the brain vesicles, undergoes fewer changes than other parts of the developing brain: the mesencephalon cavity (cerebral aqueduct) still maintains its large appearance (Figure 5, right). Towards the end of the 10th week, the most caudal of the brain compartments, the myelencephalon, becomes the medulla, whereas the metencephalon differentiates dorsally into the cerebellum and ventrally into the pons.

A sagittal scan at this period shows the echogenic basal ganglia that form the floor of the lateral ventricles, the central mass of mesencephalon, which becomes the lamina tecti of the cerebral peduncle, and the infratentorial structures – ventrally the brainstem (pons) and dorsally the cerebellum.

From the 11th week, a high axial scan reveals a BPD of 18–19 mm with the typical butterfly appearance of the echogenic choroid plexus within the lateral ventricles, and a hypoechoic cavum vergae can also be seen at the midline (Figure 6, top). Caudal inclination of 45° with the transducer to the previous axial scan shows the cerebral peduncles in the lower border of the thalamus (Figure 6, middle), and more caudally and inferiorly the characteristic appearance of the posterior fossa containing the cerebellum and the cisterna magna (Figure 6, bottom). Cerebellar width, as well cisterna magna measurements, can be evaluated from this age for the diagnosis of infratentorial dysmorphism.

From 11 weeks, it is possible clearly to obtain an anterior coronal section of the fetal face, an integral part of the CNS examination, since some intracranial abnormalities are associated with facial anomalies that can be recognized even during the first trimester of pregnancy.

From the 12th week, the head and brain assume the appearance of those of the early second-trimester fetus. Mid-coronal scanning demonstrates the basal ganglia, and the corpus striatum that forms a longitudinal ridge in the floor of the lateral ventricle, and comes in close contact with the lateral surface of the thalamus. The capsula interna breaks through the nuclear mass of the corpus striatum, dividing it into the

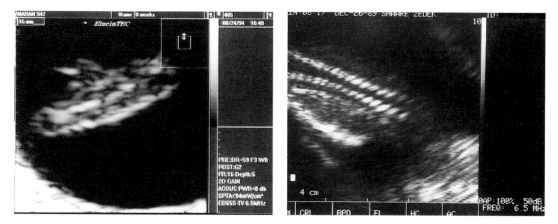

Figure 7 Coronal view (left) of the developing spine of an 8-week fetus: (right) at 12 weeks every individual vertebral body is demonstrated. From reference 38, with permission

caudate and lentiform nuclei. A further posterior coronal section shows the atria of the lateral ventricles with the posterior fossa. The cerebellum is clearly depicted under the cerebellar tentorium. In an oblique axial scan, the hypoechoic cisterna magna can be visualized and measured at a diameter of approximately 3 mm. The fourth ventricle and the sinii rectus are noted as small hypoechoic structures positioned anteriorly and posteriorly to the cerebellum.

The anatomical description of the fetal brain from the 12th week onward is beyond the scope of this chapter, and the reader is referred to the chapter on vaginal sonography during the second and third trimesters.

Imaging of the normal spine

Although a fetal spine is visualized from the end of the 8th week (Figure 7, left), only by the 11–12th week does ossification of the spine and skull demarcate the neural canal and the calvarium. Since the mineralization process is not complete until the end of the first trimester, visualization of the entire echogenic skull and spine is possible from 12 weeks (Figure 7, right). Evaluation of the fetal spine requires three sections of sonographic planes: (1) the sagittal cross-section, which demonstrates the spine as two echogenic lines representing the vertebral bodies and posterior vertebral processes; (2) the coronal cross-section, which demonstrates three lines that originate from

the posterior processes and vertebral bodies; and (3) the transverse cross-section, which demonstrates the neural canal as a closed circle, demarcated anteriorly and posteriorly by the ossification centers of the vertebral bodies and posterior processes.

IMAGING OF BRAIN ABNORMALITIES

Congenital anomalies of the CNS are common, occurring in approximately 3/1000 births. Most CNS defects can be accurately detected during routine mid-trimester sonography[1]. However, with the advent of high-resolution TVS, normal brain anatomy can be evaluated in the first trimester, with the possibility of recognizing CNS abnormalities now becoming a reality[8].

Abnormal calvarial development: anencephaly and exencephaly

Anencephaly and exencephaly are two anomalies involving the fetal cranial vault, with an incidence of about 1/1000 births. In both, absence of the cranium (acrania) is a constant finding. While exencephaly is an uncommon malformation of the cranium scarcely reported in human fetuses and mainly documented in animal studies[9], anencephaly is a more common neural tube abnormality, which historically was the first fetal

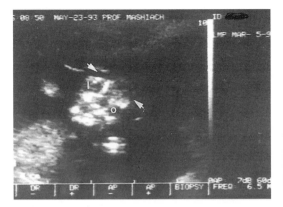

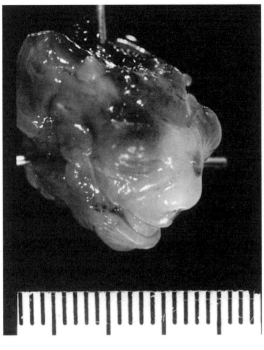

Figure 8 Coronal view of fetal face shows typical 'frog-like' appearance of anencephalus at 11 weeks' gestation: (left) note the symmetrical absence of normal brain development (arrows) as well as the absence of the frontal bones above the orbits (o) (l, lens); (right) pathological specimen confirming the early transvaginal diagnosis

malformation to be recognized by sonography. Since both conditions share common features, it was postulated that exencephaly is a rare embryological precursor of anencephaly[10]. Anencephaly is characterized by failure of the cephalic part of the neural tube to close at its cephalic end. The primary insult in this malformation is absence of the telencephalon and midbrain associated with maldevelopment of the frontal, parietal and occipital bones. From 14 weeks' gestation onwards, absence of the cranial vault on abdominal sonography establishes the diagnosis[11]. With the use of TVS, the absence of the telencephalon and the typical 'frog-eye' appearance of the fetus can be determined earlier (Figure 8). However, in some cases the typical appearance of the anencephalic fetus may be altered by the presence of a brain-like structure situated superior to the orbits, mimicking a normal brain. Goldstein and colleagues[12] found that between 11 and 12 weeks' gestation it may be difficult to diagnose this conspicuous lesion precisely, by abdominal sonography. The authors drew attention to the fact that a missed diagnosis of anencephaly at 11 to 12 weeks' gestation is possible in cases with exencephaly, due to the appearance of preserved brain tissue, a so-called angiomatous stroma, that mimics the normal brain appearance on standard abdominal ultrasound. Whether the tissue seen

above the orbits represents brain, as in early exencephaly, or the 'buoyant' angiomatous stroma associated with already degenerated brain is not the important issue, since both conditions are incompatible with life. What is imperative for the sonologist performing a standard abdominal scan is that the disorder can be overlooked in early pregnancy. Therefore, any suspected cephalic pool in the first trimester should undoubtedly be evaluated by TVS. The abnormal cranial development seen in anencephaly and exencephaly has been explained by several theories, including failure of the neural tube to close, rupture of the brainstem caused by excessive accumulation of neural tube fluid, and failure of junction of the intrinsic primitive blood vessels. Warkany[13] showed that exencephaly has early developmental stages similar to those of an anencephalic fetus; furthermore, exencephaly was frequently observed in animals with a relatively short gestational period, and when gestation was artificially prolonged in these animals it was possible to obtain the traditional appearance of anencephaly. Ganchrow and Ornoy[14] postulated that the primary event in acrania is the lack, or abnormal development of, the neurocranium, which results in exencephaly and subsequent degeneration of

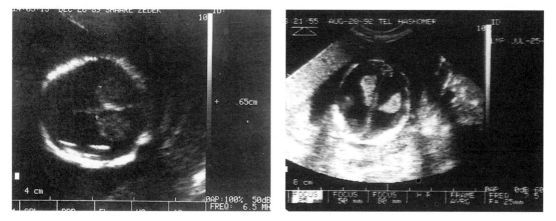

Figure 9 Axial scan: (left) showing normal large lateral ventricle at 13 weeks' gestation. From reference 38, with permission. (right) hydrocephalus at 14 weeks. Note the right angle between the choroid plexus, a very early sign of fluid accumulation within the lateral ventricles

the exposed neural tissue. These assumptions led to the theory that exencephaly is the embryological predecessor of anencephaly in the human fetus. However, according to our experience[15], supported by others[16], the persistence of exencephaly in some cases into the late second trimester, and the classical appearance of some anencephalic fetuses already at 11 weeks of gestation may contradict this theory. Therefore, we assume that although both conditions are considered to be open neural tube defects, anencephaly and exencephaly are two distinct anomalies involving different mechanisms of abnormal neurocranial development.

Intracranial abnormalities

Hydrocephaly

Hydrocephaly is characterized by an abnormal accumulation of cerebrospinal fluid (CSF) within the ventricular system. In most cases, hydrocephalus in the fetus is thought to be due to an obstruction of the aquaduct of Sylvius, which prevents the passage of CSF from the lateral and third ventricles into the fourth ventricle, resulting in ventriculomegaly with increased intraventricular pressure.

Much experience has been gained using standard abdominal sonography to evaluate early ventricular enlargement. For many years it was thought that hydrocephalus could not be diagnosed before 22–24 weeks[17], as until then lateral ventricles are normally large in relation to the width of the cerebral hemispheres. Measurements of lateral ventricle width in relation to hemispheric width were developed to confirm early *in utero* diagnosis. The disadvantage of the lateral ventricle to hemispheric ratio measurements is the large standard deviation, particularly between 12 and 16 weeks (Figure 9, left). Transvaginal sonography allows detailed visualization of the lateral ventricle and choroid plexus and their measurement from 11 weeks, thus enabling the detection of early morphological changes in these structures. As *in utero* hydrocephalus results mainly from obstruction with increased intraventricular CSF pressure, the large echogenic choroid plexus that normally fills the atrium and body of the lateral ventricle shrinks and detaches from its medial wall, dangling into the lumen of the dilated lateral ventricle. The dangling choroid plexus forms an angle with the contralateral choroid plexus to a degree that depends on the severity of the ventricular enlargement (Figure 9, right). These morphological changes in the configuration of the choroid plexus and the lateral ventricles facilitate *in utero* diagnosis of ventriculomegaly very early in pregnancy[18–20]. However, our experience, as well as that of others[21], indicates that in hydrocephalic fetuses ventriculomegaly and obstruction is not manifested during the first trimester of pregnancy. We recently had the opportunity of studying a fetus at risk for X-linked

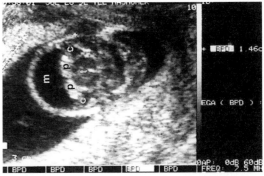

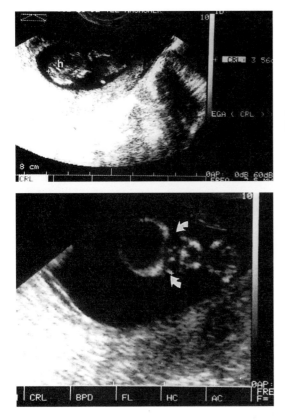

Figure 10 Alobar holoprosencephaly in the first trimester: (top left) longitudinal scan demonstrating 35 mm CRL fetus compatible with 10.4 weeks' gestation. The fetal head (h) is on the left; (top right) magnification using a high-frequency transducer of 7.5 MHz shows mid-coronal view of the same fetus as above. A single, wide, fluid-filled ventricle is seen. The third ventricle is absent, the thalami (t) are fused at the floor of the monoventricle (m), and there are no detectable midline echoes. The cerebral cortici (c) are displaced laterally; p, choroid plexus; (bottom left) anterior coronal view through the fetal face reveals hypotelorism; note the narrow interorbital distance (arrows) which is decreased. From reference 29, with permission

hydrocephalus from the 9th week of gestation on a weekly basis. Only at the 15th week did morphological changes in the configuration of the lateral ventricle and the choroid plexus appear, enabling a definitive *in utero* diagnosis.

Holoprosencephaly

Holoprosencephaly is a rare, developmental abnormality of the brain, resulting from absent or incomplete cleavage of the forebrain (prosencephalon) into the two cerebral hemispheres and lateral ventricles. Depending on the degree and the stage at which morphological development is inhibited, DeMyer categorized holoprosencephaly into alobar, semilobar and lobar types[22].

Alobar-type holoprosencephaly is the most severe lesion in which no cleavage of the prosencephalon has occurred. Instead of a ventricular system with distinct lateral and third ventricles, a monoventricle cavity is present. The thalamus and corpus striatum are fused in the midline, while the midbrain, brainstem and cerebellum are

structurally normal. Associated with this type is a variety of facial abnormalities (cleft lip and palate, cyclopia) and chromosomal aberrations, usually trisomy 13. With less severe cleavage abnormalities of the prosenecephalon, an intermediate type, semilobar holoprosencephaly, results. In this type, although a frontal monoventricle is present, posterior partial formation of occipital lobes occurs. In the mildest form, lobar holoprosencephaly, the two hemispheres and lateral ventricles are better separated, the hemispheres may be fused, and the lateral ventricles widely intercommunicate, due to absence of the septum pellucidum.

Several chromosomal abnormalities are associated with alobar holoprosencephaly, the most frequent being trisomy 13. Other abnormal karyotypes are trisomy 18, 13q–, and 18q–. Severe facial abnormalities may complicate alobar holoprosencephaly. Hypotelorism, cyclopia, arhinia with proboscis and median cleft lip/palate strengthens the diagnosis of alobar holoprosencephaly[23].

Due to poor infant prognosis, a specific *in utero* diagnosis of holoprosencephaly is essential. Until

1984, the earliest gestational age at the time of diagnosis was 27 weeks[24]. Nyberg and co-workers[25] reported *in utero* diagnosis during the early second trimester; Bronshtein and Weiner[26] and Birnholz[27] were the first to describe a transvaginal approach to diagnose holoprosencephaly, the former at 14 weeks' gestation, and the latter at 12.1 weeks' gestation. Nelson and King[28] reported first-trimester diagnosis of this anomaly; however, vague intracranial findings were presented. We observed a case, in which identification of a large monoventricular cavity, no midline echo or third ventricle, fused thalami, and hypotelorism could be seen at 10.5 weeks[29] (Figure 10).

Embryologically, holoprosencephaly develops as early as 6–10 weeks' gestation. Therefore, it was not surprising that a high-resolution transvaginal transducer enabled an early *in utero* diagnosis. In this review, we have shown that at the beginning of the 10th week the telencephalon, consisting of two lateral outpockets representing the cerebral hemispheres, is clearly identified. This is due to the echogenic choroid plexus that fills the bodies of the lateral ventricles almost completely. Caudally, the hypoechoic thalamus, which is the dominant portion of the developing diencephalon, can also be observed at this stage of gestation. Failure to identify this classical pattern, together with the appearance of facial abnormality, provided an accurate specific prenatal diagnosis so early in

pregnancy. In the differential diagnosis of a fetus with a large intracranial frontal cyst at such a stage of gestation, other abnormalities, in addition to alobar holoprosencephaly, should be considered. It would be difficult to differentiate alobar holoprosencephaly from hydranencephaly, since absence of the midline echo is consistent in both conditions[30]. However, midline structures such as falx cerebri, interhemispheric fissure and a third ventricle are present in hydranencephaly and absent in alobar holoprosencephaly. In our case, hydranencephaly could be excluded by demonstration of a displaced cerebral cortex and hypotelorism that are typical of alobar holoprosencephaly.

Dandy–Walker malformation

The Dandy–Walker malformation represents a complex of developmental anomalies of the rhombencephalon, characterized by abnormal cystic dilatation of the posterior fossa with aplasia or hypoplasia of the cerebellum. Obstructive hydrocephaly is a common feature in this syndrome. Because of associated facial, cardiac and limb anomalies, it has been suggested that Dandy–Walker malformation originates before the 6–7th week of embryonic development. The prenatal diagnosis of the Dandy–Walker malformation depends on the demonstration of a posterior fossa cyst communicating with the 4th ventricle, or enlarged cisterna magna. Midline measurements of the cisterna magna are easily obtained from the cerebellar vermis to the inner table of the occiput. Mahoney and co-workers[31] found that between 14 and 35 weeks the mean cisterna magna depth is 5 mm, with a range of 1–10 mm and one standard deviation of 3 mm. Although the usefulness of prenatal sonography in the detection and diagnosis of Dandy–Walker malformation has been well described in the literature, early diagnosis before the 20th week of gestation has been reported only once previously[32]. In that case, an abnormal cystic posterior fossa with failure to demonstrate the cerebellum at 11 weeks' gestation were the earlier sonographic markers for establishing the diagnosis (Figure 11). The further development of ventriculomegaly at 15 weeks'

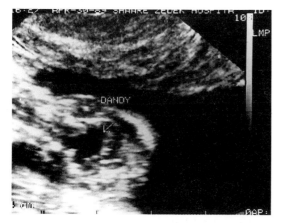

Figure 11 Scan of 11-week fetus showing the junction between the spine and the head at the coronal plain. Note a hypoechoic cystic lesion (DANDY) indicating early Dandy–Walker malformation. From reference 32, with permission

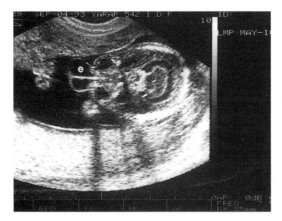

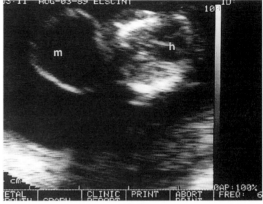

Figure 12 Scan of 13-week fetus demonstrating inter-orbital encephalocele (e) in a case with alobar holoprosencephaly

Figure 13 Transverse section through thorax at the level of the heart (h) in a 12-week fetus showing myelomeningocele (m) sac floating in the amniotic fluid

gestation in that case shed light on the pathogenic mechanism in Dandy–Walker malformation. For many years it was postulated that Dandy–Walker malformation resulted from congenital atresia of the foramina of Magendie and Luschka, with obstructive hydrocephalus predominantly affecting the fourth ventricle[33]. Because subsequent experimental and clinicopathological investigations observed that not all cases were associated with atretic foramina of Magendie and Luschka[34], it was suggested that it involved the rhombencephalon[35]. Gardner and associates[36] proposed that the pathogenesis of Dandy–Walker malformation is due to an imbalance between the production of CSF in the lateral and third ventricles, compared to its production in the fourth ventricle. As over-production of the CSF would be maximal at the level of the fourth ventricle, early dilatation and compression with secondary cerebellar hypoplasia results. According to this hypothesis, the early enlargement of the fourth ventricle would be responsible for the cyst seen in the posterior fossa. Consequently, the only early *in utero* manifestations in fetuses affected by the disease would be the posterior fossa abnormalities. The early appearance of a posterior fossa cyst in our case at the 11th week of gestation, and the subsequent development of hydrocephalus at the 15th week of gestation, support Gardner's hypothesis.

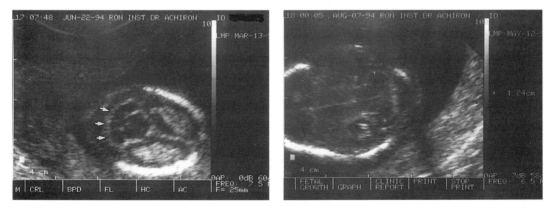

Figure 14 Scan of 13-week fetus of a mother at risk for neural tube defect: no spinal dysmorphism was noted; however, exaggerated convexity (banana sign) of the cerebellum (arrows) was noted (left), compared with normal appearance of 12 mm cerebellum (caliper) in a normal fetus (right) at the same gestational age

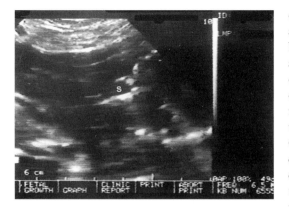

Figure 15 Scan demonstrating unequivocal lumbar spina bifida (s), which was missed at the previous scan at 13 weeks' gestation

Spinal dysraphism (encephalocele, myelomeningocele)

The primary cause for this neural-tube lesion is an ossification defect in the spinal vertebrae. Any region along the spine can be involved in this pathological process. Encephalocele denotes a defect of the rostral portion of the neural tube, in which herniation of cerebral tissue and meninges most commonly occurs posteriorly and in the midline. The earliest ultrasonographic diagnosis of encephalocele was made at our Institute at 13 weeks' gestation (Figure 12). In contrast, the earliest open neural tube defect of the spine was diagnosed by us at the 12th week due to the appearance of bulging thoracal meningeal membranes that could easily be recognized during TVS a long time before screening α-fetoprotein would detect the lesion (Figure 13). Although the spinal defects occur before 6 menstrual weeks, no accurate diagnosis of a lower open neural-tube defect without a bulging sac has been reported to date. Our experience, similar to that of others[37], indicates that in cases with low neural-tube defects, the cerebellar dysmorphism as the banana sign precedes the demonstration of the spinal lesion in about 2–3 weeks. Recently we had the opportunity of examining a woman taking valporic acid, in whom, at 13 weeks' gestation, the only sign that indicated a lower spinal defect was the exaggerated convexity of the cerebellum (Figure 14), while the direct visualization of the spinal defect could not be obtained until the 15–16th week (Figure 15).

SUMMARY

Detection of fetal anomalies during early fetal life is an exciting breakthrough in the field of prenatal diagnosis. This chapter affirms that transvaginal sonography is a feasible and useful diagnostic tool for accomplishing this goal. With pictures obtained by the transvaginal route, it is possible to investigate the fetal central nervous system in the first trimester, enhancing the early prenatal diagnosis of fetal malformations.

References

1. Benacerraf, B.R. (1990). Fetal CNS anomalies. *Ultrasound Q.*, **8**, 1–42
2. Timor-Tritsch, I.E., Farine, D. and Rosen, M.G. (1988). A close look at the embryonic development with the high frequency transvaginal transducer. *Am. J. Obstet. Gynecol.*, **159**, 676–81
3. Langman, J. (1975). *Medical Embryology*, pp. 318–63. (Baltimore: Williams & Wilkins)
4. England, M.A. (1988). Normal development of the CNS. In Levene, M.I., Bennett, M.J. and Punt, J. (eds.) *Fetal and Neonatal Neurology and Neurosurgery*, pp. 3–27. (Edinburgh: Churchill Livingstone)
5. Blaas, F.G., Eik-Nes, S.H., Kiserud, T. and Hellevik, L.R. (1994). Early development of the forebrain and midbrain: a longitudinal ultrasound study from 7 to 12 weeks of gestation. *Ultrasound Obstet. Gynecol.*, **4**, 183–92
6. Cyr, D.R., Mack, L.A., Nyberg, D.A., Shepard, T.H. and Shuman, W.P. (1988). Fetal rhomencephalon: normal ultrasound findings. *Radiology.*, **166**, 691–2
7. Jenkins, G.B. (1921). Relative weight and volume of the component parts of the brain of the human embryo at different stages of development. *Contr. Embryol. Carneg. Instn.*, **13**, 41–60
8. Rottem, S., Bronshtein, M., Thaler, I. and Brandes, J.M. (1989). First trimester transvaginal sonographic diagnosis of fetal anomalies. *Lancet*, **1**, 445–6
9. Elwood, J.M. and Elwood, J.H. (1980). *Epide-*

miology of Anencephalus and Spina Bifida, pp. 15–26. (New York: Oxford University Press)

10. Lemire, R.J., Bechwith, J.B. and Warkany, J. (1978). Experimental exencephaly and anencephaly. In Lemire, R.J., Bechwith, J.B. and Warkany, J. (eds.) *Anencephaly*, pp. 85–111. (New York: Raven Press)

11. Johnson, A., Losure, T.A. and Weiner, S. (1985). Early diagnosis of fetal anencephaly. *J. Clin. Ultrasound*, **13**, 503–5

12. Goldstein, R.B., Filly, R.A. and Callen, P.A. (1989). Sonography of anencephaly: pitfalls in early diagnosis. *J. Clin. Ultrasound*, **17**, 397–402

13. Warkany, J. (1971). Anencephaly. In Warkany, J. (ed.) *Congenital Malformations: Notes and Comments*, pp. 189–200. (Chicago: Year Book Medical Publishers)

14. Ganchrow, D. and Ornoy, A. (1979). Possible evidence for secondary degeneration of CNS in the pathogenesis of anencephaly and brain dysraphia: a study in young human fetuses. *Virchows Arch.*, **384**, 285–94

15. Achiron, R., Malinger, G., Tadmor, O., Diamant, Y. and Zakut, H. (1990). Exencephaly and anencephaly: a distinct anomaly or an embryologic precursor: *in utero* study by transvaginal sonography. *Israel J. Obstet. Gynecol.*, **1**, 60–3

16. Bronshtein, M. and Ornoy, A. (1991). Acrania: anencepahaly resulting from secondary degeneration of a closed neural tube: two cases in the same family. *J. Clin. Ultrasound*, **19**, 230–4

17. Hudgins, R.J., Edwards, M.S.B., Goldstein, R., Callen, P.W., Harrison, M.R., Filly, R.A. and Golbus, M.S. (1988). Natural history of fetal ventriculomegaly. *Pediatrics*, **82**, 692–7

18. Cardoza, J.D., Goldstein, R.B. and Filly, R.A. (1988). Exclusion of fetal ventriculomegaly with a single measurement: the width of the lateral ventricular atrium. *Radiology*, **169**, 711–14

19. Goldstein, R.B., La Pidus, A.S., Filly, R.A. and Cardoza, J. (1990). Mild lateral cerebral ventricular dilatation *in utero*: clinical significance and prognosis. *Radiology*, **176**, 237–42

20. Mahony, B.S., Nyberg, D.A., Hirsch, J.H., Petty, C.N., Hendricks, S.K. and Mack, L.A. (1988). Mild idiopathic lateral ventricular dilatation *in utero*: sonographic evaluation. *Radiology*, **169**, 715–21

21. Bronshtein, M. and Ben-Shlomo, I. (1991). Choroid plexus dysmorphism detected by transvaginal sonography: the earliest sign of fetal hydrocephalus. *J. Clin. Ultrasound*, **19**, 547–53

22. DeMyer, W. (1977). Holoprosencephaly. In Vinken, P.J. and Bruyn, G.W. (eds.) *Handbook of Clinical Neurology*, vol. 30, pp. 431–78. (Amsterdam: Elsevier)

23. Cohen, M., Jirasek, J., Guzman, R., Gorlin, R. and Peterson, M. (1971). Holoprosencephaly and facial dysmorphia: nosology, etiology, and pathogenesis. *Birth Defects*, **7**, 125–35

24. Chervenak, F.A., Isaacson, G., Mahoney, M.J., Tortora, M., Mesologites, T. and Hobbins, J.C. (1984). The obstetric significance of holoprosencephaly. *Obstet. Gynecol.*, **63**, 115–21

25. Nyberg, D.A., Mack, L.A., Bronshtein, M., Hirsch, J. and Pagon, R.A. (1987). Holoprosencephaly: prenatal sonographic diagnosis of fetal anomalies. *Am. J. Radiol.*, **149**, 1051–8

26. Bronshtein, M. and Weiner, Z. (1991). Early sonographic diagnosis of alobar holoprosencephaly. *Prenat. Diagn.*, **11**, 459–62

27. Birnholz, J.C. (1992). Smaller parts scanning of the fetus. *Radiol. Clin. N. Am.*, **30**, 977–91

28. Nelson, L.H. and King, M. (1992). Early diagnosis of holoprosencephaly. *J. Ultrasound Med.*, **11**, 57–9

29. Achiron, R., Achiron, A., Lipitz, S., Mashiach, S. and Goldman, B. (1994). Holoprosencephaly: alobar. *Fetus*, **4**, 9–12

30. Lin, Y.S., Chang, F.M. and Liu, C.H. (1992). Antenatal detection of hydranencephaly at 12 weeks, menstrual age. *J. Clin. Ultrasound*, **20**, 62–4

31. Mahony, B.S., Callen, P., Filly, R. and Heoddick, K. (1984). The fetal cisterna magna. *Radiology*, **153**, 773–6

32. Achiron, R., Achiron, A. and Yagel, S. (1993). First trimester transvaginal sonographic diagnosis of Dandy–Walker malformation. *J. Clin. Ultrasound*, **21**, 62–4

33. Taggart, J.K. and Walker, A.E. (1942). Congenital atresia of the foramens of Luschka and Magendie. *Arch. Neurol. Psychiatry*, **48**, 583–8

34. Benda, C.E. (1954). The Dandy–Walker or the so-called atresia of the foramen Magendie. *J. Neuropathol. Exp. Neurol.*, **13**, 14–29

35. Raybaud, C. (1982). Cystic malformations of the posterior fossa: abnormalities associated with the development of the roof of the fourth ventricle and adjacent meningeal structures. *J. Neuroradiol.*, **9**, 103–8

36. Gardner, E., O'Rahilly, R. and Prolo, D. (1975). The Dandy–Walker and Arnold–Chiari malformations: clinical, developmental and teratological considerations. *Arch. Neurol.*, **32**, 393–407

37. Blumenfeld, Z., Siegler, E. and Bronshtein, M. (1993). The early diagnosis of neural tube defects. *Prenat. Diagn.*, **13**, 863–71

38. Achiron, R. and Achiron, A. (1991). Transvaginal ultrasonic assessment of the early fetal brain. *Ultrasound Obstet. Gynecol.*, **1**, 336–44

Transvaginal fetal neurosonography: the second and third trimesters of pregnancy

6

A. Monteagudo and I. E. Timor-Tritsch

INTRODUCTION

In infants or adults, ultrasound scans are directed towards specific organs or organ systems according to the type of complaint or symptomatology. In contrast to this, regardless of the primary reason for a fetal scan, almost every time a prenatal scan is performed, all organs are scrutinized sonographically. Therefore, the obstetric sonologist or sonographer has to be familiar with the normal and abnormal appearance of all fetal organs, including the fetal brain.

During the second and third trimesters of the pregnancy, the fetal brain can be imaged with the use of both transabdominal and transvaginal sonography. Transvaginal sonography was introduced and popularized during the last decade[1–3]. In 1989, Benacerraf and Estroff[4] were the first to publish a report on the use of transvaginal sonography to measure the low or deeply engaged fetal head. Subsequently, in 1991, Monteagudo and colleagues[5] reported the use of transvaginal sonography to perform a systematic study of the fetal brain.

The widespread and customary approach for scanning of the fetal brain was, and in many places still continues to be, the transabdominal route[6–10]. It became evident that the vaginal scanning technique yields better pictures that better serve the diagnostic process[5, 11, 12]. However, due to certain limitations in obtaining all the desired sections and planes, transabdominal and transvaginal sonography are found to complement each other, and should therefore both be employed to image the fetal brain. It is important to use both techniques, especially when a fetal brain anomaly is encountered. When an anomaly is detected, in addition to our task to describe the lesion, it is also important to attempt to establish the most likely diagnosis or differential diagnosis. Determining that a structure or an organ is normal is a far more difficult task than confirming the presence of an anomaly. Therefore, the added information provided by transvaginal sonography (TVS), as a result of its higher resolution, allows us to assess normalcy with greater accuracy and confidence.

This chapter describes in detail the sonographic anatomy of the normal fetal brain during the second and third trimesters of pregnancy. This anatomy will be described by means of the classical coronal and sagittal sections as used in neonatal brain scans and as seen with transvaginal sonography.

THE TRANSVAGINAL– TRANSFONTANELLE SCANNING TECHNIQUE

Transvaginal sonography of the fetal brain can be performed any time during gestation if the fetus is in a cephalic presentation. Performing TVS is the easiest way to access the fontanelles of the fetal head, especially the anterior fontanelle, which is the largest. Neonatal sonographers were the first to realize that by performing transfontanelle brain sonography, the resolution of their images improved dramatically[13–16]. When performing TVS during the second and third trimesters of pregnancy, the same safety guidelines employed for the use of a speculum or the bimanual examination should be observed. In the event of a breech presentation, the sagittal and coronal views may be obtained transabdominally. In a few cases in which a fetal intracranial anomaly is suspected and the transabdominal examination is sub-optimal, an external cephalic version may be indicated. In these cases, the appropriate institutional guidelines to perform the external cephalic version must be followed. The advantages of the additional and more

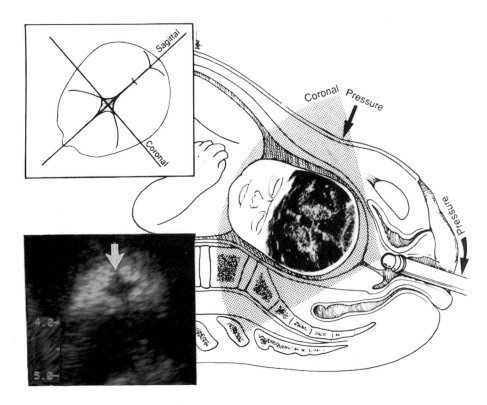

Figure 1 Ink drawing depicting the transvaginal–transfontanelle technique of imaging the fetal brain. By applying gentle pressure on the fetal head through the abdominal wall and by angling the probe, an 'in-axis' view of the fetal brain through the anterior fontanelle is imaged. Upper inset: the sagittal and coronal planes can be obtained by rotating the probe 90° from the initial plane. Lower inset: the actual tangential image of the anterior fontanelle. Modified after reference 5

accurate information obtained by TVS has to be weighed against the potential risks of the external cephalic version.

The ideal transvaginal probe for performing transvaginal-transfontanelle imaging of the fetal brain is an end-firing 5.0–7.5-MHz probe with a rounded tip, which is placed in one of the vaginal fornices, preferably the posterior fornix. Curvilinear probes, with offset angles and asymmetrical shapes are technically difficult to align with the fetal fontanelle. Also, when such a probe is rotated around its axis over the fetal head, it may be uncomfortable to the patient. The probe is covered with a sheath, sonic gel is applied, and the probe is slowly advanced through the vagina until the entire fetal head is imaged. Once the transvaginal probe is in place, clear images can usually be obtained by moving the probe until its tip is lined

up with the fetal anterior fontanelle (Figure 1). Although most commonly we are able to scan through the anterior fontanelle, at times the posterior fontanelle is the one used. On occasion, after placing the transducer probe in the posterior fornix of the vagina, the image obtained is of poor quality. This is most probably due to the fact that neither fontanelle is lined up with the probe and the scanning is taking place through the cranial bones. To correct this situation, the fetal head may need to be manipulated through the maternal abdomen with the free hand of the sonologist or sonographer. This rectifies deviations in the alignment, or prevents the fetal head from constantly moving out of focus. Once a clear image is obtained, scanning begins.

The coronal and the sagittal planes are obtained by rotating the probe 90° around its axis over the anterior fontanelle. For example, if a coronal section is apparent on the monitor, by rotating the probe 90° the sagittal section will be imaged. Serial coronal sections are obtained by slowly sweeping the probe in an anterior-to-posterior fashion (away from the face and towards the occiput or vice versa) and serial sagittal sections by angling the probe laterally towards the right and left ears of the fetus.

Before we engage in a more detailed discussion of the specific anatomic brain structures, several general comments need to be made.

First, it is important to note that the brain is a symmetric organ. The only exception may be the topography of the hemispheric gyri and sulci. On the various coronal sections, the two sides have to be symmetrical unless pathology causes asymmetry. However, in the literature, at least one article[17] indicates that there seems to be asymmetry of the neonatal brain regarding the body of the lateral ventricles, and the left lateral ventricle was found to be larger than the right.

Second, there are several prominent structures that make scanning the fetal brain easier. These structures are extremely echogenic, making their detection obvious and thereby enabling easy orientation within the brain itself. The following structures appear as high echoes: the choroid plexus (starting at 9 weeks), the soft membranous covers of the brain (pia mater and arachnoid, mentioned as leptomeninges) and finally the internal linings of the ventricles.

The cortex of the hemispheres as well as the cerebellum assumes rapid growth after 28–30 weeks' gestation[18, 19]. Therefore, the many invaginations (sulci) carry the covering pia mater into the depths of the cortex. These foldings of the echoic pia mater are easily imaged. The rich network of small vessels intimately following the pia mater enhances its echogenicity. This process is accentuated within the cerebellum. Here, the gyri and sulci are numerous and deep, therefore the cerebellum appears as an extremely bright echogenic structure.

Finally, the subarachnoid space, brain cisterns and the vessels or structures crossing them are imaged. In the subarachnoid space, bridging vessels appear as bright echoes giving the subarachnoid space a 'speckled' appearance. In the cisterna

magna, a cyst-like structure is commonly imaged. This represents the leptomeninges traversing this space[20]. These bridging vessels and leptomeninges are observed, because the cerebrospinal fluid accentuates them.

The anatomy that we describe is by no means inclusive of all the structures that can be seen by TVS, but is a fair representation of the major anatomical landmarks.

NORMAL INTRACRANIAL ANATOMY

The normal intracranial anatomy will be presented in great detail in a series of coronal and sagittal sections. In the coronal plane the anatomy will be described from the most anterior to the most posterior section. Although the anatomy can be delineated in three planes – anterior, midline and posterior – many more planes can be imaged, depending on how thin or thick the sections of the brain are made. If the reader is able to master all these three coronal sections, he or she will be able (a) to assess if normal development has so far occurred, and (b) to note and identify most of the congenital abnormalities that affect the developing fetal brain.

The sagittal anatomy will be described in two planes: midline sagittal and parasagittal sections. Combining all of these five planes results in a thorough study of the fetal brain. There are many textbooks, atlases and articles that deal with the normal and abnormal anatomy of the neonatal brain. These publications are a source of invaluable information, because the anatomy is described in the coronal and sagittal planes and can be applied to the fetal brain as viewed by TVS. A few of these are added to the reference list[21–26].

It is also important to mention that with this technique as with any newly acquired skill there is a learning curve. In the beginning, not all sections described will be consistently imaged, but as experience and confidence is gained, the number of scans in which all planes are imaged will steadily increase. In our first publication[5], involving 70 fetuses, we documented a learning curve. In that study, we were able to image all sections in approximately 75% of the fetuses. In addition, we found that the most difficult section to obtain was the posterior coronal section, which we imaged in approximately 59% of the fetuses.

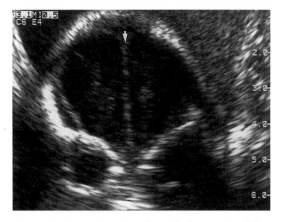

Figure 2 Coronal section through the anterior lobes of the fetal brain. The interhemispheric fissure (arrow) of this 22-week fetus appears relatively straight

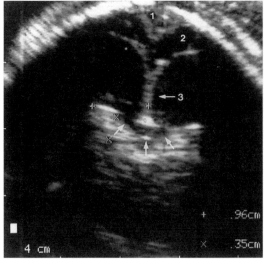

Figure 3 Mid-coronal image of a 22-week fetus. 1, Superior sagittal sinus; 2, subarachnoid space; 3, interhemispheric fissure. White arrows point to the hypoechoic corpus callosum. Calipers are measuring the distance between the interhemispheric fissure and the lateral edge of the ventricle and depth of the ventricle (see Figure 19)

Coronal sections

First coronal section

The first coronal section passes through the parenchyma of the frontal lobes (Figure 2). The frontal lobes of the brain are separated into the right and left by the interhemispheric fissure. The interhemispheric fissure appears as a bright echogenic midline structure. During the first half of pregnancy, this midline echo looks like a relatively straight line. As the pregnancy progresses, it becomes increasingly more branched due to the growth spurt of the fetal brain during the early third trimester. In this section, the imaged bony component of the face has the appearance of a 'steer's head'.

It is important to mention that after the 20th week of gestation in a 'normal brain', this section never shows the frontal horns. This is due to growth of the frontal lobes, which takes place at the expense of the frontal horns of the lateral ventricles. If the frontal horns are imaged in this coronal section, ventriculomegaly or hydrocephalus should be suspected.

Below the bright echogenic rim of the cranium, several structures can be imaged in a slightly more posterior section. Immediately below the cranium, the superior sagittal sinus can be seen as a slightly triangular structure through which, with the use of a high frame rate or color Doppler, blood flow can be observed. Below the superior sagittal sinus, the subarachnoid space appears as a hypoechoic area above the cerebral cortex. In some sections, the subarachnoid space has a 'speckled' appearance. This is due to the multiple vessels that transverse this space, which becomes less prominent with the progressive brain growth as term is reached (Figure 3).

Mid-coronal section

The mid-coronal section is very important, because it not only contains parts of the lateral ventricular system, but also has the corpus callosum and cavum septi pellucidi, which are important midline structures (Figure 4). At the base of the interhemispheric fissure and at right angles to it, the hypoechoic corpus callosum is located. Although the corpus callosum starts developing early in the second trimester, it is not consistently imaged until the 20th week of gestation. Also, in the midline the cingulate gyrus can be seen above the corpus callosum. The cingulate gyrus is consistently imaged after 25 weeks' gestation (Figure 5). To the right and left of the interhemispheric fissure, the

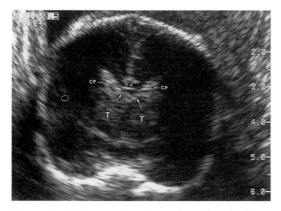

Figure 4 Mid-coronal section of a 22-week fetus. CC, corpus callosum; CP, choroid plexus; T, thalamus. Arrows point to the foramina of Monro

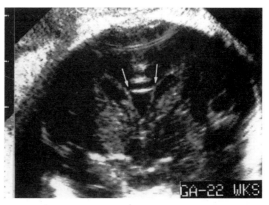

Figure 6 The cavum septum pellucidum is the central triangularly shaped structure in this scan of a 22-week fetus. The lateral ventricles are separated from the cavum by parallel sheets of tissue (white arrows)

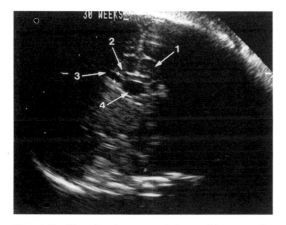

Figure 5 The cingulate gyrus is imaged between the sulcus of the cingulate gyrus and that of the corpus callosum in this mid-coronal section of a 30-week fetus. The cavum septum pellucidum appears as a prominent midline hypoechoic structure. 1, cingulate gyrus; 2, corpus callosum; 3, lateral ventricle; 4, cavum septum pellucidum

anterior horns of the lateral ventricles appear as linear, bilateral fluid-filled structures. As the fetus matures, the lateral ventricles become narrower and are sometimes quite difficult to image. The ventricles approximate each other in the midline and contain the echogenic choroid plexus. The choroid plexus fills the cavities of the lateral ventricles. The right and left arms of the choroid plexus fuse in the midline after passing through the foramina of Monro and then continue into the third ventricle, forming the shape of the letter 'Y'.

Between the anterior horns and below the corpus callosum in the midline, the cavum septi pellucidi is seen. The cavum is separated from the ventricles by a thin sheet of tissue (septum) (Figure 6). The thalami are located below the cavum septi pellucidi. In the midline between the thalami, the third ventricle can occasionally be imaged as a thin, longitudinal narrow slit. In brain scans of normal fetuses, the third ventricle is usually not imaged. When it is imaged, one should suspect an abnormality such as ventriculomegaly or hydrocephalus. If it is imaged in an unusually high position, below the interhemispheric fissure, absence of the corpus callosum and of the cavum septi pellucidi must be ruled out[27].

Posterior coronal section

In the most posterior coronal section that can sometimes be imaged, the occipital horns of the lateral ventricle, the cerebellum and the tentorium above the cerebellum are imaged (Figure 7). The occipital horns appear as perfectly rounded sonolucent structures, giving the impression of an 'owl's eye or face'. In the posterior fossa, the cerebellum is imaged. Above the cerebellum, the sonolucent fourth ventricle can be imaged. Below the cerebellum, an equally sonolucent cisterna magna is present. In the majority of cases of open spinal defects, the cisterna magna will be obliterated in this section.

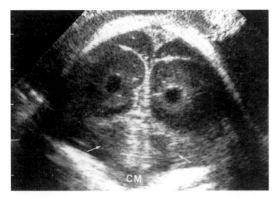

Figure 7 Posterior coronal section of a 19.5-week fetus. The occipital horns of the lateral ventricles appear as round sonolucent structures. The white arrows point to the cerebellum. The bright central echoes represent the area of the vermis. CM, cisterna magna

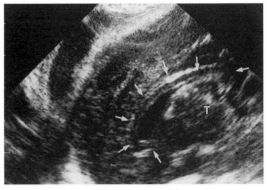

Figure 9 The corpus callosum of this 31-week fetus is delineated by small white arrows. Below the corpus callosum the prominent and sonolucent cavum septum pellucidum is imaged. T, thalamus

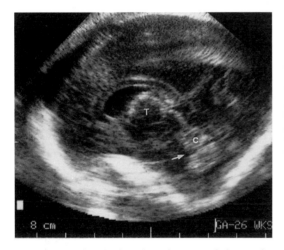

Figure 8 Mid-sagittal section of a 26-week fetus. The semicircular corpus callosum and the sonolucent cavum septum pellucidum are the two prominent structures in the center of the image. The cerebellum appears hyperechoic and is indented by the hypoechoic fourth ventricle (white arrow). T, thalamus; C, cerebellum

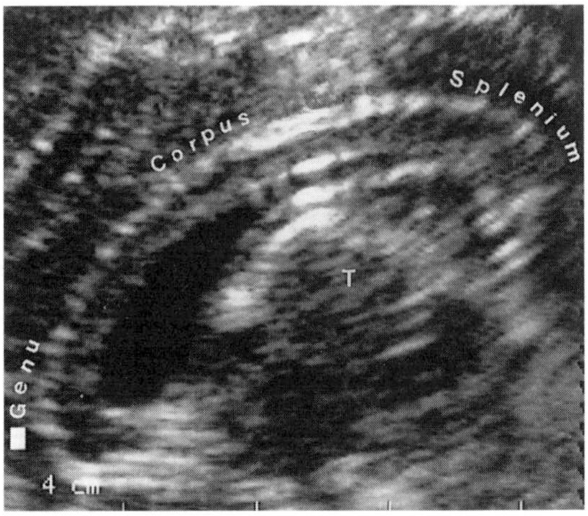

Figure 10 Mid-sagittal section of a 30-week fetus showing only the corpus callosum and cavum septum pellucidum. The three parts of the corpus callosum – the genu (knee), corpus (body) and splenium (tail) – are imaged. T, thalamus

Sagittal and parasagittal sections

Mid-sagittal section

The mid-sagittal section reveals two simple-to-locate structures, namely the corpus callosum and the sonolucent cavum septi pellucidi (Figure 8). The corpus callosum develops in an anterior-to-posterior fashion and it is fully developed by

18–20 weeks' gestation. The corpus callosum is a prominent hypoechoic, semilunar midline structure located above the cavum septi pellucidi (Figure 9). It has three parts: the anterior or knee (genu), middle portion or body (corpus) and a posterior part or tail (splenium) (Figure 10). Therefore, by simply looking at the shape of the corpus callosum, one can become orientated as to which direction the fetus is facing. Above and

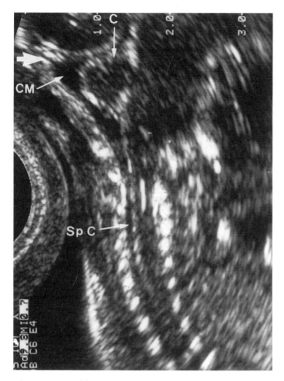

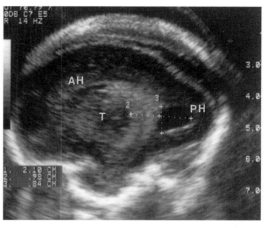

Figure 12 In this parasagittal section the fetus is facing towards the left side of the image. AH, anterior horn; PH, posterior horn; T, thalamus. Inset: measurements of the lateral ventricle (refer to text and Figure 19)

Figure 11 Mid-sagittal view of the posterior fossa. The large arrowhead points to the location of the tentorium of the cerebellum, below which the cisterna magna (CM) is seen. The cerebellum has two different types of echogenicity. There is an outer border which is hyperechoic, but the inner cerebellar parenchyma is homogeneous with low-level echoes. Sp C, spinal canal

parallel to the corpus callosum, the cingulate gyrus can be seen progressively more easily as gestation advances. Below the corpus callosum, the cavum septum pellucidum appears as a large prominent hypoechoic structure. The posterior part of the cavum is referred to as the cavum vergae. As the fetus reaches term, the cavum begins to close in a posterior-to-anterior fashion, with the cavum vergae being the first to be obliterated. Cysts may occur within the cavum septum pellucidum or cavum vergae, and have been associated with hydrocephalus[28].

Located above and covering the thalamus, the bright echogenic tela choroidea (choroid plexus) of the third ventricle can be imaged. As we follow the structures towards the posterior fossa, below the tentorium, the cerebellum and the hyperechoic vermis appear. The cisterna magna is hypoechoic

and surrounds these structures (Figure 11). The triangularly shaped hypoechoic fourth ventricle can be seen at times indenting the cerebellum anteriorly (Figure 8). Abnormalities of the posterior fossa, such as an arachnoid cyst or a megacisterna magna can be diagnosed with relative ease on this section.

Parasagittal section

By tilting the transvaginal probe slightly to the right or left, a parasagittal section is obtained. This section reveals the anterior horn and body of the lateral ventricles, with the choroid plexus within this area of the lateral ventricle, and the occipital horn, which is a prominent sonolucent structure (Figure 12). The anterior and posterior horns form the shape of the mirror image of the letter 'C', the open end of which points anteriorly towards the fetal face (another easy way to become orientated as to which way the fetus is facing). Because of their lateral position, the temporal horns can be seen only if one angles the transducer to obtain an extremely lateral section, usually impossible by TVS. It should therefore be mentioned that if all parts of the lateral ventricles (anterior, posterior and temporal horns) are imaged on the same parasagittal section, ventriculomegaly or hydrocephalus must be suspected.

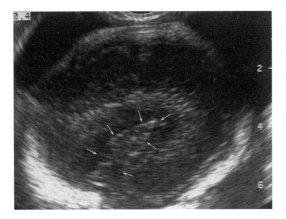

Figure 13 An extreme parasagittal section of a 26-week fetus. The white arrows demarcate the edges of the Sylvian fissure

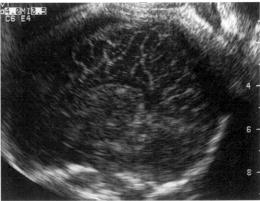

Figure 14 Mid-sagittal section of a 36-week fetus. The multiple hyperechoic lines covering the hemispheres are the gyri and sulci

The caudothalamic groove can be imaged in this section. As pregnancy nears term, involution of the germinal matrix occurs and it is no longer imaged. Its appearance is that of a bright echogenic arc, which separates the head of the caudate nucleus anteriorly from the more posterior thalamus. This is the area that is considered to be the origin of most intracranial hemorrhages in preterm neonates[29]. If the probe is tilted even more towards the fetal ears, the resulting lateral sagittal section reveals a gaping Sylvian fissure, the insula, and the brain parenchyma of the parietal lobe (Figure 13). As pregnancy progresses and the fetal brain continues to grow, this fissure will eventually become increasingly narrow (slit-like), resembling that of the neonatal brain.

In both the midline and parasagittal sections, the gyri and sulci can be imaged. During the first and second trimester of the pregnancy, the surface of the brain is smooth, but with the growth spurt that occurs around 28–30 weeks' gestation, the number of gyri and sulci increases rapidly[18, 19]. The sonographic appearance of the brain surface then changes from a smooth one to one with an interlacing network of hyperechoic lines (Figure 14).

DETECTION OF VENTRICULOMEGALY AND HYDROCEPHALUS

Transvaginal sonography is an excellent tool for imaging of the brain in the presence of any con-genital brain malformation, but in the presence of ventriculomegaly and hydrocephalus it can provide information not readily available with conventional transabdominal sonography. When scanning a fetus with *in utero* ventriculomegaly and/or hydrocephalus, it is important to be able to image both hemispheres with equal clarity and side by side. This is difficult to achieve with transabdominal sonography, due mainly to artifacts[30–32] and attenuation of the sound wave as it travels to and through the fetal cranium. The clarity of the TVS pictures of the fetal brain is due to the fact that the brain is scanned through the anterior fontanelle. Therefore, the end result of adding TVS to the conventional transabdominal scan is that the fetal brain is imaged in the three scanning planes (axial, coronal and sagittal) enabling the sonologist or sonographer to reconstruct a more accurate three-dimensional image of the abnormality.

Another advantage of performing TVS of the fetal brain is that the pediatric neuroradiologist, neurologist and neurosurgeon are more familiar with the coronal and sagittal sections, as generated by the neonatal ultrasound examination, than with the axial views of the fetal brain. Therefore, looking at the familiar coronal and sagittal images makes it easier for all of those involved in the present and future care of the baby with a congenital anomaly, such as hydrocephalus, to plan the delivery route and future surgical procedures.

Hydrocephalus or ventriculomegaly refers to dilatation of the fetal lateral ventricles with or

Table 1 Congenital hydrocephalus. Adapted from reference 35

Non-communicating hydrocephalus
Aqueductal stenosis
Dandy–Walker malformation
Masses

Communicating hydrocephalus
Arnold–Chiari malformation
Encephalocele
Leptomeningeal inflammation
Lissencephaly
Congenital absence of arachnoid granulations

---

without enlargement of the cranium. In hydrocephalus, the dilatation of the cerebral ventricles is the result of an increased amount of cerebrospinal fluid with an accompanying increase in intraventricular pressure. Fetuses with hydrocephalus usually have a head circumference and/or biparietal diameter that is larger than appropriate for their dates. The greater the discrepancy, the worse is the degree of hydrocephalus present. In contrast, ventriculomegaly refers to dilatation of the fetal lateral ventricles. In these cases, the fetal head circumference may be within the normal range for gestational age[9,33]. Although most cases of ventriculomegaly or hydrocephalus are bilateral, unilateral hydrocephalus is a rare condition that can affect the fetus. It usually results from unilateral obstruction of the foramen of Monro[34,35].

The estimated incidence of hydrocephalus is 0.5–3 per 1000 live births. The incidence of isolated hydrocephalus is between 0.4 and 0.9 per 1000 live births[36]. The most common cause of hydrocephalus is obstruction of the cerebrospinal fluid along its route of circulation. The cerebrospinal fluid is produced by the choroid plexus of the lateral ventricles and its flow is unidirectional. In the neonate, it is estimated that the choroid plexus produces approximately 650 ml of cerebrospinal fluid per day[37]. It circulates from the lateral ventricles to the third ventricle, aqueduct of Sylvius, fourth ventricle through the foramina of Magendie or Luschka to the basal cisterns, and eventually to the subarachnoid space, where it is absorbed by the arachnoid granulations. Obstruction to the flow of cerebrospinal fluid along this pathway will result in ventriculomegaly and hydrocephalus. If obstruction to flow occurs as the fluid flows out of the ventricles, the resulting pathology is termed non-communicating hydrocephalus. When the obstruction occurs at the level of the subarachnoid space, the resulting hydrocephalus is termed communicating (Table 1).

In neonates, among cases of congenital hydrocephalus, aqueductal stenosis is the most common cause, accounting for 43% of all cases. In aqueductal stenosis, there is obstruction to flow of the cerebrospinal fluid leaving the fourth ventricle. In approximately 70% of these cases, a lesion obstructing this flow can be demonstrated[38]. This is followed by communicating hydrocephalus, which accounts for 38%, and Dandy–Walker malformation, which accounts for 13%[39]. Other causes that account for about 6% of all cases include agenesis of the corpus callosum, arachnoid cysts and aneurysm of the vein of Galen. In approximately 30% of the cases of hydrocephalus, polyhydramnios is present[40].

Early diagnosis of *in utero* ventriculomegaly or hydrocephalus remains a diagnostic challenge. It is extremely difficult to make the diagnosis of ventriculomegaly or hydrocephalus in the first and sometimes even in the early second trimester, unless the condition is very severe. In the early second trimester, the relative size of the lateral ventricle in relation to the brain parenchyma is quite high, but as the fetus approaches term this relationship diminishes. At term the normal fetal lateral ventricle appears 'slit-like', while at 20 weeks the appearance is more 'plump' but still within the normal limits for the gestational age. Therefore, when assessing if ventriculomegaly or hydrocephalus is present, the gestational age of the fetus must be taken into consideration.

Using TVS, ventriculomegaly or hydrocephalus can be diagnosed by either qualitative or quantitative methods[41–49].

Qualitative methods of diagnosis

'Gestalt approach'

For this diagnosis, an experienced sonographer and/or sonologist looks at the brain and decides whether it appears dilated or not.

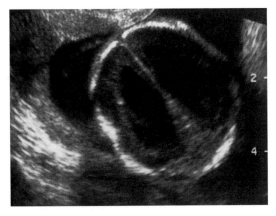

Figure 15 Coronal section through the frontal lobes of the fetal brain. The anterior horns are very prominent in this 18.5-week fetus with hydrocephalus, in contrast to Figure 2, in which the anterior horns of the lateral ventricle were not imaged

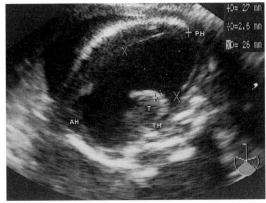

Figure 16 Parasagittal section of an 18.5-week fetus with hydrocephalus. Note that all three components of the lateral ventricle are imaged. The choroid plexus is thin and distorted. AH, anterior horn; PH, posterior horn; TH, temporal horn; T, thalamus. Inset are the measurements of the lateral ventricle (refer to Figures 19–23)

Change in shape of lateral ventricles

There are suggestive changes in the shape of the lateral ventricles. In the presence of hydrocephalus, the anterior horns will be imaged in the first coronal section; normally in this section, only brain parenchyma is present (Figure 15). In the mid-coronal section, there may be progressive rounding and bulging of the superior and lateral aspects of the frontal horns, pointed inferiorly. Its appearance resembles that of an inverted 'teardrop' with the rounded segment on top, and the tapered end pointing towards the third ventricle. On the parasagittal plane, all three components of the lateral ventricle (anterior, posterior and temporal horns) will be imaged in the same section (Figure 16). In the absence of ventriculomegaly or hydrocephalus, only the anterior and posterior (occipital) horns are imaged.

Appearance of choroid plexus

In cases of ventriculomegaly or hydrocephalus, the choroid plexus becomes thinner, probably due to the increase in cerebrospinal fluid pressure. In addition, during real-time scanning, the choroid plexus may be seen 'dangling' or floating freely within the dilated ventricle (Figure 17).

Imaging of third ventricle

The third ventricle may be easily imaged and possesses a measurable diameter. As mentioned previously, the normal third ventricle, due to its narrow diameter, is rarely imaged during scanning (Figure 18).

Quantitative methods of diagnosis

Quantitative methods for assessment of ventriculomegaly or hydrocephalus have been based on widely accepted nomograms of the fetal lateral ventricles[50–56]. All of the commonly used nomograms of the fetal lateral ventricles were generated by using measurements obtained transabdominally in the axial plane. Therefore, when the fetal brain is scanned transvaginally in coronal and sagittal sections, these nomograms cannot be applied. Using TVS, we recently developed and published nomograms of the fetal lateral ventricles[57,58]. The main difference between our nomograms and those previously published is that we performed all our measurements transvaginally, using coronal and sagittal sections. Nine nomograms were developed from 347 fetuses of 14–40 weeks' gestation. Seven measurements of the fetal lateral ventricles were used to generate the nomograms (Figures 19–28).

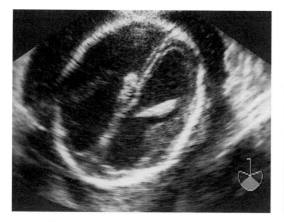

Figure 17 Axial section of an 18.5-week fetus showing the 'dangling' choroid plexus within the dilated lateral ventricles

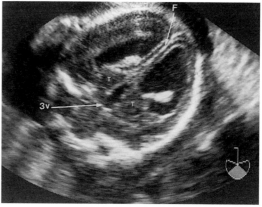

Figure 18 Mid-coronal section showing the dilated anterior horns of the lateral ventricle, dangling choroid plexus, and the prominent third ventricle (3v). F, falx cerebri; T, thalami

Table 2 Measurements of the lateral ventricles by transvaginal sonography. Reproduced with permission from ref. 58

	Measurement number	Description
Parasagittal plane	1	thalamus–choroid plexus interface to the tip of the occipital horn (TCP–TOH)
	2	choroid plexus thickness (CPT)
	3	occipital horn height (OHH)
Midline coronal plane	4	midline to upper edge of lateral ventricle (MUELV)
	5	depth of lateral ventricle (DLV)
Posterior coronal plane	6	width of occipital horn (WOH)
	7	height of occipital horn (HOH)
Ratio		thalamus to tip of occipital horn (TCP–TOH)/choroid plexus thickness (CPT)
Ratio		occipital horn height (OHH)/choroid plexus thickness (CPT)

In addition, two ratios were calculated from three of the seven measurements (Table 2). Serial follow-up of 36 patients carrying fetuses with hydrocephalus was carried out. As expected, all parts of the lateral ventricles increased with progressing ventriculomegaly or hydrocephaly. The only exception was the thickness of the choroid plexus, which decreased as ventriculomegaly progressed[57,58].

The earliest changes occurring in the size of the lateral ventricle during the development of ventriculomegaly or hydrocephalus are as follows. Dilatation of the posterior (occipital) horn of the lateral ventricle occurs first and the anterior horns are the last to increase in size[43,59]. This dilatation occurs in the direction of least resistance to increasing cerebrospinal fluid pressures. In the occipital horns, the increase in size will be detected in the up-and-down direction, in other words towards the crown or base of the skull[42,43,56,58,60]. In addition, there is compression or thinning of the choroid plexus as a result of increasing cerebrospinal fluid pressure[49,61–63]. The normal choroid plexus usually fills the antrum of the lateral ventricle totally. Its appearance is 'fluffy', similar to cotton. In cases of ventriculomegaly, the choroid plexus is compressed and floats within the dilated

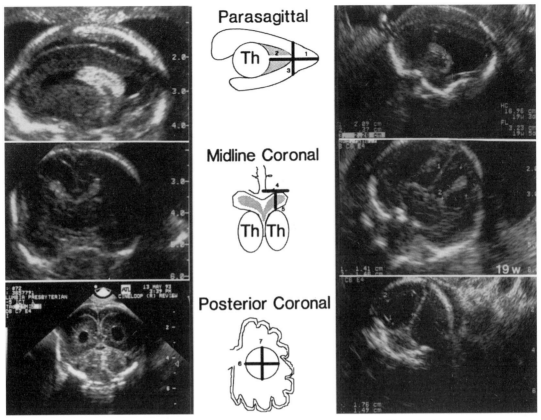

Normal   Ventriculomegaly

Figure 19 A composite picture showing the planes and location of the seven transvaginal measurements used to generate the nomograms. The left column shows a 'normal' brain scan, the right column a fetus with ventriculomegaly. The middle column shows ink drawings of the three scanning planes (parasagittal, mid-coronal and posterior coronal) used to generate the transvaginal nomograms. (19 w, gestational age of the fetus in the image). Reproduced with permission from ref. 58

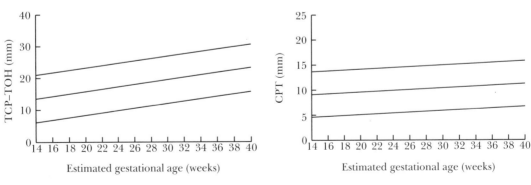

Figure 20 Nomogram for measurement number 1, in the parasagittal plane: thalamus–choroid plexus interface to the tip of occipital horn (TCP–TOH) (refer to Figure 19). The mean regression line and 2 standard deviations are shown

Figure 21 Nomogram for measurement number 2, in the parasagittal plane: choroid plexus thickness (CPT)

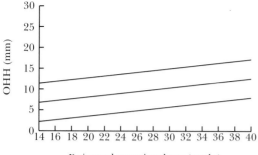

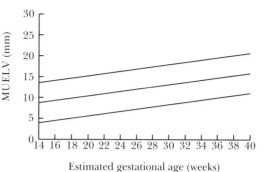

Figure 22 Nomogram for measurement number 3, in the parasagittal plane: occipital horn height (OHH)

Figure 23 Nomogram for measurement number 4, in the midline coronal plane: midline to upper edge of lateral ventricle (MUELV)

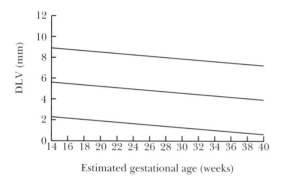

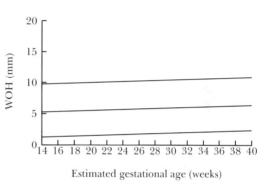

Figure 24 Nomogram for measurement number 5, in the midline coronal plane: depth of lateral ventricle (DLV)

Figure 25 Nomogram for measurement number 6, in the posterior coronal plane: width of occipital horn (WOH)

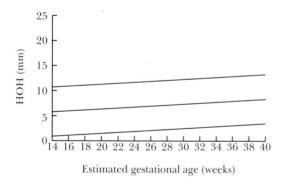

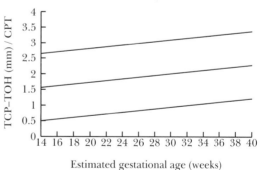
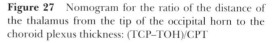

Figure 26 Nomogram for measurement number 7, in the posterior coronal plane: height of occipital horn (HOH)

Figure 27 Nomogram for the ratio of the distance of the thalamus from the tip of the occipital horn to the choroid plexus thickness: (TCP–TOH)/CPT

ventricle ('dangling choroid plexus sign')[49] and in addition it is pulled by gravity towards the dependent part of the fetal head.

The outcome of prenatally detected hydrocephalus is closely related to the presence or absence of associated anomalies. The reported incidence of anomalies in this group is 70–83%[64–68]. In the presence of other anomalies, the prognosis for the fetus/neonate is poor, and developmental delay varying from mild to severe can be expected[64].

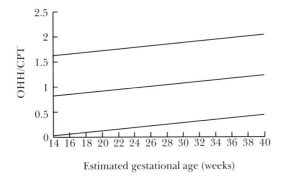

Figure 28 Nomogram for the ratio of the occipital horn height to the choroid plexus thickness: OHH/CPT

Isolated hydrocephalus has a better prognosis for the neonate and the reported incidence of 'normal' outcome is 54.5–80%[64, 69].

Recently, increasing concern over the significance of mild or borderline cases of fetal ventriculomegaly has emerged[70-73]. Although in this group of fetuses the incidence of other anomalies is lower than in the group of fetuses with obvious ventriculomegaly or hydrocephalus, a search for subtle anomalies is warranted. Another important issue in this group of fetuses is that of the association with chromosomal abnormality, especially trisomy 21. The calculated risk for trisomy 21 has been estimated at 3%[73]. In addition, 'normalization' of the lateral ventricular size has been reported. However, in view of the small number of cases, it is hard to assess what percentage of fetuses with mild ventriculomegaly will have resolution of their lesion *in utero*[72, 73].

When a fetus with suspected ventriculomegaly is scanned by means of TVS, the most practical and efficient section to obtain is a right or left parasagittal section. In this section, one can make qualitative observations of the lateral ventricle and the choroid plexus, and obtain measurements and plot the values in the described nomograms. But what are the disadvantages of obtaining *only* this one view? The main disadvantage is that TVS is not used to its full potential. It is important to note that there are several associated brain malformations that may occur together with ventriculomegaly or hydrocephalus. Among these are agenesis of the corpus callosum and cavum septum pellucidum, which can be readily observed with TVS.

CONCLUSION

Transvaginal sonography has become the 'gold standard' imaging modality in gynecology and early pregnancy. Due to its inherent limitations, applications of transvaginal sonography during the second and third trimesters of pregnancy have been relatively limited and extremely specific in their goals. One of the important uses of transvaginal sonography during the second and third trimesters of pregnancy is high-resolution imaging of the fetal intracranial structures in the sagittal and coronal planes. Although these planes can usually be obtained with transabdominal sonography as well, there are often technical difficulties in imaging, due to maternal or fetal factors that preclude adequate visualization. We believe that this new approach will become part of the routine fetal neurological examination, especially in the presence of a previous history of a fetal nervous system anomaly or predisposing factors for such conditions.

References

1. Timor-Tritsch, I.E. and Rottem, S. (1991). *Transvaginal Sonography*, 2nd edn. (New York: Elsevier)
2. Goldstein, S.R. (1988). *Endovaginal Sonography*. (New York: Alan R. Liss)
3. Fleischer, A.C. and Kepple, D.M. (1992). *Transvaginal Sonography. A Clinical Atlas*. (Philadelphia, J.B. Lippincott)
4. Benacerraf, B.R. and Estroff, J.A. (1989). Transvaginal sonographic imaging of the low fetal head in the second trimester. *J. Ultrasound Med.*, **8**, 325
5. Monteagudo, A., Reuss, M.L. and Timor-Tritsch, I.E. (1991). Imaging the fetal brain in the second and third trimester using transvaginal sonography. *Obstet. Gynecol.*, **77**, 27–32

6. Pasto, M.E. and Kurtz, A.B. (1986). Fetal neuro-sonography. Ultrasonography of the normal fetal brain. *Neuroradiology*, **28**, 380–5

7. Filly, R.A., Cardoza, J.D., Goldstein, R.B. and Barkovich, A.J. (1989). Detection of fetal central nervous system anomalies: a practical level of effort for a routine sonogram. *Radiology*, **172**, 403–8

8. Nyberg, D.A. (1989). Recommendations for obstetric sonography in the evaluation of the fetal cranium. *Radiology*, **172**, 309–11

9. Filly, R.A., Goldstein, R.B. and Callen, P.W. (1991). Fetal ventricle: importance in routine obstetric sonography. *Radiology*, **181**, 1–7

10. Romero, R., Pilu, G., Jeanty, P., Ghidini, A. and Hobbins, J.C. (1988). The central nervous system. In *Prenatal Diagnosis of Congenital Anomalies*, pp. 1–21. (Norwalk, CT: Appleton & Lange)

11. Timor-Tritsch, I.E., Monteagudo, A. and Warren, W.B. (1991). Transvaginal ultrasonographic definition of the central nervous system in the first and early second trimesters. *Am. J. Obstet. Gynecol.*, **164**, 497–503

12. Timor-Tritsch, I.E. and Monteagudo, A. (1991). Transvaginal sonographic evaluation of the fetal central nervous system. *Obstet. Gynecol. Clin. N. Am.*, **18**, 713–48

13. Ben-Ora, A., Eddy, L., Hatch, G. and Solida, B. (1980). The anterior fontanelle as an acoustic window to the neonatal ventricular system. *J. Clin. Ultrasound*, **8**, 65–7

14. Dewbury, K.C. and Aluwihare, A.P.R. (1980). The anterior fontanelle as an ultrasound window for study of the brain: a preliminary report. *Br. J. Radiol.*, **53**, 81–4

15. Slovis, T.L. and Kuhns, L.R. (1981). Real-time sonography of the brain through the anterior fontanelle. *Am. J. Roentgenol.*, **136**, 277–86

16. Cremin, B.J., Chilton, S.J. and Peacock, W.J. (1983). Anatomical landmarks in anterior fontanelle ultrasonography. *Br. J. Radiol.*, **56**, 517

17. Horbar, J.D., Leahy, K.A. and Lucey, J.F. (1983). Ultrasound identification of lateral ventricular asymmetry in the human neonate. *J. Clin. Ultrasound*, **11**, 67–9

18. Chi, J.G., Dooling, E.C. and Gilles, F.H. (1977). Gyral development of the human brain. *Ann. Neurol.*, **1**, 86

19. Dorovini-Zis, K. and Dolman, C.L. (1977). Gestational development of brain. *Arch. Pathol. Lab. Med.*, **101**, 192

20. Knutzon, R.K., McGahan, J.P., Salamat, M.S. and Brant, W.E. (1991). Cisterna magna septa: a normal anatomical finding. *J. Ultrasound Med.*, **11**, S13

21. Rumack, C.M., Johnson, M.L. (eds.) (1984). *Perinatal & Infant Brain Imaging: Role of Ultrasound and Computed Tomography*. (Chicago: Year Book Medical Publishers)

22. Naidich, T.P., Yousefzadeh, D.K. and Gusnard, D.A. (1986). The neonatal head. Sonography of the normal neonatal head. Supratentorial structures: state-of-the-art imaging. *Neuroradiology*, **28**, 408–27

23. Grant, E.G. (1986). *Neurosonography of the Pre-term Neonate*. (New York: Springer-Verlag)

24. Grant, E.G., Schellinger, D., Borts, F.T., McCullough, D.C., Friedman, G.R., Sivasubramanian, K.N. and Smith, Y. (1981). Real-time sonography of the neonatal and infant head. *Am. J. Roentgenol.*, **136**, 265–70

25. Johnson, M.L. and Rumack, C.M. (1980). Ultrasonic evaluation of the neonatal brain. *Radiol. Clin. N. Am.*, **18**, 117–31

26. Pigadas, A., Thompson, J.R. and Grube, G.L. (1981). Normal infant brain anatomy: correlated real-time sonograms and brain specimens. *Am. J. Neuroradiol.*, **2**, 339–44

27. Pilu, G., Sandri, F., Perolo, A., Pittalis, M.C., Grisdia, G., Cocchi, G., Forshini, M.P., Salvioli, G.P. and Bovicelli, L. (1993). Sonography of fetal agenesis of the corpus callosum: a survey of 35 cases. *Ultrasound Obstet. Gynecol.*, **3**, 318–29

28. Bronshtein, M. and Weiner, Z. (1992). Prenatal diagnosis of dilated cava septi pellucidi et vergae: associated anomalies, differential diagnosis, and pregnancy outcome. *Obstet. Gynecol.*, **80**, 838–42

29. Bowie, J.D., Kirks, D.R., Rosenberg, E.R. and Clair, M.R. (1983). Caudothalamic groove: value in identification of germinal matrix hemorrhage by sonography in preterm neonates. *Am. J. Roentgenol.*, **141**, 1317–20

30. Laing, F.C. (1983). Commonly encountered artifacts in clinical ultrasound. *Semin Ultrasound*, **4**, 27

31. Stanley, J.H., Harrell, B. and Horger, E.O. (1986). Pseudoepidural reverberation artifact: a common ultrasound artifact in fetal cranium. *J. Clin. Ultrasound*, **14**, 251–4

32. Bowerman, R.A. and DiPietro, M.A. (1987). Erroneous sonographic identification of fetal lateral ventricles: relationship to the echogenic periventricular 'blush'. *Am. J. Neuroradiol.*, **8**, 661–4

33. Rumack, C.M. and Johnson, M.L. (1984). Hydrocephalus. In Rumack, C.M. and Johnson, M.L. (eds.) *Perinatal & Infant Brain Imaging. Role of Ultrasound & Computed Tomography*, pp. 155–74. (Chicago: Year Book Medical Publishers)

34. Patten, R.M., Mack, L.A. and Finberg, H.J. (1991). Unilateral hydrocephalus: prenatal sonographic diagnosis. *Am. J. Roentgenol.*, **156**, 359–63

35. Chari, R., Bhargava, R., Hammond, I., Ventureyra, E.C. and Lalonde, A.B. (1993). Antenatal unilateral hydrocephalus. *Can. Assoc. Radiol. J.*, **44**, 57–9

36. Habib, Z. (1981). Genetics and genetic counselling in neonatal hydrocephalus. *Obstet. Gynecol. Surv.*, **36**, 529

37. Freeman, J.N. and Brann, A.W. Jr. (1977). Central nervous system disturbances. In Behrman, R. (ed.) *Neonatal Perinatal Medicine*, 2nd edn., pp.787–836. (St Louis: CV Mosby)

38. Milhorat, T.H. (1987). Hydrocephaly. In Myrianthopoulos, N.C. (ed.) *Handbook of Clinical Neurology. Malformations*, vol. 50, pp. 285–300. (Amsterdam: Elsevier Science Publishers)

39. Burton, B.K. (1979). Recurrence risks for cogenital hydrocephalus. *Clin. Genet.*, **16**, 47

40. Vintzileos, A.M., Ingardia, C.J. and Nochimson, D.J. (1983). Congenital hydrocephalus: a review and protocol for perinatal management. *Obstet. Gynecol.*, **62**, 539

41. London, D.A., Carroll, B.A. and Enzmann, D.R. (1980). Sonography of ventricular size and germinal matrix hemorrhage in premature infants. *Am. J. Roentgenol.*, **1**, 295

42. Sauerbrei, E.E., Digney, M., Harrison, P.B. and Cooperberg, P. (1981). Ultrasonic evaluation of neonatal intracranial hemorrhage and its complications. *Radiology*, **139**, 677

43. Poland, R.L., Slovis, T.L. and Shankaran, S. (1985). Normal values for ventricular sizes as determined by real time sonographic techniques. *Pediatr. Radiol.*, **15**, 12

44. Rumack, C.M. and Johnson, M.L. (1982). Real-time ultrasound evaluation of the neonatal brain. *Clin. Diagn. Ultrasound*, **10**, 179

45. Shackelford, G.D. (1986). Neurosonography of hydrocephalus in infants. *Neuroradiology*, **28**, 452

46. Naidich, T.P., Schott, L.H. and Baron, R.L. (1982). Computed tomography in evaluation of hydrocephalus. *Radiol. Clin. N. Am.*, **20**, 143

47. Naidich, T.P., Epstein, F., Lin, J.P., Kricheff, I.I. and Hochwald, G.M. (1976). Evaluation of pediatric hydrocephalus by computed tomography. *Radiology*, **119**, 337

48. Edwards, M.K. and Brown, D.L. (1982). Hydrocephalus and shunt function. Semin. *Ultrasound*, **3**, 242

49. Cardoza, J.D., Filly, R.A. and Podrasky, A.E. (1988). The dangling choroid plexus: a sonographic observation of value in excluding ventriculomegaly. *Am. J. Roentgenol.*, **151**, 767–70

50. Jeanty, P., Dramaix-Wilmet, M., Delbeke, D., Rodesch, F. and Struyven, J. (1981). Ultrasonic evaluation of fetal ventricular growth. *Neuroradiology*, **21**, 127

51. Pretorius, D.H., Drose, J.A. and Manco-Johnson, M.L. (1986). Fetal lateral ventricular ratio determination during the second trimester. *J. Ultrasound Med.*, **5**, 121

52. Cardoza, J.D., Goldstein, R.B. and Filly, R.A. (1988). Exclusion of fetal ventriculomegaly with a single measurement of the width of the lateral ventricular atrium. *Radiology*, **169**, 711

53. Pilu, G., Reece, E.A., Goldstein, I., Hobbins, J.C. and Bovicelli, L. (1989). Sonographic evaluation of the normal developmental anatomy of the fetal cerebral ventricles: II. The atria. *Obstet. Gynecol.*, **73**, 250–6

54. Siedler, D.E. and Filly, R.A. (1987). Relative growth of higher fetal brain structures. *J. Ultrasound Med.*, **6**, 573–6

55. Denkhaus, H. and Winsberg, F. (1979). Ultrasonic measurement of the fetal ventricular system. *Radiology*, **131**, 781–7

56. Johnson, M.L., Dunne, M.G., Mack, L.A. and Rashbaum, C.L. (1980). Evaluation of fetal intracranial anatomy by static and real-time ultrasound. *J. Clin. Ultrasound*, **8**, 311–18

57. Monteagudo, A., Timor-Tritsch, I.E. and Moomjy, M. (1993). Nomograms of the fetal lateral ventricles using transvaginal sonography. *J. Ultrasound Med.*, **5**, 265–9

58. Monteagudo, A., Timor-Tritsch, I.E. and Moomjy, M. (1994). In utero detection of ventriculomegaly during the second and third trimesters by transvaginal sonography. *Ultrasound Obstet. Gynecol.*, **4**, 193–8

59. Epstein, F., Naidich, T., Kricheff, I., Chase, N., Lin, J. and Ransohoff, J. (1977). Role of computerized axial tomography in diagnosis, treatment and follow-up of hydrocephalus. *Child's Brain*, **3**, 91–100

60. Fiske, C.E. and Filly, R.A. (1982). Ultrasonic evaluation of the normal and abnormal fetal neural axis. *Radiol. Clin. N. Am.*, **20**, 285–96

61. Benacerraf, B.R. and Birnholz, J.C. (1987). The diagnosis of fetal hydrocephalus prior to 22 weeks. *J. Clin. Ultrasound*, **15**, 531–6

62. Bronshtein, M. and Ben-Shlomo, I. (1991) Choroid plexus dysmorphism: a sonographic sign of fetal hydrocephalus. *J. Clin. Ultrasound*, **19**, 547–53

63. Chinn, D.H., Callen, P.W. and Filly, R.A. (1983). The lateral cerebral ventricle in early second trimester. *Radiology*, **148**, 529–31

64. Drugan, A., Krause, B., Canady, A., Zador, I.E. and Sacks, A.J. (1989). The natural history of prenatally diagnosed cerebral ventriculomegaly. *J. Am. Med. Assoc.*, **261**, 1785–8

65. Pretorius, D.H., Davis, K., Manco-Johnson, M.L., Manchester, D., Meier, P.R. and Clewell, W.H. (1985). Clinical course of fetal hydrocephalus: 40 cases. *Am. J. Roentgenol.*, **144**, 827–31

66. Chevernak, F.A., Berkowitz, R.L., Tortora, M. and Hobbins, J.C. (1985). The management of fetal hydrocephalus. *Am. J. Obstet. Gynecol.*, **151**, 933–42

67. Nyberg, D.A., Mack, L.A., Hirch, J., Pagon, R.O. and Shepard, T.H. (1987). Fetal hydrocephalus: sonographic detection and clinical significance of associated anomalies. *Radiology*, **82**, 692–7

68. Hudgins, R.J., Edwards, M.S., Goldstein, R., Callen, P.W., Harrison, M.R., Filly, R.A. and Golbus, M.S. (1988). Natural history of fetal ventriculomegaly. *Pediatrics*, **82**, 692–7

69. Glick, P.L., Harrison, M.R., Nakayama, D.K., Edwards, M.S., Filly, R.A., Chinn, D.H., Callen, P.W., Wilson, S.L. and Golbus, M.S. (1984). Management of ventriculomegaly in the fetus. *J. Pediatr.*, **105**, 97–105

70. Mahony, B.S., Nyberg, D.A., Hirsch, J.H., Petty, C.N., Hendricks, S.K. and Mack, L.A. (1988). Mild idiopathic lateral cerebral ventricular dilatation *in utero*: sonographic evaluation. *Radiology*, **169**, 715–21

71. Goldstein, R.B., LaPidus, A.S., Filly, R.A. and Cardoza, J. (1990). Mild lateral cerebral dilation *in utero*: clinical significance and prognosis. *Radiology*, **176**, 237–42

72. Bromley, B., Frigoletto, F.D. and Benacerraf, B.R. (1991). Mild fetal lateral cerebral ventriculomegaly: clinical course and outcome. *Am. J. Obstet. Gynecol.*, **164**, 863–7

73. Achiron, R., Schimmel, M., Achiron, A. and Mashiach, S. (1993). Fetal mild idiopathic lateral ventriculomegaly: is there a correlation with fetal trisomy? *Ultrasound Obstet. Gynecol.*, **3**, 89–92

Color Doppler assessment of early fetal cerebral circulation

7

A. Kurjak, S. Kupesic and D. Zudenigo

INTRODUCTION

At the present, color Doppler sonography is a unique non-invasive method for measurement of fetal cerebral blood flow changes in physiological and pathophysiological states of pregnancy. Fetal brain vascularity has been excessively analyzed during the second and third trimesters of pregnancy with this technique[1,2]. Studies on cerebral blood flow in this period of pregnancy in fetuses with intrauterine growth retardation (IUGR) have confirmed the results of experimental studies in fetal sheep which have shown that hypoxic fetuses redistributed their blood flow and gave preferential supply to the brain, myocardium and adrenals.

All these studies used the transabdominal approach, which did not enable a precise and reproducible investigation of cerebral blood flow in early pregnancy. The explosive progress of transvaginal ultrasound has recently enabled us to obtain anatomical images of even the small embryo or fetus in early pregnancy. As a result, the new clinical field, which was termed 'sonoembryology', was established. Transvaginal sonography combined with color Doppler ultrasound offered a new approach for the investigation of the human embryofetal circulation. Fetal blood flow in early pregnancy has consequently become the object of investigation in numerous institutions.

The purpose of this chapter is to summarize current understanding of the anatomy and physiology of the early cerebral circulation and to assess the nature of these circulatory modifications on normal pregnancy development.

ANATOMY AND REGULATION OF CEREBRAL CIRCULATION

Each cerebral hemisphere is supplied by an anterior, middle and posterior cerebral artery, the first two of which arise by the division of the internal carotid artery, the posterior being the terminal branch of the basilar artery. The circle of Willis (circulus arteriosus) is a seven-sided anastomosis of the main cerebral vessels completed by the short anterior communicating artery, located between the anterior cerebral arteries and, on each side, by the posterior communicating arteries, connecting the internal carotid artery with the posterior cerebral arteries.

The middle cerebral artery (MCA) is the largest branch of the circle of Willis and runs laterally in the Sylvian fissure as a continuation of the intracranial internal carotid artery. The middle cerebral artery sends branches to the corpus striatum as well as to the internal capsule. In its lateral portion it gives rise to the lenticular striate artery. It then continues its course backwards and upwards over the surface of the insula and the inferior frontal gyrus. The middle cerebral artery is extremely important in normal brain development and evolution. It has the highest volume of flow of all the vascular branches arising from the circle of Willis, carrying about 80% of the flow to the hemisphere. It consists of four segments: M1, M2 (segment of bifurcation or trifurcation), M3 and M4 (this segment runs temporally and frontally). The diameter of the MCA remains constant during various physiological and pathophysiological changes in brain metabolism and function.

Autoregulation of the cerebral circulation can be defined as the presence of a relatively constant blood flow despite moderate variations in perfusion pressure. It represents the mechanism that protects the brain from hypoxia (low pressure) and edema (high pressure)[2]. This definition of autoregulation is of cardinal importance in the context of the so-called 'brain-sparing effect'.

TRANSVAGINAL COLOR DOPPLER SONOGRAPHY

The central nervous system (CNS), mainly occupying the head, which is a comparatively simple anatomical structure, is the easiest part of the fetus for sonographic depiction. In terms of the embryo or fetus in early pregnancy, the ratio of the head to the whole body is as high as one-half to one-third. Accordingly, the CNS occupies the main part of the morphological observations of fetal development.

Between 7 and 8 menstrual weeks, the fetal cephalic pole is clearly distinguishable from the fetal torso, whereas in the developing brain the ventricular system has not yet partitioned, and the forebrain appears as a hypoechoic vesicle below the calvarial roof. Towards the end of the 8th week, the brain is divided by an echogenic line representing the falx cerebri.

At 9 weeks, the head begins to assume its round shape, and the falx cerebri becomes more prominent. On oblique scan it is possible to visualize the cerebral peduncles. At the beginning of the 10th week, the rostral brain vesicle, the telencephalon with its two lateral outpocketings representing the cerebral hemispheres, can be clearly seen. A transverse anatomic section for evaluation of the fetal brain at this gestational age is optimal. When this plane has been established, the transducer moves up and down to obtain details of the various anatomic levels. The most prominent intrahemispheric structures seen on a high transverse scan through the fetal head are the lateral ventricles. These are identified by the echogenic choroid plexus, which almost completely fills the bodies of the lateral ventricles. Caudally, a hypoechoic thalamus, the dominant portion of the developing diencephalon, can be visualized. Anteriorly to the thalami on the same scan plane, the cavum septum pellucidum appears as a central echo-free area adjacent to the frontal horns.

The mesencephalon, which is morphologically the most primitive of the brain vesicles, undergoes fewer changes than other parts of the developing brain. From the basal plate of the midbrain, swelling and enlargement of the marginal layer form the cruras cerebri or cerebral peduncles. The most caudal of the brain compartments, the myelencephalon, becomes the medulla, whereas the metencephalon differentiates ventrally into the pons and dorsally into the cerebellum, which can clearly be visualized and measured from the end of the 10th week.

From 11 weeks on, it is possible to obtain both coronal and sagittal sections of the fetal brain and face. On paramedian sagittal scan, the echogenic choroid plexus completely fills the body of the lateral ventricle; the thalamus, lamina tecti, brainstem and cerebellum appear as hypoechoic structures.

A mid-coronal scan shows an echogenic line above the thalamus, compatible with the corpus callosum; on the lower border of the thalamus the cerebral peduncles are visible. The hippocampi appear laterally to the cerebral peduncle. On a more posterior coronal plane, the posterior fossa with the cisterna magna appears as a hypoechoic structure at the site of spinal cord entry into the skull. Axial scans at 11 weeks can show the spongy appearance of the echogenic choroid plexus within the body of the lateral ventricles.

From the 12th week on, the fetal brain scan demonstrates the corpus striatum, which forms a longitudinal ridge in the floor of the lateral ventricle, and comes in close contact with the lateral surface of the thalamus. The capsula interna breaks through the nuclear mass of the corpus striatum, dividing it into the caudate and lentiform nuclei. A further caudal coronal section demonstrates the occipital lobes lateral to the cerebellar tentorium, with the occipital horns of the ventricles and the echogenic choroid plexus. The cerebellum is visualized under the cerebellar tentorium, and the vermis can be identified. On the same plane, the hypoechoic cisterna magna can be measured at a diameter of approximately 3 mm. The fourth ventricle and the sinii rectus are noted on axial scan as small hypoechoic structures in front of and behind the cerebellum[3].

The internal carotid artery and MCA are located at the base of the skull. The distance between these two arteries is a few millimeters or even less. Therefore, it is very difficult to distinguish blood flow between these two arteries. Based on its position only, arterial blood flow could be presumed to be the MCA.

The intracranial circulation becomes visible as early as the 8th week of gestation[4–7]. At this time, discrete pulsations of the internal carotid arteries are detectable at the base of the skull. During the 9th and the 10th gestational weeks, color patterns representing blood flow can be visualized in the anterolateral quadrant of the skull base. From the 10th gestational week, arterial pulsations can be detected on transverse section, lateral to the mesencephalon and cephalic flexure.

There are few transvaginal color Doppler studies of cerebral blood flow in early pregnancy. In the study of Wladimiroff and colleagues[8], flow velocity waveform recordings were made in the umbilical artery, fetal descending aorta and intracerebral arteries in 30 normal pregnancies between 11 and 13 weeks of gestation. No distinction could be made between the internal carotid, MCA or anterior cerebral artery waveforms. Technically acceptable flow velocity waveforms were obtained from intracerebral arteries in 21 fetuses (70%). Although flow velocity waveforms in the descending aorta and umbilical artery display absent end-diastolic flow, flow velocity waveforms in the intracerebral arteries are characterized by forward flow throughout the cardiac cycle. These results suggest a relatively lower vascular resistance at the fetal cerebral level in early gestation.

Van Zalen-Sprock and associates[9] analyzed blood flow in the fetal aorta, umbilical artery and cerebral arteries in 18 pregnant women between 6 and 16 weeks of gestation. Flow velocity waveforms of the umbilical artery were characterized by absence of end-diastolic velocities until the 12th week, while in the aorta, end-diastolic velocity was absent until the 14th week. The cerebral arteries showed positive end-diastolic velocity in all fetuses after the 10th week of gestation. The trend in the pulsatility index of the umbilical artery as well as of the aorta showed a strong decrease towards the 16th week. In the cerebral artery, the trend of the pulsatility index showed a mild gradual decrease towards the 16th week of pregnancy.

These data suggest a low vascular impedance in the fetal brain, not dependent on changes in vascular resistance of the fetal trunk or uteroplacental circulation. This apparently independent and autoregulatory mechanism thus provides an adequate blood supply to the growing fetal brain.

In our study[5], middle cerebral artery blood flow was analyzed in 106 pregnant women.

Table 1 Transvaginal color Doppler visualization rate for the intracranial circulation (middle cerebral artery) in early normal and complicated pregnancy (n = 106)

Gestational age (weeks)	Visualization rate (%)
8	50
9	71
10	83
11–18	100

Gestational age ranged from the 7th to the 18th gestational week. Women were divided into two groups. The first group included 75 clinically normal singleton pregnancies. Another 31 patients were admitted to the hospital because of vaginal bleeding. Seventeen of these complicated pregnancies ended in spontaneous abortion. The visualization rate of the MCA is displayed in Table 1.

A characteristic waveform profile, i.e. a systolic component with absent end-diastolic frequencies, was observed from the 8th to the 11th gestational week. The end-diastolic component of the blood flow was inconsistently seen from the 11th to the 13th gestational week, earlier than has been found in other fetal vessels. From the 13th gestational week onwards, end-diastolic flow within the MCA was consistently observed. A significant decrease of pulsatility index (PI) was observed in both groups of women and it was present 2 weeks earlier than has been noted in other parts of the fetal circulation[4] (Figure 1). However, there was no significant difference of PI between normal pregnancies and pregnancies complicated by vaginal bleeding, regardless of pregnancy outcome[5] (Figure 2). Our data are in accordance with the results of the groups of Wladimiroff and Van Zalen-Sprock and prove that cerebral vessels are a separate hemodynamic system that is independent of the other parts of the fetal circulation from the beginning of the pregnancy. Due to this mechanism, the fetal brain is probably well protected from hypoxia even in early pregnancy. Recently, more sophisticated equipment has enabled us to detect continuous diastolic flow in the MCA of embryos between 9 and 10 weeks of gestation. Color Plates B–D demonstrate the absence of diastolic flow in the fetal aorta and umbilical artery in the fetus with increased end-diastolic flow in the MCA.

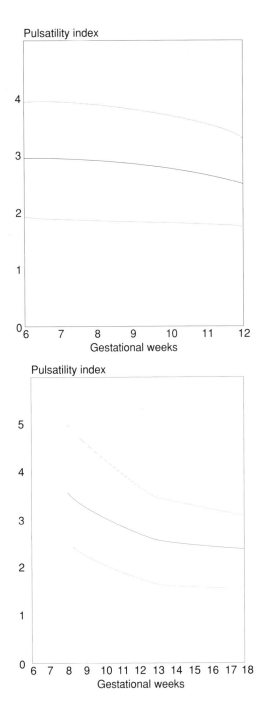

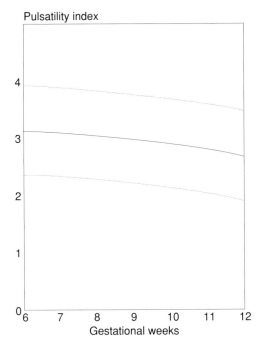

Figure 1 Reference range (mean ± 1SD) of the pulsatility index obtained from the umbilical artery (top left), fetal aorta (top right) and middle cerebral artery (bottom) in normal early pregnancy

index was found between normal pregnancies and those with threatened abortion that had a normal pregnancy outcome. In those with threatened abortion, there was no significant difference in vascular impedance between pregnancies with normal outcome and those that ended in spontaneous abortion.

Our results suggest that in cases of threatened abortion, there are no significant hemodynamic changes that could cause hypoxia and eventually affect fetal cerebral blood flow.

FETAL CHOROID PLEXUS VASCULARIZATION

The fetal choroid plexus plays a large role in brain development. It is proportionally larger than that of an adult human being and fills more of the space in the ventricles. The choroid plexus and arachnoid membrane act together as barriers between the blood and cerebrospinal fluid (CSF).

In our recent study[10], early cerebral blood flow was assessed in 90 women with normal intrauterine pregnancy and 60 women with symptoms of threatened abortion. In eight women with threatened abortion, subsequent abortion of a live fetus occurred. No difference in terms of the pulsatility

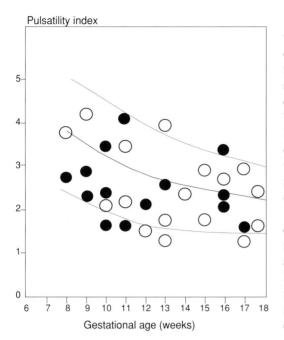

Figure 2 Pulsatility index values plotted on reference ranges for 31 pregnancies complicated by vaginal bleeding. Seventeen pregnancies ended in spontaneous abortion (open circles); and 14 continued as a normal pregnancy (filled circles)

In effect, the choroid plexus is like a 'kidney' for the brain[11]. It is not a simple excretory organ for creating CSF, but also provides the fluid with nutrients extracted from the blood. The choroid plexus also has an important role in the cleaning of the CSF of waste substances that exist in the brain tissues as by-products of metabolic reactions. In early to midpregnancy, fetal choroid plexus cells contain significant amounts of glycogen and serve as a storage site.

The choroid plexus of the lateral ventricles receives blood from the anterior and posterior choroidal arteries. A small anterior branch arises at the origin of the middle cerebral artery. The remainder of the blood supply comes from a posterior communicating artery. The choroid vein runs along the whole length of the outer border of the choroid plexus, receiving veins from the hippocampus major, the fornix and corpus callosum, and unites behind the anterior extremity of the choroid plexus with the vein of the corpus striatum.

The vascular network of the choroid plexus vessels is characteristic. Each frond consists of capillaries and other small blood vessels surrounded by a single layer of epithelial cells[11]. One side of each cell, called the basolateral surface, is in contact with blood plasma that filters through the 'leaky' wall of the choroid plexus capillaries. Hence, the behavior of the choroid plexus is quite different from that of the cerebral capillaries, which constitute the blood–brain barrier and mediate the diffusion of substances from the blood directly into the interstitial fluid.

Studies evaluating the function of the fetal choroid plexus are limited. A current debate revolves around the role of choroid plexus cysts and their association with fetal trisomy[12–14]. Because trisomies are associated with mental retardation, we undertook a study to define the normal development of blood flow in the fetal choroid plexus[15].

Our study comprised 102 patients with healthy pregnancies between 9 and 16 weeks' gestation. Imaging was performed transvaginally, except in the pregnancies of longer duration with unfavorable fetal positions. Color flow imaging was used to identify vessels in the cranium and within the choroid plexus. Pulsed Doppler signals were obtained from an internal carotid–middle cerebral artery and from choroid plexus vessels. The pulsatility index was calculated from the Doppler spectral envelope.

A major cerebral vessel could be seen at 9 weeks' gestation. Choroid plexus vessels were first seen at 10 weeks 3 days. Subtle color and pulsed Doppler signals could be obtained at the inner edge of the lateral ventricle choroid plexus. The pulsed Doppler waveform profile of choroid plexus blood vessels was characteristic. The systolic component of blood flow within a cardiac cycle was not pronounced, while the slope from the systolic peak till the end of the cycle was very mild (Color Plate E).

In most of the cases, it appeared that there was end-diastolic flow, but because of the wall filters, it was not displayed. Very low velocities are an additional reason that the end-diastolic component could not be obtained before 12 gestational weeks. The visualization rates for the cerebral and choroid plexus vessels are shown in Figure 3. With

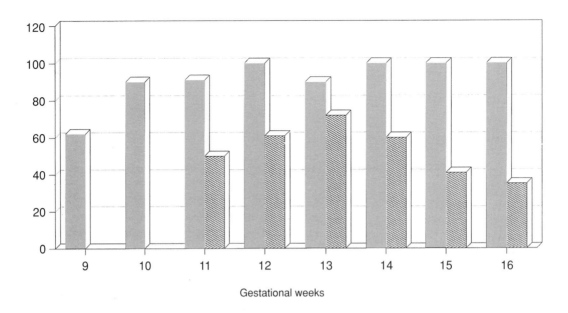

Figure 3 Visualization rate (%) of cerebral artery (gray bars) and choroid plexus vessels (hatched bars). Note peaking and decline of choroid plexus imaging

current technology, there is good success in observing and measuring these vessels. Visualization rates range from 35 to 75% for plexus vessels, and 65 to 100% for cerebral vessels. The visualization of the cerebral vessels improves with each gestational week. Choroid plexus vessels are most easily seen at 13 weeks, and then visualization rates decline. Visualization of the vessels of the choroid plexus increases and decreases as the gland develops and shrinks. As the majority of studies have been performed vaginally, this decline cannot be attributed to differences in the approach.

Figure 4 portrays the evolution of the flow velocity levels in the two measured structures. In both cases, a steady decline in resistance and a probable increase in flow (assuming no increase in blood pressure and change in pulse rate) is evident. The pulsatility index for the cerebral arteries at this gestational period averaged 2.6 ± 0.6. The result for the choroid plexus was 1.66 ± 0.5 ($p < 0.001$).

Our results showed significant flow velocity differences between the larger cerebral vessels and the smaller choroidal vessels. This is characteristic of other organs as well. For example, the larger vessels encounter the resistance of the entire organ,

but the smaller vessels supply smaller areas with a more uniform vascular network.

Visualization of pulsatility flow in the choroid plexus was possible at 10 weeks 3 days' gestation. This coincides with morphological development. Four stages of differentiation have been observed in the development of the human telencephalic plexus. The period occupied by this study is stage II, at 9–17 weeks. During this period, the plexus is characterized by low columnar epithelium with apical nuclei. The epithelial cells have abundant glycogen and villi are sparse. The stroma is composed of extremely loose mesenchyme, with a small amount of connective tissue fibers. Tubules then begin to appear. Also present are definite vascular walls, capillaries located subepithelially, and large blood vessels in the central interstitium. The plexus is extremely large in its relation to the size of the ventricles. As pregnancy continues, the epithelium becomes cuboidal, the glycogen diminishes, tubules are numerous, capillaries and vessels proliferate, large vessels decrease, and overall size diminishes[16].

Cystic structures are seen in approximately 30% of histological specimens from aborted fetuses[16]. The cysts form when the stroma proliferates,

Pulsatility index

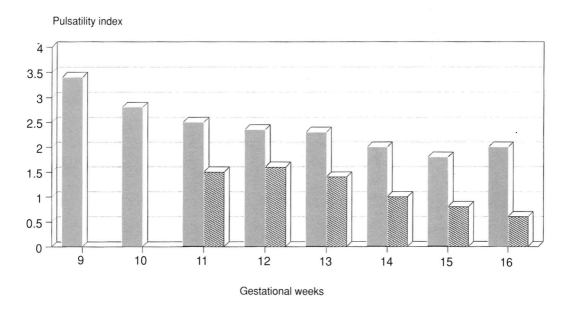

Gestational weeks

Figure 4 Evolution of intracranial flow velocity. Pulsatility indices decline progressively, suggesting decreasing of resistance to flow velocity. Gray bars, cerebral artery; hatched bars, choroid plexus

causing folding and agglutination of the neuroepithelium. Congenital hypoplasia of the lateral ventricular choroid plexus causes severe hydrocephaly. Tumors of the choroid plexus include angioma, berry aneurysm, epidermoidal tumors, lipomas, nodular hyperplasia, adenoma (ependymoma), meningiomas and carcinoma.

The choroid plexus is largest when the brain is undergoing its maximum neurogenesis. This study shows that vascularization also proceeds in parallel fashion. Further study of this structure might prove useful in the evaluation of fetal and neonatal brain maturation.

CONCLUSION

The introduction of the transvaginal color Doppler technique has opened new frontiers in the investigation of the early uteroplacental and fetal circulation. The early fetal cerebral circulation is of great importance for normal development of the fetal brain, and the first color Doppler studies showed that it was independent of the other parts of the fetal circulation. Therefore, it can be concluded that the fetal brain is well protected from hypoxia, even in early pregnancy. Investigation of choroid plexus vascularization has confirmed that the choroid plexus is an organ with specific and separated hemodynamic characteristics. This could contribute to a better understanding of the function of the choroid plexus in early brain development.

Indeed, the possibility of precise and reproducible investigation of early fetal cerebral circulation provided by transvaginal color Doppler will undoubtedly contribute to better understanding of the physiology and pathophysiology of early pregnancy.

References

1. Mari, G. and Deter, R.L. (1992). Middle cerebral artery flow velocity waveforms in normal and small-for-gestational age fetuses. *Am. J. Obstet. Gynecol.*, **166**, 1262–70

2. Marsal, K., Gudmundsson, S. and Stale, H. (1994). Cerebral circulation in the perinatal period. In Kurjak, A. and Chervenak, F. (eds.) *The Fetus as a Patient*, pp. 477–90. (Carnforth, UK: Parthenon Publishing)

3. Achiron, R. and Achiron, A. (1991). Transvaginal ultrasonic assessment of the early fetal brain. *Ultrasound Obstet. Gynecol.*, **1**, 336–44

4. Kurjak, A., Predanic, M. and Predanic, A. (1993). Fetal intracranial circulation. In Kurjak, A. (ed.) *An Atlas of Transvaginal Color Doppler*, p. 71. (Carnforth, UK: Parthenon Publishing)

5. Kurjak, A., Predanic, M., Kupesic, S., Funduk-Kurjak, B., Demarin, V. and Salihagic, A. (1992). Transvaginal color Doppler study of middle cerebral artery blood flow in early normal and abnormal pregnancy. *Ultrasound Obstet. Gynecol.*, **2**, 424–8

6. Kurjak, A., Zudenigo, D. and Kupesic, S. (1994). Early pregnancy hemodynamics assessed by transvaginal color Doppler. In Kurjak, A. and Chervenak, F. (eds.) *The Fetus as a Patient*, pp. 435–54. (Carnforth, UK: Parthenon Publishing)

7. Kurjak, A., Zudenigo, D., Predanic, M. and Kupesic, S. (1994). Recent advances in the Doppler study of early fetomaternal circulation. *J. Perinat. Med.*, **22**, 419–39

8. Wladimiroff, J.W., Huisman, T.W.A. and Stewart, P.A. (1992). Intracerebral, aortic, and umbilical artery flow velocity waveforms in the late-first-trimester fetus. *Am. J. Obstet. Gynecol.*, **166**, 46–9

9. Van Zalen-Sprock, M.M., van Vugt, J.M.G., Colenbrander, G.J. and van Geijn, H.P. (1994). First-trimester uteroplacental and fetal blood flow velocity waveforms in normally developing fetuses: a longitudinal study. *Ultrasound Obstet. Gynecol.*, **4**, 284–8

10. Kurjak, A., Zudenigo, D., Predanic, M., Kupesic, S. and Funduk, B. (1994). Transvaginal color Doppler study of fetomaternal circulation in threatened abortion. *Fet. Diagn. Ther.*, **9**, 341–7

11. Spector, R. and Johanson, C.E. (1989). The mammalian choroid plexus. *Sci. Am.*, **6**, 48–53

12. Chudleigh, P., Pearce, J. and Campbell, S. (1984). The prenatal diagnosis of transient cysts of the fetal choroid plexus. *Prenat. Diagn.*, **4**, 435–8

13. Platt, L., Carlson, D., Medearis, A., Nelson, N.L. and Johnson, P. (1991). Fetal choroid plexus cysts in the second trimester: a cause for concern. *Am. J. Obstet. Gynecol.*, **164**, 1632–5

14. Nelson, N.L., Callen, P.W. and Filly, R.A. (1992). The choroid plexus pseudocyst: sonographic identification and characterization. *J. Ultrasound Med.*, **11**, 597–601

15. Kurjak, A., Schulman, H., Predanic, A., Predanic, M.,Kupesic, S. and Zalud, I. (1994). Fetal choroid plexus vascularization assessed by color and pulsed Doppler. *J. Ultrasound Med.*, **13**, 841–4

16. Netsky, M.G. and Shuangshoti, S. (1975). *The Choroid Plexus in Health and Disease*. (Charlottesville: University Press of Virginia)

Doppler assessment of fetal brain circulation during late pregnancy

8

K. Maršál, G. Gunnarsson and A. Maesel

INTRODUCTION

It is of great interest to study the changes of blood flow in the brain of human fetuses and to elucidate the pathophysiological mechanisms behind perinatal brain damage in relation to the immediate and long-term outcome of pregnancies. Experience from experimental studies on fetal sheep indicating that hypoxic fetuses redistribute their blood flow and give preferential supply to the brain [1–3] stimulated ultrasound experts to examine whether the phenomenon of 'brain sparing' could be identified in human fetuses and, possibly, used for clinical purposes. The first successful recording of blood velocities from the fetal common carotid artery was reported in 1984 using a combined linear array real-time and pulsed Doppler ultrasound method [4]. Already in this first report, a difference was observed between normally grown fetuses and fetuses that were small-for-gestational age (SGA), the latter having a lower pulsatility index (PI) in the blood velocity recorded from the common carotid artery. That finding, indicating lower peripheral vascular resistance in the cerebral circulation, was then confirmed by the examinations of the fetal internal carotid artery [5] and middle cerebral artery [6], when combined pulsed Doppler and sector real-time scanners became available.

More recently, the technical development of Doppler ultrasound with color flow imaging enabled studies of other fetal cerebral vessels, e.g. the anterior and posterior cerebral arteries [7]. Thus, it became possible to evaluate the cerebral circulation *in utero*, both antenatally and during labor. As in other vessel areas in the fetus, the present Doppler technique does not allow an accurate quantitative measurement of cerebral blood flow. Blood velocity waveform analysis offers only an indirect measure of the hemodynamic situation in the fetal brain. Still, the information obtained is of considerable interest.

In this chapter, an account is given of the published Doppler ultrasound studies examining the cerebral circulation antenatally and during labor.

FETAL CEREBRAL VELOCIMETRY DURING LATE PREGNANCY

Uncomplicated pregnancies

Each cerebral hemisphere is supplied by anterior, middle and posterior cerebral arteries, the first two arising by the division of the internal carotid artery, the posterior being the terminal branch of the basilar artery. The circle of Willis is a seven-sided anastomosis of the main cerebral vessels completed by the short anterior communicating artery, located between the anterior cerebral arteries and, on each side, by the posterior communicating arteries connecting the internal carotid artery with the posterior cerebral arteries. The color Doppler technique enables visualization of the circle of Willis and identification of its branches (Color Plate F).

Middle cerebral artery

Since the use of color-coded Doppler for localizing intracranial vessels became common, most authors choose to study the middle cerebral artery, since this vessel is usually the most accessible major cerebral vessel *in utero* [7] (Figure 1). A prerequisite for a successful recording of Doppler signals is that the fetal head is not too far engaged in the maternal pelvis. In a longitudinal study, Meerman and associates [8] did not show a statistically significant

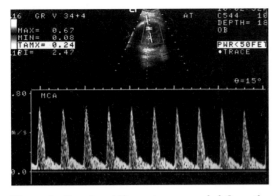

Figure 1 Doppler shift spectrum recorded from the middle cerebral artery of a healthy fetus at 34 weeks of gestation

decrease in PI, although their findings suggested an increase in cerebral blood flow with advancing gestational age. Similarly, Noordam and co-workers[9] did not find a significant negative correlation between the PI and gestational age. They explained this finding by the fact that all measurements were performed on fetuses younger than 34 weeks of gestation. Several authors have studied the fetal middle cerebral artery and found an increasing PI until the late second trimester of pregnancy, followed by a decline in the third trimester[10–13] (Figure 2; Table 1). Mari and Deter[12] have proposed a theory for the rise in pulsatility

in the second trimester and decline in the third trimester – they attributed the low PI values at the beginning and the end of pregnancy to increased metabolic requirements and therefore lower cerebral vascular impedance to blood flow. Gunnarsson and Maršál[13] speculated that this phenomenon might be due to an evolutionary pattern in the blood supply of the developing brain, where the blood supply changes from a centrifugal to a centripetal pattern as the cerebral hemispheres develop and the germinal matrix decreases.

In a longitudinal study, Arström and colleagues[14] have studied the fetal middle cerebral artery and did not find any detectable blood flow velocities in end-diastole before 28 weeks of gestation. This finding conflicts with the reports in some more recent studies[13] and might be due to the ultrasound equipment used.

The possible dependence on fetal activity of the velocity waveform shape has been examined for the fetal internal carotid artery[15] and middle cerebral artery[16]. The middle cerebral artery PI was found to be lower in active than inactive fetuses before 28 weeks of gestation. The difference was less pronounced during the third trimester. In healthy term fetuses, the change in activity evoked by a vibroacoustic stimulation did not influence the middle cerebral artery PI[17].

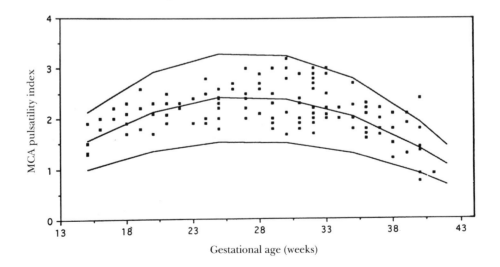

Figure 2 Pulsatility index of middle cerebral artery (MCA) plotted against gestational age. (Reproduced, with permission, from reference 12)

Table 1 Relation between the middle cerebral artery pulsatility index (PI) and gestational age (GA) in normal fetuses

Authors	Regression equation	Coefficient of determination (r^2)
Arström et al.[14]	$PI = 5.13 - 0.09 \times GA$	0.52
Kofinas et al.[16]	$PI = 3.477 - 0.055 \times GA$	0.40
Noordam et al.[9]*	$PI = 2.65 - 0.03 \times GA$	0.04
van den Wijngaard et al.[10]	$PI = -3.44 + 0.36 \times GA - 0.006 \times GA^2$	—
Arduini and Rizzo[11]	$PI = -0.006 + 0.144 \times GA - 0.003 \times GA^2$	0.52
Mari and Deter[12]	$PI = -1.97 + 0.327 \times GA - 0.006 \times GA^2$	0.45
Gunnarsson and Maršál[13]	$PI = -2.703 + 0.369 \times GA - 0.006 \times GA^2$	0.48

*Includes only fetuses younger than 34 weeks of gestation

Anterior cerebral artery and posterior cerebral artery

The success rate in recording blood velocity signals from the fetal anterior and posterior cerebral arteries was found to be 98% and 87%, respectively[9]. Both the anterior and posterior cerebral arteries show a fall in PI in the third trimester of pregnancy[9,18]. The PI of the proximal anterior cerebral artery has been shown to be significantly different from the PI in the middle cerebral artery and not significantly different from the PI in the internal carotid artery[18]. This emphasizes the necessity of knowing exactly which vessel is being examined.

Complicated pregnancies

Intrauterine growth retardation

The finding of proportionally increased diastolic velocity and decreased PI of blood velocity waveforms recorded from the cerebral vessels of growth retarded fetuses suggests a decreased resistance and, consequently, increased flow in the cerebral vascular bed (Figure 3). This is in agreement with the above-mentioned animal experimental studies[1-3]. In the human SGA fetuses, as compared with control fetuses, a reduction in PI was described for the common carotid artery[4], internal carotid artery[19], middle cerebral artery[6] and anterior and posterior cerebral arteries[10]. Noordam and colleagues[9] compared the power of the various velocity waveform variables and different cerebral vessels for discriminating between SGA

and control fetuses. All examined vessels – internal carotid artery, middle, anterior and posterior cerebral vessels – showed significantly lower PI in SGA fetuses. However, the most sensitive discriminator was the end-diastolic velocity in the middle and anterior cerebral arteries, showing a highly significant increase[9].

In SGA fetuses, the ratio of the mean flow velocity in the common carotid artery and that of the fetal descending aorta predicted a pathological fetal heart rate (FHR) tracing with a sensitivity of 94% and a specificity of 60%[20]. In a combined cordocentesis and Doppler velocimetry study, the best predictor of asphyxia was an index comprising the aortic mean velocity and the common carotid artery PI[21]. Both the common carotid

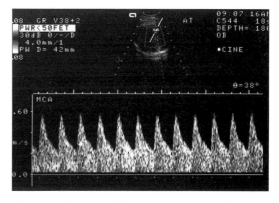

Figure 3 Doppler shift spectrum recorded from the middle cerebral artery of a growth-retarded, 38-week-old fetus. Note the pronounced increase in the diastolic flow velocities as an expression of the redistribution of flow (brain-sparing phenomenon)

artery PI and the ratio between the common carotid PI and the PI in the aorta or umbilical artery have been shown to differ significantly between normal fetuses and growth-retarded fetuses and fetuses with imminent asphyxia[22].

The flow velocity waveforms in the middle cerebral artery in human pregnancies with intrauterine growth retardation (IUGR) have been studied by many authors, all reports presenting according results[9, 10, 12, 23–29]. Vyas and colleagues[30] performed Doppler velocimetry and cordocentesis in 81 SGA fetuses and found a significant correlation between fetal hypoxemia and the degree of reduction in the fetal middle cerebral artery PI. The maximum reduction in PI was found when the fetal pO_2 was 2–4 SD below the gestational-age-related mean of the normal population. When the oxygen deficit was greater, there was a tendency for the PI to rise. Arduini and co-workers[24] found that a maximum vasodilatation in fetal cerebral arteries was reached 2 weeks before the onset of antepartum late FHR decelerations, whereas significant changes in the peripheral and umbilical vessel PI occurred close to the onset of abnormal FHR patterns. Mari and Deter[12] stated that the SGA fetus with a normal middle cerebral artery PI was at lower risk than the fetus with abnormal PI values. In another comparative study, hypoxemia at delivery appeared to be better recognized by the fetal middle cerebral artery flow velocity waveform than by the FHR analysis[28]. However, the specificity of the method was low. Favre and colleagues[29] found that fetal cerebral velocimetry showed a poor sensitivity and a low positive predictive value for prediction of IUGR and fetal acidosis. Using the technique of receiver operating characteristic curves, Noordam and associates[9] demonstrated that umbilical artery PI was superior to any of the Doppler velocity parameters of the fetal cerebral vessels as an indicator of IUGR.

In an attempt to improve diagnostic accuracy, some authors have studied the ratio between Doppler waveform indices in the fetal middle cerebral artery and umbilical artery. Gramellini and co-workers[26] reported the diagnostic accuracy [(true positives + true negatives)/total number of cases] in predicting adverse perinatal outcome for the cerebral:umbilical ratio to be 90%, as compared with 79% for the middle cerebral artery and 83% for the umbilical artery. These results, although encouraging, await confirmation.

The fetal internal carotid artery has also been extensively studied in the context of IUGR[5, 9, 14, 24, 31–36]. Arduini and colleagues[31] used fetal cerebral Doppler ultrasonography as a screening tool at 26–28 weeks of gestation in high-risk pregnancies and found the ratio of PI between the umbilical artery and the internal carotid artery to be an accurate predictor of growth retardation (specificity 92%; sensitivity 78%; positive predictive value 82%; negative predictive value 90%; accuracy 88%). In the study by McCowan and Duggan[33] on 28 SGA fetuses, there was a highly significant association between an abnormal internal carotid waveform and a poor outcome; this was particularly pronounced at a gestational age of less than 34 weeks, where the sensitivity, specificity and predictive values were all 100%. The authors pointed out that whether or not this information should be used clinically is not clear, as the abnormal umbilical and internal carotid waveforms were sometimes present for weeks before delivery occurred, due to fetal causes. In a study of 44 cases of IUGR with eight perinatal deaths, Wladimiroff and associates[36] did not find any correlation between the indicators of fetal well-being (Apgar score at 1 min, FHR patterns, umbilical arterial pH) and the internal carotid artery PI.

Fetal hydrocephalus

In cases of fetal hydrocephaly, blood flow velocity waveforms in the fetal internal carotid artery have been studied. Degani and co-workers[37] described four fetuses with hydrocephalus diagnosed at 24–33 weeks of gestation. The velocimetry results showed an inverse relation to the degree of ventriculomegaly in all four fetuses. A sharp decrease and later a total cessation of blood flow during diastole was observed. Three out of four pregnancies were electively terminated; no neurological follow-up on the surviving infant was presented. Van den Wijngaard and colleagues[38] presented data on nine fetuses with bilateral symmetrical hydrocephalus and four with unilateral hydrocephaly. An elevated internal carotid artery PI was demonstrated in five cases. The fetal outcome was poor: only one infant seemed to be developing normally at 1 year of age. There was no relation between the PI and fetal outcome. Finally, Kirkinen and associates[39] studied flow velocity waveforms from the internal carotid artery in nine hydrocephalic fetuses during the second and third trimesters of pregnancy. Normal, increased and decreased values of waveform indices were found in these cases; one of the fetuses presented retrograde diastolic flow. Cerebral blood flow patterns in hydrocephalic fetuses seemed to vary from case to case, presenting no typical changes in late pregnancy. There was no obvious correlation between the degree of ventricular dilatation and the velocity waveform.

The published cases do not justify any definitive conclusions to be drawn about the prognostic significance of cerebral blood flow measurements in cases of fetal hydrocephaly. For the assessment of the prognosis, the most important factors are other malformations possibly associated with the cerebral abnormalities[39].

Polyhydramnios

Mari and associates[40] examined flow velocity waveforms in the middle cerebral artery of fetuses before and after amniotic fluid decompression in symptomatic polyhydramnios. After amniocentesis, the PI of the middle cerebral artery was reduced in all fetuses. The authors concluded that the impact of acute amniotic fluid decompression on the fetal circulation as reflected in the marked PI changes, suggests a possible role of cerebral velocimetry in avoiding large acute changes in pressure during therapeutic amniocentesis.

Oligohydramnios

Van den Wijngaard and colleagues[41] described flow velocity waveforms in the fetal internal carotid artery in five cases of oligohydramnios due to bilateral renal agenesis. End-diastolic flow velocity was reduced, absent or even reversed, resulting in raised PI in all five cases. The authors hypothesized that prolonged severe oligohydramnios may hamper cerebral blood flow, because of fetal head compression.

Subdural hematoma

Ben-Chetrit and co-workers[42] diagnosed antenatally a posterior fossa subdural hematoma in a fetus at 30 weeks of gestation. Doppler velocimetry studies of the middle cerebral artery at that time showed an abnormally high resistance pattern with reverse end-diastolic flow. The ultrasonic assessment of the fetus indicated associated quadriplegia. No cause for the lesion was demonstrated antenatally or at pathological examination postpartum. In the authors' opinion, this case demonstrates the advantage of the determination of cerebral blood flow in the evaluation of cases with suspected high intracranial pressure.

Fetal asphyxia

Two reports on the terminal patterns of the fetal cerebral blood velocity have been published. Chandran and associates[43] followed a case with proteinuric pre-eclampsia superimposed on essential hypertension and IUGR diagnosed at 22 weeks of gestation. Starting 14 days before fetal death, the middle cerebral artery was examined on four occasions. A progressive fall in PI was followed by an increase registered 12h before fetal death. A similar increase in the middle cerebral PI preceding fetal death has also been reported in a case of a pregnant woman with lupus anticoagulant[44]. Pre-terminal brain edema has been suggested as the underlying cause of this phenomenon[30].

FETAL CEREBRAL VELOCIMETRY DURING LABOR

Fetal cerebral blood flow during labor has not been studied as extensively as during the antenatal and neonatal periods. This is partly due to the practical and ethical problems involved in performing Doppler measurements in labor. For the same reason, most human studies during labor describe normal physiological changes.

Uterine contractions, molding of the skull and metabolic changes during labor are some of the factors possibly influencing fetal cerebral blood flow. It is known that uterine contractions reduce the blood flow velocities in uterine vessels[45–47]. However, the umbilical circulation seems to remain unaffected by the contractions[45, 46, 48, 49]. An experimental animal study has shown that external mechanical compression of the fetal skull leads to a reduction of cerebral blood flow followed by a redistribution of flow with preferential supply to the brainstem[50]. In humans, it has been shown that pressure applied to the maternal abdomen increases the vascular resistance in fetal cerebral vessels[51]. Clinical Doppler studies of the fetal cerebral circulation in labor have given very varying results. One possible explanation for this is the difficulty in controlling the intensity of uterine contractions. These might have a more pronounced effect on the fetal cerebral circulation in the active phase of labor than in the earlier stage of labor.

Due to anatomical circumstances, e.g. the fetal skull being located behind the symphysis of the mother, transabdominal measurement of fetal cerebral flow velocity waveforms is difficult to perform during the second stage of labor. The transvaginal approach might be a solution to this problem.

Several published studies have compared the fetal cerebral PI values during and between contractions. An increase in vascular resistance was described during uterine contractions in the fetal internal carotid artery[52] and in the anterior cerebral artery[53]. However, other authors found no difference in the anterior cerebral artery[54] and in the middle cerebral artery[55]. An interesting finding in the study by Yagel and colleagues[56] showed a reduction of 40% in the vascular resistance in the fetal middle cerebral artery during labor. The authors speculated that this was a protective process aiming to prevent fetal cerebral hypoxia. Their finding was further supported by a study demonstrating that the fetal aortic blood flow increased with the progress of labor[57].

During normal vaginal delivery, at the moment of birth, a decompression of the fetal skull occurs. At this moment, very high time-averaged maximum velocity and low resistance values were found in the middle cerebral artery of healthy neonates, suggesting high cerebral blood flow[58]. In a study of infants delivered by means of Cesarean section, Ipsiroglu and associates[59] reported the highest blood velocities among those infants, where the obstetrician had difficulties in delivering the head.

The mode of delivery is known to influence various neonatal parameters, most of them reflecting the stress occurring during vaginal delivery. Levels of catecholamines are lower in babies delivered by means of elective Cesarean section than in those delivered vaginally[60]. Furthermore, the body temperature of newborn infants is lower after Cesarean section[61]. The mode of delivery did not seem to influence the time-averaged blood flow velocity in cerebral arteries of healthy term neonates shown by Shuto and co-workers[62], nor in our own study comparing the time-averaged blood velocity in the middle cerebral artery after vaginal delivery and after elective Cesarean section (A. Maesel and colleagues, in preparation).

SUMMARY

The Doppler ultrasound technique, combining the spectral and color Doppler mode, has made it possible to evaluate the fetal cerebral blood circulation non-invasively *in utero*. The analysis of blood velocity waveforms gives information on the resistance in the cerebral vascular bed, and the changes in time-averaged blood velocity reflect the changes in blood flow. For the main fetal cerebral vessels, i.e. the middle cerebral artery, anterior and posterior cerebral arteries, and common and internal carotid arteries, reference values of velocity waveform indices have been established. In general, during the last trimester of pregnancy, the values of waveform indices (pulsatility index, resistance index) in all fetal cerebral vessels decrease. In Doppler studies performed during labor in healthy fetuses, no significant influence of uterine contractions on fetal cerebral circulation was observed. Immediately after birth, a decrease in the vascular resistance and an increase in the mean velocity was observed in the middle cerebral artery. There was no difference in the mean blood velocity between the infants born vaginally and those born by means of Cesarean section. In growth-retarded fetuses, especially those developing signs of hypoxia, the waveform indices of cerebral vessels are often low, indicating the redistribution of flow – the brain-sparing effect. The first clinical reports suggest that Doppler velocimetry of fetal cerebral vessels might be useful as a clinical test with regard to the prediction of fetal outcome. However, the possible place of cerebral velocimetry in clinical management has not yet been decided.

References

1. Rudolph, A.M. and Heymann, M.A. (1967). The circulation of the fetus *in utero. Circ. Res.*, **21**, 163–84

2. Cohn, H.E., Sacks, E.J., Heymann, M.A. and Rudolph, A.M. (1974). Cardiovascular responses to hypoxemia and acidemia in fetal lambs. *Am.J. Obstet. Gynecol.*, **120**, 817–24

3. Peeters, L.L.H., Sheldon, R.E., Jones, M.D., Makowski, E.L. and Meschia, G. (1979). Blood flow to fetal organs as a function of arterial oxygen content. *Am. J. Obstet. Gynecol.*, **135**, 637–46

4. Maršál, K., Lingman, G. and Giles, W. (1984). Evaluation of the carotid, aortic and umbilical blood velocity waveforms in the human fetus. In *Society for the Study of Fetal Physiology, XI. Annual Conference*, p. C33. (Oxford: Nuffield Institute of Fetal Physiology)

5. Wladimiroff, J.W., Tonge, H.M. and Stewart, P.A. (1986). Doppler ultrasound assessment of cerebral blood flow in the human fetus. *Br. J. Obstet. Gynaecol.*, **63**, 471–5

6. Kirkinen, P., Müller, R., Huch, R. and Huch, A. (1987). Blood flow velocity waveforms in human fetal intracranial arteries. *Obstet. Gynecol.*, **70**, 617–21

7. Arbeille, P.H., Tranquart, F., Berson, M., Roncin, A., Saliba, E. and Pourcelot, L. (1989). Visualization of the fetal circle of Willis and intracerebral arteries by color-coded Doppler. *Eur. J. Obstet. Gynecol. Reprod. Biol.*, **32**, 195–8

8. Meerman, R.J., van Bel, F., van Zwieten, P.H.T., Oepkes, D. and den Ouden, L. (1990). Fetal and neonatal cerebral blood velocity in the normal fetus and neonate – a longitudinal Doppler ultrasound study. *Early Hum. Dev.*, **24**, 209–17

9. Noordam, M.J., Heydanus, R., Hop, W.C.J., Hoekstra, F.M.E. and Wladimiroff, J.W. (1994). Doppler colour flow imaging of fetal intracerebral arteries and umbilical artery in the small for gestational age fetus. *Br. J. Obstet. Gynaecol.*, **101**, 504–8

10. van den Wijngaard, J.A.G.W., Groenenberg, I.A.L., Wladimiroff, J.W. and Hop, W.C.J. (1989). Cerebral Doppler ultrasound of the human fetus. *Br. J. Obstet. Gynaecol.*, **96**, 845–9

11. Arduini, D. and Rizzo, G. (1990). Normal values of pulsatility index from fetal vessels: a cross-sectional study on 1556 healthy fetuses. *J. Perinat. Med.*, **18**, 165–72

12. Mari, G. and Deter, R.L. (1992). Middle cerebral artery flow velocity waveforms in normal and small-for-gestational-age fetuses. *Am. J. Obstet. Gynecol.*, **166**, 1262–70

13. Gunnarsson, G. O. and Maršál, K. (1994). Blood flow velocity waveforms in the middle cerebral, renal and femoral arteries of human fetuses. *Acta Obstet. Gynecol. Scand.*, in press

14. Arström, K., Eliasson, A., Hareide, J.H. and Maršál, K. (1989). Fetal blood velocity waveforms in normal pregnancies. A longitudinal study. *Acta Obstet. Gynecol. Scand.*, **68**, 171–8

15. Wladimiroff, J.W. and Cheung, K. (1989). Vibratory acoustic stimulation and the flow velocity waveform in the fetal internal carotid artery. *Early Hum. Dev.*, **19**, 61–6

16. Kofinas, A.D., Cavanaugh, S., McGuines, T., Simon, N.V., King, K. and Clay, D. (1994). The effect of fetal heart rate and fetal activity on the middle cerebral artery flow velocity waveforms in normal human fetuses from 18 to 42 weeks gestation. *J. Matern. Fetal Invest.*, **9**, 93–9

17. Maesel, A., Sladkevicius, P., Valentin, L. and Maršál, K. (1994). Effect of vibroacoustic stimulation on blood circulation in the middle cerebral and umbilical arteries in healthy term fetuses. *J. Matern. Fetal Invest.*, **9**, 69–72

18. Mari, G., Moise, K.J., Deter, R.L., Kirshon, B., Carpenter, R.J. and Huhta, J.C. (1989). Doppler assessment of the pulsatility index in the cerebral circulation of the human fetus. *Am. J. Obstet. Gynecol.*, **160**, 698–703

19. Wladimiroff, J.W., Tonge, H.M., Stewart, P.A. and Reuss, A. (1986). Severe intrauterine growth retardation; assessment of its origin from fetal arterial flow velocity waveforms. *Eur. J. Obstet. Gynecol. Reprod. Biol.*, **22**, 23–8

20. Arabin, B., Siebert, M. and Saling, E. (1989). The prospective value of Doppler blood flow measurement in uteroplacental and fetal blood vessels – a comparative study of multiple parameters. *Geburtsh. Frauenheilk.*, **49**, 457–62

21. Bilardo, C.M., Nicolaides, K.H. and Campbell, S. (1990). Doppler measurements of fetal and uteroplacental circulations: relationship with umbilical

venous blood gases measured at cordocentesis. *Am. J. Obstet. Gynecol.*, **162**, 115–20

22. Lingman, G. and Maršál,, K. (1989). Noninvasive assessment of cranial blood circulation in the fetus. *Biol. Neonate*, **56**, 129–35

23. Echizenya, N., Kagiya, A., Tachizaki, T. and Saito, Y. (1989). Significance of velocimetry as a monitor of fetal assessment and management. *Fetal Ther.*, **4**, 188–94

24. Arduini, D., Rizzo, G. and Romanini, C. (1992). Changes of pulsatility index from fetal vessels preceding the onset of late decelerations in growth-retarded fetuses. *Obstet. Gynecol.*, **79**, 605–10

25. Satoh, S., Koyanagi, T., Fukuhara, M., Hara, K. and Nakano, H. (1989). Changes in vascular resistance in the umbilical and middle cerebral arteries in the human intrauterine growth-retarded fetus, measured with pulsed Doppler ultrasound. *Early Hum. Dev.*, **20**, 213–20

26. Gramellini, D., Folli, M.C., Raboni, S., Vadora, E. and Merialdi, A. (1992). Cerebral–umbilical Doppler ratio as a predictor of adverse perinatal outcome. *Obstet. Gynecol.*, **79**, 416–20

27. Veille, J.C. and Cohen, I. (1990). Middle cerebral artery blood flow in normal and growth-retarded fetuses. *Am. J. Obstet. Gynecol.*, **162**, 391–6

28. Chandran, R., Serra-Serra, V., Sellers, S.M. and Redman, C.W. (1993). Fetal cerebral Doppler in the recognition of fetal compromise. *Br. J. Obstet. Gynaecol.*, **100**, 139–44

29. Favre, R., Schonenberger, R., Nisand, I. and Lorenz, U. (1991). Standard curves of cerebral Doppler flow velocity waveforms and predictive values for intrauterine growth retardation and fetal acidosis. *Fetal Diagn. Ther.*, **6**, 113–19

30. Vyas, S., Nicolaides, K.H., Bower, S. and Campbell, S. (1990). Middle cerebral artery flow velocity waveforms in fetal hypoxaemia. *Br. J. Obstet. Gynaecol.*, **97**, 797–803

31. Arduini, D., Rizzo, G., Romanini, C. and Mancuso, S. (1987). Fetal blood flow velocity waveforms as predictors of growth retardation. *Obstet. Gynecol.*, **70**, 7–10

32. Arduini, D. and Rizzo, G. (1992). Prediction of fetal outcome in small for gestational age fetuses: comparison of Doppler measurements obtained from different fetal vessels. *J. Perinat. Med.*, **20**, 29–38

33. McCowan, L.M.E. and Duggan, P.M. (1992). Abnormal internal carotid and umbilical artery Doppler in the small for gestational age fetus predicts an adverse outcome. *Early Hum. Dev.*, **30**, 249–59

34. Rizzo, G., Arduini, D., Luciano, R., Rizzo, C., Tortorolo, G., Romanini, C. and Mancuso, S. (1989). Prenatal cerebral Doppler ultrasonography and neonatal neurologic outcome. *J. Ultrasound. Med.*, **8**, 237–40

35. Wladimiroff, J.W., van den Wijngaard, J.A.G.W., Degani, S., Noordam, M.J., van Eyck, J. and Tonge, H.M. (1987). Cerebral and umbilical arterial blood flow velocity waveforms in normal and growth retarded pregnancies. *Obstet. Gynecol.*, **69**, 705–9

36. Wladimiroff, J.W., Noordam, M.J., van den Wijngaard, J.A.G.W. and Hop, W.C.J. (1988). Fetal internal carotid and umbilical artery blood flow velocity waveforms as a measure of fetal well-being in intrauterine growth retardation. *Pediatr. Res.*, **24**, 609–12

37. Degani, S., Lewinski, R., Shapiro, I. and Sharf, M. (1988). Decrease in pulsatile flow in the internal carotid artery in fetal hydrocephalus. *Br. J. Obstet. Gynaecol.*, **95**, 138–41

38. van den Wijngaard, J.A.G.W., Reuss, A. and Wladimiroff, J.W. (1988). The blood flow velocity waveform in the fetal internal carotid artery in the presence of hydrocephaly. *Early Hum. Dev.*, **18**, 95–9

39. Kirkinen, P., Muller, R., Baumann, H., Briner, J., Lang, W., Huch, R. and Huch, A. (1988). Cerebral blood flow velocity waveforms in hydrocephalic fetuses. *J. Clin. Ultrasound*, **16**, 493–8

40. Mari, G., Wasserstrum, N. and Kirshon, B. (1992). Reduction in the middle cerebral artery pulsatility index after decompression of polyhydramnios in twin gestation. *Am. J. Perinatol.*, **9**, 381–4

41. van den Wijngaard, J.A.G.W., Wladimiroff, J.W., Reuss, A. and Stewart, P.A. (1988). Oligohydramnios and fetal cerebral blood flow. *Br. J. Obstet. Gynaecol.*, **95**, 1309–11

42. Ben-Chetrit, A., Anteby, E., Lavy, Y., Zacut, D. and Yagel, S. (1991). Increased middle cerebral artery blood flow impedance in fetal subdural hematoma. *Ultrasound Obstet. Gynecol.*, **1**, 357–8

43. Chandran, R., Serra, S.V., Sellers, S.M. and Redman, C.W.G. (1991). Fetal middle cerebral artery flow velocity waveforms – a terminal pattern. Case report. *Br. J. Obstet. Gynaecol.*, **98**, 937–8

44. Mari, G. and Wasserstrum, N. (1991). Flow velocity waveforms of the fetal circulation preceding fetal death in a case of lupus anticoagulant. *Am. J. Obstet. Gynecol.*, **164**, 776–8

45. Fleischer, A., Anyaegbunam, A.A., Schulman, H., Farmakides, G. and Randolph, G. (1987). Uterine and umbilical artery velocimetry during normal labor. *Am. J. Obstet. Gynecol.*, **157**, 40–3

46. Brar, H.S., Platt, L.D., DeVore, G.R., Horenstein, J. and Medearis, A.L. (1988). Qualitative assessment of maternal uterine and fetal umbilical artery blood flow and resistance in laboring patients by Doppler velocimetry. *Am. J. Obstet. Gynecol.*, **158**, 952–6

47. Janbu, T., Koss, K.S., Nesheim, B.-I. and Wesche, J. (1985). Blood velocities in the uterine artery in humans during labor. *Acta Physiol. Scand.*, **124**, 153–61

48. Fairlie, F.M., Lang, G.D. and Scheldon, C.D. (1989). Umbilical artery flow velocity waveforms in labor. *Br. J. Obstet. Gynaecol.*, **96**, 151–7

49. Stuart, B., Drumm, J., FitzGerald, D.E. and Duignan, N.M. (1981). Fetal blood velocity waveforms in uncomplicated labor. *Br. J. Obstet. Gynaecol.*, **88**, 865–9

50. O'Brien, W.F., Davis, S.E., Grissom, M.P., Eng, R.R. and Golden, S.M. (1984). Effect of cephalic pressure on fetal cerebral blood flow. *Am. J. Perinatol.*, **1**, 223–6

51. Vyas, S., Campbell, S., Bower, S. and Nicolaides, K.H. (1990). Maternal abdominal pressure alters fetal cerebral blood flow. *Br. J. Obstet. Gynaecol.*, **97**, 740–2

52. Fendel, H., Funk, A., Jorn, H. and Gans, A. (1990). Cerebral blood flow during labor. *Z. Geburtsh. Perinatol.*, **194**, 272–4

53. Dougall, A., Lang, G.D. and Evans, D.H. (1989). Fetal anterior cerebral flow velocity waveforms during labor. In Gennser, G., Maršál, K., Svenningsen, N. and Lindström, K. (eds.) *Fetal and Neonatal Physiological Measurements*, pp. 301–4. (Malmö: Department of Obstetrics and Gynecology, Malmö General Hospital)

54. Mirro, R. and Gonzalez, A. (1987). Perinatal anterior cerebral artery Doppler flow indexes: methods and preliminary results. *Am. J. Obstet. Gynecol.*, **156**, 1227–31

55. Maesel, A., Lingman, G. and Maršál, K. (1990). Cerebral blood flow during labor in the human fetus. *Acta Obstet. Gynecol. Scand.*, **69**, 493–5

56. Yagel, S., Anteby, E., Lavy, Y., Ben, C.A., Palti, Z., D., H.-C. and Ron, M. (1992). Fetal middle cerebral artery blood flow during normal active labor and in labor with variable decelerations. *Br. J. Obstet. Gynaecol.*, **99**, 483–5

57. Lindblad, A., Bernow, J. and Maršál, K. (1987). Obstetric analgesia and fetal aortic blood flow during labor. *Br. J. Obstet. Gynaecol.*, **94**, 306–11

58. Maesel, A., Sladkevicius, P., Valentin, L. and Maršál, K. (1994). Fetal cerebral blood flow velocity during labor and in the early neonatal period. *Ultrasound Obstet. Gynecol.*, **4**, 1–5

59. Ipsiroglu, O.S., Stöckler, S., Häusler, M.C.H., Kainer, F., Rosegger, H., Weiss, P.A.M. and Winter, R. (1993). Cerebral blood flow velocities in the first minutes of life. *Eur. J. Pediatr.*, **152**, 269–71

60. Lagercrantz, H. and Bisoletti, P. (1973). Catecholamine release in the newborn infant at birth. *Pediatr. Res.*, **11**, 889–93

61. Christensson, K., Siles, C., Cabrera, T., Belaustequi, A., De La Fuente, P., Lagercrantz, H., Pyol, P. and Winberg, J. (1993). Lower body temperature in infant delivered by caesarean section than in vaginally delivered infants. *Acta Paediatr.*, **82**, 128–32

62. Shuto, H., Yasuhara, A., Sugimoto, T., Iwase, S., Kobayashi, Y. and Nakamura, M. (1987). Longitudinal determination of cerebral blood flow velocity in neonates with the Doppler technique. *Neuropediatrics*, **18**, 218–21

Magnetic resonance imaging of the fetal brain

9

M. Resta, P. Spagnolo, V. D'Addario, P. Greco and G. Caruso

INTRODUCTION

Ultrasound is the imaging method of choice for prenatal diagnosis. However, even expert sonologists, in some circumstances, may be helped by alternative imaging procedures. Computed axial tomography (CT) should not be used, as it involves ionizing radiation. Magnetic resonance imaging (MRI), however, is a technique to be considered as an alternative imaging procedure in pregnancy.

MRI fetal diagnosis has been reported since the early 1980s[1–3]. There were preliminary results in high-risk patients with and without fetal abnormalities[4–6]. These examinations were performed with MRI equipment of medium field strength and the fetal activity, sometimes, impaired the image quality. To avoid artifacts created by fetal movement, ultrasound-guided intramuscular or intravenous fetal muscular blockade was proposed[7–15]. However, this technique is invasive, and due to the improvement of MRI software with very short sequences, the fetal paralysis could be abandoned or at least reserved for selected cases[9–11, 16].

In this chapter, the basic concepts of MRI, the examination techniques, the normal anatomy of the fetus at different gestational ages and the MRI findings of fetal pathology will be reviewed.

MAGNETIC RESONANCE IMAGING

The macroscopic tissue magnetization is normally parallel to the external magnetic field generated by a superconductive magnet (less commonly by a permanent or resistive magnet) and this is termed 'longitudinal macroscopic magnetization'. When the proton Larmor radiofrequency (RF) pulse is broadcast to the patient, the tissue magnetic moment is tipped on the transverse plane, and this is called 'excitation'. The RF pulse is sent by a transmitter coil, the same as subsequently acts as a receiver. When the longitudinal macroscopic magnetization has been tipped over, it generates a transverse macroscopic magnetization and a signal or echo, proportional to this component on the transverse plane, which can be recorded by the receiver coil. Actually, the magnetic moment of the tissue returns, in some seconds, to its longitudinal direction and this process is named 'relaxation'. The vectors return to the longitudinal plane both in the transverse direction (transverse relaxation) and, more slowly, in the longitudinal direction (longitudinal relaxation). The transverse relaxation time is called T2 and the longitudinal relaxation time is called T1.

The T1 and T2 vary in the different tissues. Generally speaking, when the T1 of the tissue is long (i.e. fluid components such as cerebrospinal fluid (CSF) and amniotic fluid), the signal recorded is hypointense, and when the T1 is short, such as in fat tissue, the signal is hyperintense. When the T2 of the tissue is short, the signal recorded will be iso-hypointense and when the T2 is long, the signal will be hyperintense.

MRI techniques are generally classified into two main categories: the spin echo sequences (SE) produced by pairs of RF pulses, and the gradient echo sequences (GRE), formed by a single RF pulse in conjunction with gradient field reversal of gradient[17, 18].

It is not the aim of this chapter to illustrate all the different MRI techniques or different pulse sequence strategies, but it should be remembered that in the GRE technique, one can record the MRI signal by the use of a steady-state free precession in fast imaging with steady-state precession (FISP), in gradient recalled acquisition in steady-state mode (GRASS) and in fast low-angle shot

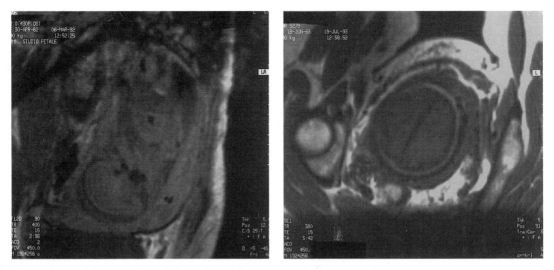

Figure 1 Fetal brain surface. Left: sagittal oblique maternal FLASH 2D T1 weighted image at 25 weeks of pregnancy. The fetal brain in parasagittal view presents a pachygyric aspect. Right: coronal oblique maternal SE T1 weighted image at 35 weeks of pregnancy. The fetal head is in axial view. Near the term of pregnancy the fetal brain presents the typical aspect of the newborn with gyri and sulci

(FLASH)[17]. The FLASH and FISP GRE techniques are particularly important in fetal MRI studies, permitting a very short acquisition time, and minimizing the fetal activity artifacts.

EXAMINATION TECHNIQUES

The most effective procedure for avoiding fetal activity is a transient fetal paralysis with fetal curarization[7-15]. This invasive technique, however, can cause serious complications, such as cord hematoma and abortion[19]. For this reason, fetal curarization should be reserved only for cases of high fetal activity, such as in polyhydramnios, in the early second trimester of pregnancy and in breech presenation, because of the influence of maternal diaphragmatic movements.

Different neuromuscular blocking agents can be used (atracurium, pancuronium bromide, vecuronium, etc.) but the most commonly used drug is pancuronium bromide at the dosage of 0.1–0.3 mg/kg of estimated fetal weight. This allows a transient fetal paralysis lasting for 40–90 min.

When the prenatal MRI is performed without fetal curarization, several solutions can be proposed. Since the fetal activity is reduced in hypoglycemia, the examination should be performed in the morn-

ing after fasting[20]. Maternal posture, such as the left lateral position, is another simple but effective solution to reduce fetal activity and maternal breathing movements[21]. The intravenous maternal administration of a sedative, such as diazepam[22], should be reserved only for distressed patients.

The MRI examination starts with the very short acquisitions of three scout images on the axial, sagittal and coronal planes to identify the fetal position. On the scout images, the slice orientations are selected, often using oblique sections. The SE, GRE and inversion recovery (IR) techniques[2, 4, 15, 23–27] have been proposed to obtain T1, T2 and T2* weighted images. In the experience of the authors working with high field strength equipment, the T1 weighted images are the preferable sequences, in order to reduce motion image degradation, thanks to the shorter acquisition time. On the other hand, the T2 weighted images are useless in the fetal brain, because of the lack of myelination of the white matter.

SE pulse sequences with short repetition time (TR) and short echo time (TE) (slice thickness 3–5 mm, slice interval 0.1 mm, matrix 192–224 × 256, FOV 400–500, acquisitions 1–3, average imaging time 3–5 min, are preferred to obtain T1 weighted images of the paralyzed fetus.

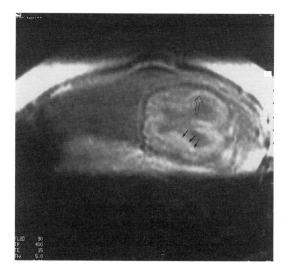

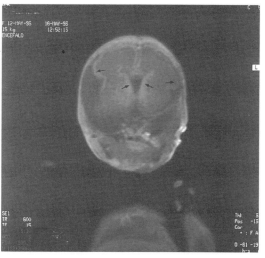

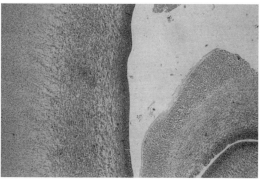

Figure 2 Germinal matrix in prenatal, postmortem MRI and histology. Top left: axial maternal FLASH 2D T1 weighted image at 22 weeks of pregnancy. The fetal head is in axial view. The germinal matrix presents a hyperintense signal (arrows) similar to the neocortex (open arrow). Top right: SE coronal T1 weighted image on an aborted fetus. The high signal of the germinal matrix and neocortex is well evident (arrows). Bottom: post-mortem histology of fetus at top right (HH stain). The neuronal population of the germinal matrix is well evident close to the ventricular edge

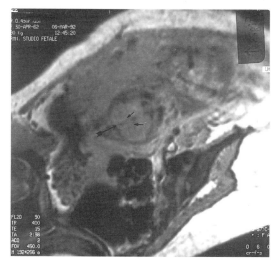

Figure 3 Normal corpus callosum in normal fetal brain. Oblique axial maternal FLASH 2D T1 weighted image at 25 weeks of pregnancy. The fetal head is in coronal view. The corpus callosum does not present the typical hyperintense signal of the adult. However, it can be recognized indirectly upon the frontal horns (small arrows) and below the interhemispheric fissure (large arrow). Note also the wide Sylvian fissure vertically orientated

Without fetal curarization, the best results can be obtained by using the GRE technique employing FLASH 2D or FISP 2D sequences (TR 400, TE 15, FA 90°, slice thickness 3–5 mm, slice interval 0.1 mm, matrix 192–224 × 256, FOV 400–500, acquisitions 2–3, average imaging time 3–5 min). The other sequences employed with the GRE technique are the 'breath hold' FLASH 2D (FA 80–90°, TR 150–200, TE 6–10, acquisitions 1–2, FOV 350–500), or FISP (FA 40°, TR 150, TE 10, acquisitions 1–2, FOV 350–500), with acquisition times ranging from 20 to 40 s with eight T1 weighted sections.

In order to minimize the artifacts produced by motion and flow from maternal vessels, the application of multiple saturation bands is always suggested. Improvement of the image quality can be expected from the availability of turbo SE and turbo GRE ultrafast imaging.

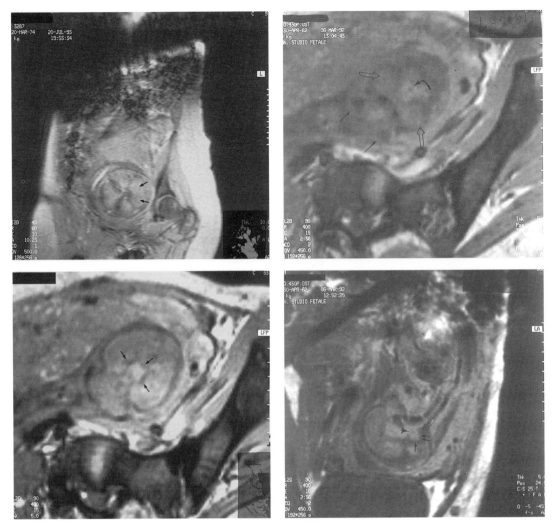

Figure 4 Fetal posterior fossa structures. Top left: coronal oblique maternal FLASH 2D T1 weighted image at 35 weeks of pregnancy. Fetal head in axial view. Cerebellar hemispheres are well evident (arrows). However, the fourth ventricle is not imaged, because of the small size of the brain and large thickness of the slices (10 mm). Top right: axial oblique maternal FLASH 2D T1 weighted image at 25 weeks of pregnancy. The fetal head is in axial view. The cerebellar hemispheres, the middle cerebellar peduncles and fourth ventricle (curved arrow), are depicted. Note also the eyeballs (black arrows), the temporal poles (open arrows) and the hypointense petrous pyramids. In this case, even though pregnancy was earlier than that at top left, the fourth ventricle is evident, because of the thinner slices. Bottom left: axial oblique maternal FLASH 2D T1 weighted image, same case as at top right, but with a more cranial slice. The mesencephalon and peripontomesencephalic cisterns (opposing arrows) are imaged. The other arrow points to the quadrigeminal cistern. Bottom right: oblique sagittal maternal FLASH 2D T1 weighted image at 35 weeks of pregnancy. The fetus is in sagittal view. The brainstem, cerebellar vermis and cervical spinal cord are very well depicted. Single arrow, superior vermian cistern; double arrows, inferior vermian cistern; arrowhead, fourth ventricle

MRI ANATOMY OF THE FETAL BRAIN

Prenatal MRI of the central nervous system (CNS), as in the adult, is its most useful application. The embryogenesis of the brain is already substantially completed at about 20 weeks of pregnancy[26, 28, 29]. However, the gyration, depending on the conclusion of the neuronal migration, is complete near

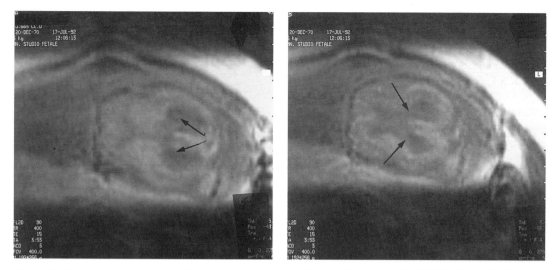

Figure 5 Lateral ventricles at second trimester of pregnancy. Left: axial maternal FLASH 2D T1 weighted image. The fetal head is in axial view. Large choroid plexuses (arrows) in the wide ventricular cavities indicate a physiological dilatation of the lateral ventricles at this age of pregnancy. Right: same case, same sequence, next slice. The arrows show well proportioned choroid plexuses

the term of pregnancy[30]. Consequently, the brain surface in early pregnancy presents a pachygyric aspect and only at term can the gyri and sulci be visualized (Figure 1).

The migration of the cortical cells starts from the germinal matrix close to the lateral ventricles, where an area of high signal, similar to the neocortex, can occasionally be depicted (Figure 2, top left and top right). Typically, the thalami and basal ganglia may show, similar to the newborn, a hyperintense signal[28]. The fetal corpus callosum[28] does not present the typical hyperintensity of the adult, because of the lack of myelination in the prenatal period[31], and it may be recognized only in indirect morphological findings (Figure 3). For the same reason, in the prenatal brain, there is no differentiation between gray and white matter and the long TR, long TE sequences for obtaining T2 weighted images are useless in prenatal MRI examination. The septum pellucidum and cavum Vergae are actual and not virtual cavities and their cystic apsect can be considered a normal finding in the prenatal period (Figure 6, top right). The orbital cavities and the eyeballs are easily but only occasionally depicted on prenatal MRI, because of the large thickness of the slices (Figure 4, top right). Posterior fossa structures such as cerebellar

hemispheres, cerebellar vermis and brainstem are already well depicted from the early second trimester[26,29] (Figure 4).

The cerebral ventricles and subarachnoid spaces appear hypointense in T1 weighted images, because of the long T1 of CSF. The lateral ventricles[28,29,32–34] show morphological and size variations during pregnancy. In the second trimester, the lateral ventricles appear characteristically wide and contain large choroid plexuses within the bodies and the atria (Figure 5; Figure 6, top left). In the absence of other CNS abnormalities, the slightly enlarged lateral ventricles do not constitute a pathological event in this period of pregnancy and the erroneous diagnosis of hydrocephalus should be avoided. On the other hand, the mild dilatation of the lateral ventricles with *small* choroid plexuses could be considered as an early finding of fetal hydrocephalus.

Near the term of pregnancy, the lateral ventricles show an aspect similar to that of the newborn. The third (Figure 6, top left) and fourth ventricles (Figure 4, top and bottom right), starting from the 20th week of pregnancy, show the morphology of the newborn. They are small in size[28,29] and for this reason, in some circumstances, they cannot be visualized on prenatal MRI (Figure 4, top left).

The first sulcus visualized on fetal MRI is the

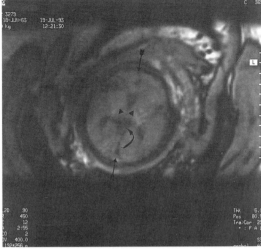

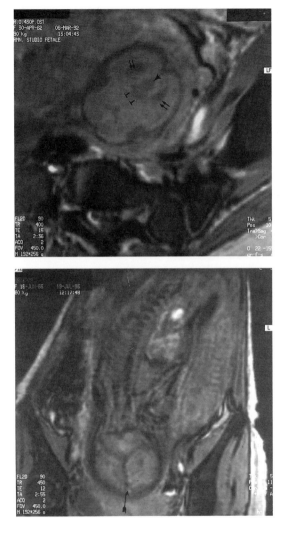

Figure 6 Ventricular cavities and fetal cisterns at different ages of pregnancy. Top left: axial oblique maternal FLASH 2D T1 weighted image at 25 weeks of pregnancy. The third ventricle is depicted as a thin line between the thalami (T). The arrowhead indicates the normally wide cisterna ambiens. Double arrows, choroid plexuses proportional to the ventricular atria. Note also the wide and open Sylvian fissure. Top right: oblique axial maternal FLASH 2D T1 weighted image at 35 weeks of pregnancy. The lateral ventricles near the term of the pregnancy are smaller than in early pregnancy, and similar to those of the newborn. The septum pellucidum is an actual cavity, but not cystic. The curved arrow is pointed at the large cisterna ambiens. The arrows indicate the anterior and posterior tract of the interhemispheric fissure. Bottom: coronal maternal FLASH 2D T1 weighted image. The fetus is in coronal view. The cisterna magna (arrowhead), the interhemispheric fissure (arrows) and the cerebellar tentorium (double arrows) are well depicted. L, fetal lung

Sylvian fissure and, in early pregnancy, this sulcus is wide and vertical (Figure 3; Figure 6, top left). The wide aspect of the subarachnoid spaces and of the fetal cisterns is a normal finding in the prenatal period, particularly at the level of the interhemispheric cistern as well as at the level of the posterior fossa (Figure 4). Because of the inclination of the fetal head, the region of the fetal neck cannot be easily visualized on the prenatal MRI. Especially when the MRI is performed with fetal curarization, the fetal head may be hyperflected on the cervical spine, taking an asynclitic position, and consequently it is very difficult to obtain appropriately orientated slices. The fetal spine and the fetal spinal cord may present a fascinating image

(Figure 6, bottom; Figure 7), but, unlike with ultrasound, they are only occasionally visualized.

MRI OF FETAL BRAIN ANOMALIES

The most severe fetal brain malformations are anencephaly and other forms of altered closure of the neural tube[35–41]. In these pathologies, ultrasound is conclusive and fetal MRI may be useful only in selected cases, to evaluate the content of a herniated sac or to differentiate some severe forms of microcephaly. This can be divided in two major categories: true microcephaly of Evrard and the microcephalic malformation

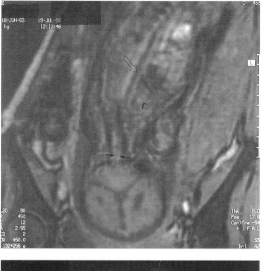

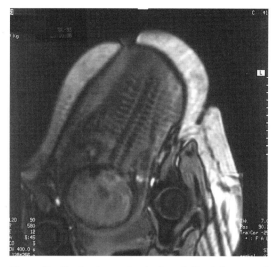

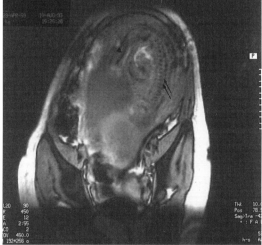

Figure 7 Fetal spine and spinal cord. Top left: coronal maternal FLASH 2D T1 weighted image at 35 weeks of pregnancy. The fetus is in coronal view. The upper spinal cord is well depicted (arrows). The thoracic aorta (open arrow) is also evident. L, lung. Top right: oblique coronal maternal FLASH 2D T1 weighted image at 35 weeks of pregnancy. The fetus is in coronal view. The spinal cord, the spinal canal and the ribs are evident. Bottom: oblique coronal maternal FLASH 2D T1 weighted image at 27 weeks of pregnancy. The fetal body is in sagittal view. The thoracic and lumbar vertebral bodies (arrows) are depicted with their characteristic hypointense signal, but the spinal cord image is unclear. A fetal femur is well evident (arrowhead)

complexes[39, 42]. In the true microcephaly of Evrard, the fetal head is small and contains a morphologically normal brain, but the MRI signal of the germinal matrix can typically be absent. Only histology, however, may confirm the suspicion from MRI, showing the depletion of the germinal zone[42] (Figure 8). In the other form, the microcephaly is part of a malformation complex and the fetal head is very small and disproportioned.

In the abnormalities of the telencephalon, such as the holoprosencephalies, fetal MRI[43–50] plays an important role only in the semilobar holoprosencephaly. Indeed, in the case of severe alobar holoprosencephaly, MRI offers superb pictures, but is substantially superfluous in comparison with ultrasound evaluation (Figure 9). Similarly, lobar holoprosencephaly is too close to the normal fetal brain and may be missed at both ultrasound and MRI examinations. In semilobar holoprosencephaly, however, the fetal MRI is generally relevant and conclusive for a correct diagnosis, by disclosing the frontal lobar fusion and a dorsal holoventricular cavity (Figure 10).

The most common midline dysraphism imaged in the prenatal period is agenesis of the corpus callosum[28, 51–55]. The ultrasound evaluation of agenesis of the corpus callosum is usually easy when the transvaginal approach is possible[64]. In some circumstances, MRI examination can be proposed for better definition of a ventriculomegaly observed during conventional ultrasound examination. In the MRI axial plane, the common findings are

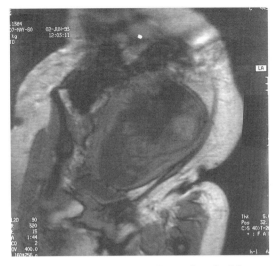
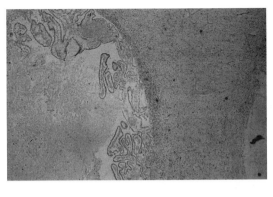

Figure 8 Microcephaly vera of Evrard. Left: oblique sagittal maternal FLASH 2D T1 weighted image at 21 weeks of pregnancy. The fetus is in sagittal view. The microcephaly is harmonic and the thorax and abdomen seem to be normal. The patient requested and obtained the termination of pregnancy. Right: histology of the same case, showing the depletion (HH stain) of the germinal matrix. Compare with Figure 2, top right

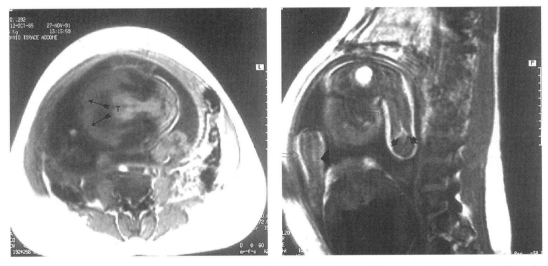

Figure 9 Severe form of alobar holoprosencephaly. Left: axial maternal FLASH 2D T1 weighted image at 28 weeks of pregnancy. The fetal head is in axial view. Note the complete fusion of the thalami (T) and of the rostral maldeveloped frontal lobes. Right: parasagittal maternal FLASH 2D T1 weighted image. The fetus is in coronal position. Perfect depiction of the fused thalami (T) and the large holoventricular cavity (open circle)

colpocephaly, i.e. the dilatation of the trigones and the occipital horns, because of the underdevelopment of the callosal fibers, and the outward dislocation of the lateral ventricles separated by the dorsally elevated third ventricle and/or by the interhemispheric cyst (Figures 11 and 12). The MRI coronal section is also very useful showing the crescent-like frontal horns, as a consequence of the compression by the Probst's bundles and the diamond aspect of the elongated and cranially dislocated third ventricle (Figure 13). Unlike in the adult, the prenatal MRI sagittal view is less

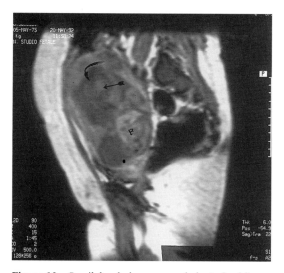 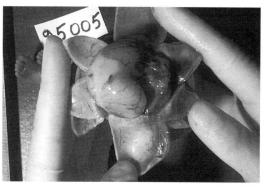

Figure 10 Semilobar holoprosencephaly. Left: oblique sagittal maternal FLASH 2D T1 weighted image. The arrow shows the anterior parenchymal fusion and the curved arrow shows the absence of the cerebral falx and a posterior cavity. Right: the open fetal head of the aborted fetus clearly confirms the MRI findings

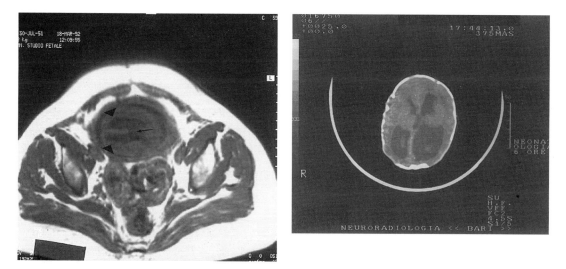

Figure 11 Agenesis of the corpus callosum. Left: axial maternal SE T1 weighted image. The fetal head is in axial view. The lateral ventricles are enlarged, particularly at the level of the occipital horns (colpocephaly) (arrowheads) and separated by the dorsally dislocated third ventricle (arrow). Right: postnatal CT scan confirms the corpus callosum dysgenesis and colpocephaly

informative, since the normal fetal corpus callosum is an unmyelinated structure similar to the fetal gray and white matter.

Among posterior fossa anomalies, the most frequent is the Dandy–Walker malformation[56,57]. All the posterior fossa cysts have recently been classified as the Dandy–Walker complex[58,59]. In the classic Dandy–Walker malformation, the fetal MRI shows a typical large cystic dilatation of the fourth ventricle (Figure 14). As in other major brain malformations, MRI appears superfluous and the sonographic diagnosis remains the more immediate and conclusive procedure. To evaluate the possible association of cerebral compromise in less severe

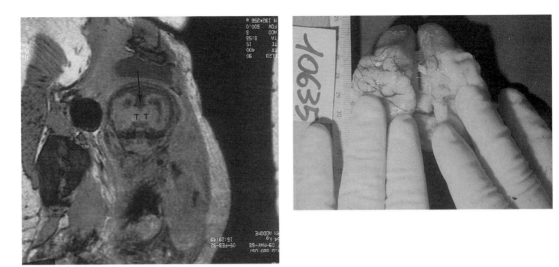

Figure 12 Complete agenesis of the corpus callosum. Left: oblique maternal sagittal FLASH 2D T1 weighted image (upside-down image). The fetal head is in coronal view. The third ventricle directly communicates with a large interhemispheric cyst (arrow) because of the agenesis of the corpus callosum. T, thalami. Right: anatomical specimen: the third ventricle is clearly seen through the interhemispheric fissure

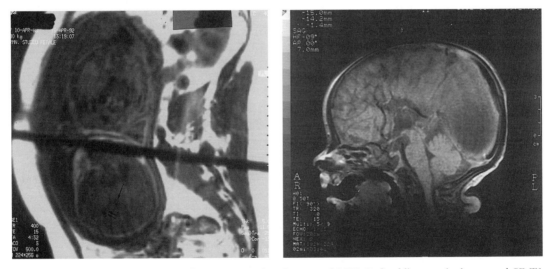

Figure 13 Agenesis of the corpus callosum. Prenatal and postnatal MRI. Left: oblique sagittal maternal SE T1 weighted image. The arrow indicates the diamond-shaped third ventricle cranially dislocated between the lateral ventricles. The right frontal horn presents the typical crescent-like aspect, due to compression by Probst's bundles (double arrows). Right: postnatal, SE sagittal T1 weighted MRI image showing agenesis of the corpus callosum

forms of the Dandy–Walker complex, such as Dandy–Walker variant, enlarged cisterna magna and retrocerebellar cysts, fetal MRI may once again be useful.

The Arnold–Chiari malformations are other important posterior fossa anomalies where prenatal MRI could be useful for a new diagnostic approach[60–62]. In the Chiari I malformation, the cerebellar amygdalae are herniated at the level of the foramen magnum and of the upper cervical

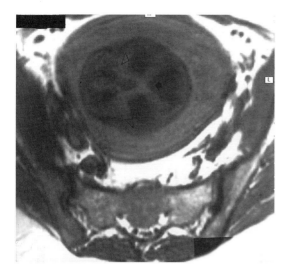

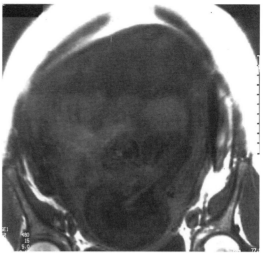

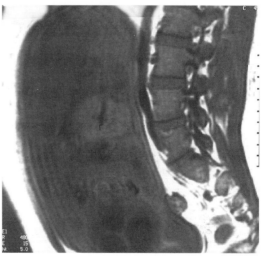

Figure 14 Dandy–Walker malformation. Top left: axial maternal SE T1 weighted image. The fetal head is in axial view. The cystic dilatation of the fourth ventricle is well evident (black arrow). The supratentorial hydrocephalus is more pronounced at the level of the temporal horns (open arrow-heads). Top right: coronal maternal SE T1 weighted image. Fetus in sagittal view. The cyst of the fourth ventricle causes a moderate compression on the brainstem (double arrows). Bottom: oblique sagittal maternal SE T1 weighted image (upside-down image). Fetus in coronal view. The black arrow is in the enlarged fourth ventricle. The arrowheads indicate the cerebellar tentorium. H, fetal heart; L, fetal liver

canal. Ventriculomegaly is not frequent and osseous malformations of the craniocervical joint are possible.

The Chiari II malformation is almost always associated with spina bifida; the cerebellar vermis, the fourth ventricle and the amygdalae are displaced downward below the foramen magnum into the cervical canal. The brainstem is elongated and kinked. Hydrocephalus is frequent but not always present. In the Chiari II malformation, the evidence of a small posterior fossa seems to be frequent. In the experience of the authors, based on about 50 MRI fetal examinations, some cases of ventriculomegaly could show a small posterior fossa and a caudal displacement of the cerebellar tonsils without any ultrasonic evidence of spinal defect. Therefore, several intermediate forms of Chiari malformation could be postulated and division of the two major types should be further considered (Figure 15).

The dilatation of the ventricular system (hydrocephalus) may be a condition associated with different cerebral malformations or an independent entity. The ultrasound diagnosis of early hydrocephalus may occasionally be doubtful, and the MRI morphological findings may be more sensitive. It is well known, in fact, that morphological criteria are more reliable than biometric criteria, and MRI evaluation offers more detailed visualization of the brain parenchyma than does ultrasound. Therefore, the slightly enlarged lateral ventricles with distorted lateral walls and inversion of the typical external concavity, associated with shrunken choroid plexuses, are MRI features strongly suspicious for early hydrocephalus. In severe hydrocephalus, the MRI evaluation does

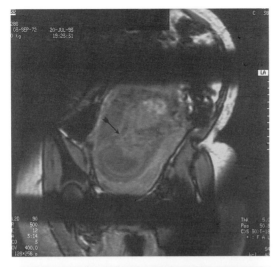

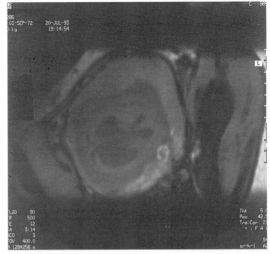

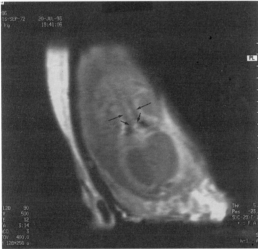

Figure 15 Chiari I malformation and hydrocephalus. Top right: oblique axial maternal FLASH 2D T1 weighted image. The fetal head is in axial view. The ventricular dilatation is more evident at the level of the atria and occipital horns. Top left: coronal oblique maternal FLASH 2D T1 weighted image. Fetus in sagittal view. The small posterior fossa is clearly evident but the caudal dislocation of the cerebellar amygdala can be only suspected (arrow). Bottom: oblique sagittal maternal FLASH 2D T1 weighted image. Fetus in coronal view. The coronal section more clearly shows the displacement of the cerebellar tonsils (small arrows). The large arrows indicate the spinal cord

not add any information to conventional ultrasound, and only the associated CNS malformations may be better appreciated[32–34] (Figure 16).

CONCLUSIONS

Ultrasound is at present the modality of choice for imaging of the fetal brain. Recently, sonographic methods have improved, due to the availability of high-resolution real-time scanners with endovaginal probes[63, 64]. However, in some circumstances such as breech presentation, maternal obesity, severe oligohydramnios and rare complex anomalies, even expert ultrasound operators may benefit from an alternative fetal brain imaging method.

MRI examination is harmless for the fetus. The energetic sources used by the MRI procedure are a static magnetic field and the radiofrequency radiation that induces no significant biological effect, with the exception of a mild increase of body temperature and heart rate[65–68].

Several authors, during the last 10 years, have proposed the potential application of prenatal MRI examination as a second-step imaging procedure after the conventional ultrasound evaluation. This is particularly true in the pathology of the central nervous system, where as in the adult population, the MRI examination has its most useful role. Actually, in the experience of the authors, in the most severe forms of fetal brain abnormalities as well as in severe hydrocephalus,

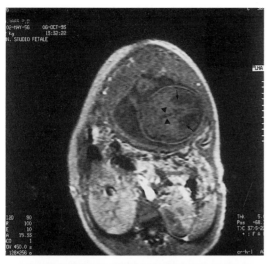

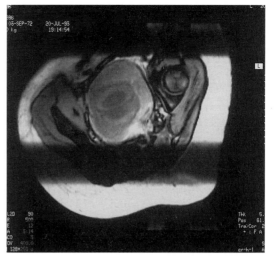

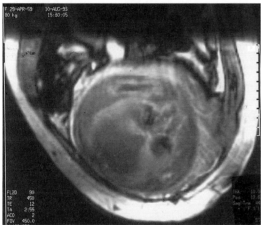

Figure 16 Isolated hydrocephalus. Top left: early second trimester of pregnancy. Oblique coronal maternal FISP T1 weighted image. The fetal head is in axial view. The third ventricle is only moderately enlarged (arrowheads) but the choroid plexuses are shrunken in the enlarged atria (arrows). The morphological findings are sufficient to diagnose a condition of early hydrocephalus. Top right: early second trimester of pregnancy. Oblique axial maternal FLASH 2D T1 weighted image. The fetal head is in axial view. The lateral wall of the lateral ventricles are deformed, with loss of their typical external concavity. This is a typical change of fetal hydrocephalus. Bottom: third trimester of pregnancy. Oblique coronal maternal FLASH 2D T1 weighted image. The fetal head is in coronal view, showing severe dilatation of the third ventricle and the frontal horns of the lateral ventricles

the MRI evaluation is clinically not of value, although it offers fascinating images, to compare with ultrasound.

However in some cases, such as in mild early hydrocephalus, in agenesis of the corpus callosum, in semilobar holoprosencephaly, in minor forms of the Dandy–Walker complex and in some distructive prenatal brain disorders, MRI is in the authors' experience a clinically useful adjunct to ultrasound examination.

ACKNOWLEDGEMENTS

The authors are very grateful to R. Soranno, S. De Ceglie, C. Dell' Orso and M. Mastromauro (MRI technicians) for their expert collaboration. Special thanks are due to Dr A. Vimercati and Dr D. Milella for their enthusiastic work in assisting the patients.

Some of the pictures included in this chapter have already been published in the authors' papers reported in the references or in the press.

References

1. Johnson, I.I., Symonds, E., Kean, A., Worthington, F., Diplain, B., Hawkes, R. and Gyngell, M. (1984). Imaging of the pregnant human uterus with nuclear magnetic resonance. *Am. J. Obstet. Gynecol.*, **148**, 1136–9

2. Smith, F.W., Adam, A.M. and Phillips, W.D.P. (1983). NMR imaging in pregnancy. *Lancet*, **1**, 61–2

3. Smith, F.W., Kent, C., Abramovich, D.R. and Sutherland, H.W. (1985). Nuclear magnetic resonance imaging: a new look at the fetus. *Br. J. Obstet. Gynaecol.*, **92**, 1024–33

4. Mc Carthy, S.M., Filly, R.A., Stark, D.D., Callen, P.W., Golbus, M.S. and Hricak, H. (1985). Magnetic resonance imaging of the fetal anomalies in utero: early experience. *Am. J. Roentgenol.*, **14**, 677–82

5. Mc Carthy, S.M., Filly, R.A., Stark, D.D., Hricak, H.H., Brandt-Zawadzki, M.N., Calle, P.W. and Higgins, C.B. (1985). Obstetrical magnetic resonance imaging: fetal anatomy. *Radiology*, **154**, 427–32

6. Mc Carthy, S.M., Stark, D.D., Filly, R. A., Callen, P.W., Hricak, H. and Higgins, C.B. (1985). Obstetrical magnetic resonance imaging: maternal anatomy. *Radiology*, **154**, 421–5

7. Daffos, F., Forestier, F., Mac Aleese, J. *et al.* (1988). Fetal curarization for prenatal magnetic resonance imaging. *Prenat. Diagn.*, **8**, 311–14

8. Moise, K.J., Carpenter, R.J., Deter, R.L., Kirshon, B. and Diaz, S.F. (1987). The use of fetal neuro-muscular blockade during intrauterine procedures. *Am. J. Obstet. Gynecol.*, **157**, 874–9

9. Resta, M., Greco, P., D'Addario, V., Florio, C., Dardes, N., Caruso, G., Spagnolo, P., Clemente, R., Vimercati, A. and Selvaggi, L. (1994). MRI in pregnancy. Study of cerebral fetal malformations. *Ultrasound Obstet. Gynecol.*, **4**, 7–20

10. Resta, M., Spagnolo, P., DiCuonzo, F., Palma, M., Greco, P., D'Addario, V., Vimercati, A., Selvaggi, L., Caruso, G. and Clemente, R. (1994). La RM del feto. Parte l: storia, tecnica d' esame ed anatomia cerebrale normale. *Rivista Neuroradiol.*, **7**, 53–65

11. Resta, M., Spagnolo, P., DiCuonzo, F., Palma, M., Greco, P., D'Addario, V., Vimercati, A., Selvaggi, L., Caruso, G. and Clemente, R. (1994). La RM del feto. Parte II: quadri patologici. *Rivista Neuroradiol.*, **7**, 557–71

12. Seeds, J.W., Corke, B.C. and Spielman, F.J. (1986). Prevention of fetal movements during invasive procedures with pancuronium bromide. *Am. J. Obstet. Gynecol.*, **155**, 818–19

13. Toma, P., Lucigrai, G., Dodero, P. and Vlituania, M. (1990). Prenatal detection of an abdominal mass by MR imaging performed while the fetus is immobilized with pancuronium bromide. *Am. J. Roentgenol.*, **154**, 1049–50

14. Wenstrom, K.D., Williamson, R.A., Weiner, C.P., Sipes, S.L. and Yuh, W.T.C. (1991). Magnetic resonance imaging of fetuses with intracranial defects. *Obstet. Gynecol.*, **77**, 529–32

15. Williamson, R.A., Weiner, C.P., Yuh, W.T.C. and Abu-Yousef, M.M. (1989). Magnetic resonance imaging of anomalous fetuses. *Obstet. Gynecol.*, **73**, 952–6

16. Mansfield, P., Stehling, M.K., Ordidge, R.J. *et al.* (1990). Echo planar imaging of the human fetus *in utero* at 0.5T. *Br. J. Radiol.*, **63**, 833–41

17. Elster, A.D. (1993). Gradient–echo MR imaging: techniques and acronyms. *Radiology*, **186**, 1–8

18. Pyket, I.L., Newhouse, J.H., Buonanno, F.S., Brady, T.J., Goldman, M.R., Kiotler, J.P. and Pohost, C.M. (1982). Principles of nuclear magnetic resonance imaging. *Radiology*, **143**, 157–68

19. Revel, M.P., Pons, J.C., Lelairder, C. *et al.* (1993). MRI of the fetus: a study of 20 cases performed without curarization. *Prenat. Diagn.*, **13**, 775–99

20. Gelmann, S.R. (1980). Fetal movements and ultrasound effects of intravenous glucose administration. *Am. J. Obstet. Gynecol.*, **137**, 459–61

21. Minors, D.S. and Waterhose, J.M. (1979). The effects of maternal posture, meals, and time of day on fetal movements, *Br. J. Obstet. Gynaecol.*, **86**, 717–23

22. Birger, M., Homburg, R. and Insler, V. (1980). Clinical evaluation of fetal movements. *Int. J. Gynaecol. Obstet.*, **18**, 337–82

23. Garden, A.S., Weindling, A.M., Griffiths, R.D. and Martin, P.A. (1991). Assessment of fetal well-being with magnetic resonance. *J. Perinat. Med.*, **19**, 435–8

24. Powell, M.C. and Worthington, B.S. (1986). MRI: a new milestone in modern OB care. *Diagn. Imaging*, **April**, 86–91

25. Smith, F.W. and Sutherland, H.W. (1986). Short T1 inversion recovery (STIR) imaging in human pregnancy. *Magn. Reson. Imaging*, **4**, 137

26. Weinreb, J.C., Lowe, T., Coen, J.N. and Kutler, M. (1985). Human fetal anatomy: MR imaging. *Radiology*, **157**, 715–20

27. Weinreb, J.C., Lowe, T.W., Santos-Ramos, R., Cunningham, F.G. and Parkey, R. (1985). Magnetic resonance imaging in obstetric diagnosis. *Radiology*, **154**, 157–61

28. Barkovich, A.J. (1990). *Pediatric Neuroimaging*, pp. 5–13. (New York: Raven Press)

29. Normann, M.G. (1992). Central nervous system. In Dimmick, J.E. and Kalousek, D.K. (eds.) *Developmental Pathology of the Embryo & Fetus*, pp. 341–8. (Philadelphia: J.B. Lippincott)

30. Barkovich, A.J., Gressens, P. and Evrard, P. (1992). Formation, maturation, and disorders of brain neocortex. *Am. J. Neuroradiol.*, **13**, 423–46

31. Dietrich, R., Bradley, W., Zaragoza, E., Otto, R.J., Taise, R.K., Wilson, G.H. and Kangarloo, H. (1988). MR evaluation of early myelination pat-

terns in normal and maldevelopmentally delayed infants. *Am. J. Neuroradiol.*, **9**, 69–76

32. Chinn, D.H., Calle, P.W. and Filly, R.A. (1983). The lateral ventricle in early second trimester. *Radiology*, **148**, 529–31

33. Fiske, C.E., Filly, R.A. and Callen, P.W. (1981). Sonographic measurement of lateral ventricle width in early ventricular dilatation. *J. Clin. Ultrasound*, **9**, 303–7

34. Hadlock, F.P., Deter, R.L. and Park, S.K. (1981). Real-time sonography: ventricular and vascular anatomy of the fetal brain in utero. *Am. J. Roentgenol.*, **136**, 133–7

35. Aleksic, S., Budzilovi, C.G., Greco, M.A., Feigin, I., Epstein, F. and Pearson, J. (1983). Iniencephaly: neuropathologic study. *Clin. Neuropathol.*, **2**, 55–61

36. Foderaro, A.E., Abu Yousef, M.M. and Benda, J.A. (1987). Antenatal ultrasound diagnosis of iniencephaly. *J. Clin. Ultrasound*, **15**, 550

37. Friedle, R.L. (1975). Anencephaly, rachischisis and encephaloceles. In *Developmental Neuropathology*, Part 2, Malformations, pp. 230–40. (New York: Springer–Verlag)

38. Lemire, R.J., Beckwith, J.B. and Warkany, J. (1978). *Anencephaly.* (New York: Raven Press)

39. Naidich, T.P., Altman, N.R., Braffman, B.H., McLone, D.G. and Zimmerman, R.A. (1992). Cephaloceles and related malformations. *Am. J. Neuroradiol.*, **13**, 655–90

40. Rakestraw, M.R., Massod, S., Ballinger, W.E. (1987) Brain heterotopia and anencephaly. *Arch. Pathol. Lab. Med.*, **111**, 858

41. Scherrer, C.C., Hammer, F., Schinzel, A. and Beiner, J. (1992). Brain stem and cervical spine cord dysraphic lesions in iniencephaly. *Pediatr. Pathol.*, **12**, 469–76

42. Evrard, P., de Saint Georges, P., Kadhim, H. and Gadisscaux, J.F. (1989). Pathology of prenatal encephalopathies. In French, J. (ed.) *Child Neurology and Developmental Disabilities*, pp. 153–76. (Baltimore: Paul H. Brookes)

43. Cohen, M.M., Jirasek, J.E. and Guzman, R.T. (1971). Holoprosencephaly and facial dysmorphia: nosology, etiology and pathogenesis. *Birth Defects*, **7**, 125–35

44. De Myer, W. (1977). Holoprosencephaly. In Vinicken, P.J. and Bruyn, G.W. (eds.) Handbook of Clinical Neurology, vol. 30, pp. 431–78. (Amsterdam: North Holland)

45. Filly, R.A., Chinn, D.H. and Callen, P.W. (1984). Alobar holoprosencephaly: ultrasonic prenatal diagnosis. *Radiology*, **151**, 455–9

46. Fitz, C.R. (1983). Holoprosencephaly and related entities. *Neuroradiology*, **25**, 225–38

47. Jellinger, K., Gross, H. and Kaltenback, E. (1981). Holoprosencephaly and agenesis of the corpus callosum: frequency of associated malformations. *Acta Neuropathol.*, **55**, 1

48. Leech, R.W. and Shuman, R.M. (1986). Holoprosencephaly and related cerebral midline anomalies: a review. *J. Child. Neurol.*, **1**, 3–18

49. Müller, F. and O'Rahilly, R. (1989). Mediobasal prosencephalic defects, including holoprosencephaly and cyclopia, in relation to the development of the human forebrain. *Am. J. Anat.*, **40**, 409

50. Nyberg, D.A., Mack, L.A., Bronstein, A., Hirsch, J. and Pagon, R.A. (1987). Holoprosencephaly: prenatal sonographic diagnosis *Am. J. Neuroradiol.*, **8**, 871–8

51. Barkovich, A.J. and Norman, D. (1985). Anomalies of the corpus callosum: correlation with further anomalies of the brain. *Am. J. Neuroradiol.*, **9**, 493–501

52. Barkovich, A.J. (1990). Apparent atypical callosal dysgenesis: analysis of MR findings in six cases and their relationship to holoprosencephaly. *Am. J. Neuroradiol.*, **11**, 333–40

53. Barkovich, A.J., Lyon, G. and Evrard, P. (1992). Formation, maturation, and disorders of white matter *Am. J. Neuroradiol.*, **13**, 447–61

54. Ettlinger, G. (1977). Agenesis of the corpus callosum. In Vinicken, P.J. and Bruyn, G.W. (eds.) *Handbook of Clinical Neurology*, vol. 30, pp. 431–78. (Amsterdam: North Holland)

55. Kendall. B.E. (1983). Dysgenesis of the corpus callosum. *Neuroradiology*, **25**, 239–56

56. Hirsch, J.F., Pierre Kahn, A. and Renier, D. (1984). The Dandy–Walker malformation. *J. Neurosurg.*, **61**, 515–22

57. Raybaud, C. (1982). Cystic malformations of the posterior fossa: abnormalities associated with development of the roof of the fourth ventricle and adjacent meningeal structures. *J. Neuroradiol.*, **9**, 103–33

58. Barkovich, A.J., Kjos, B.O., Normann, D. and Edwards, M.S. (1988). New concepts of posterior fossa cysts in children (abst.). *Am. J. Neuroradiol.*, **9**, 1016

59. Barkovich, A.J., Kjos, B.O., Norman, D. and Edwards, M.S. (1989). Revised classification of posterior fossa cysts and cyst-like malformations based upon the results of multiplanar MR imaging. *Am. J. Neuroradiol.*, **10**, 977–88

60. Barkovich, A.J., Wippold, F.J., Shermann, J.L. *et al.* (1986). Significance of cerebellar tonsillar ectopia on MR. *Am. J. Neuroradiol.*, **7**, 795–9

61. McLone, D.G. and Naidich, T.P. (1992). Developmental morphology of the subarachoid space, brain vasculature, and contiguous structures, and the cause of the Chiari II malformation. *Am. J. Neuroradiol.*, **13**, 463–82

62. Naidich, T.P. (1986). Cranial CT signs of the Chiari II malformation. *J. Neuroradiol*, **8**, 233–9

63. Benaceraff, B.R. and Estroff, J.A. (1989). Transvaginal sonographic imaging of the low fetal head in the second trimester. *J. Ultrasound Med.*, **8**, 325

64. Monteagudo, A., Reuss, M.L. and Timor-Tritsch, I.E. (1991). Imaging of the fetal brain in the

second and third trimester using transvaginal sonography. *Obstet. Gynecol.*, **77**, 27–32

65. Kido, D.K., Morris, T.W., Erickson, J.L., Plewes, D.B. and Simon, J.H. (1987). Physiologic changes during high field strength MR imaging. *Am. J. Nucl. Radiol.*, **8**, 263–6

66. Shellock, F.G. and Crues, J.V. (1988). Temperature changes caused by MR imaging of the brain with a head coil. *Am. J. Nucl. Radiol.*, **9**, 287–91

67. Wolff, S., Crooks, L.E., Brown, P. *et al.* (1980). Tests for DNA and chromosomal damage induced by nuclear magnetic resonance imaging. *Radiology*, **136**, 707–10

68. Wolff, S., James, T.L., Young, G.B., Margulis, A.R., Bodycote, J. and Afzal. V. (1985). Magnetic resonance imaging: absence of in vitro cytogenetic damage. *Radiology*, **155**, 163–5

Fetal neurology

10

J. C. Birnholz

Measuring the transverse diameter of the fetal skull was one of the pioneer clinical applications of ultrasound[1], building upon much earlier experience in pathology and radiology. A transducer was placed over a presumed location of the fetal head and moved in contact with the maternal abdomen while a search was conducted for a distinctive pattern of large echoes (the calvarium) with a midline complex (the apposing surfaces of the cortex adjoining the interhemispheric fissure) on an A-mode display. B-mode imaging depicted the oval shape of the base of the calvarium on a calibrated display screen, speeding the search process and providing standards for measurement of specific cranial dimensions. This imaging capability led directly to a primary screening application for ultrasound in detecting (or excluding) exencephaly acrania (i.e. anencephaly) in the second trimester[2]. The dual introductions of imaging devices with high speed and wide dynamic range in the mid-1970s gave operators the ability to study fetal dynamics, to locate specific scan planes, to optimize instrument settings expeditiously and to traverse the barrier of the skull to view the brain itself[3]. A large literature has developed about the uses of ultrasound for visualizing cerebral anatomy, tracking the time course of the appearance of some cerebral morphological features, recognizing malformations, and attempting to monitor the emergence of central nervous system control mechanisms. This chapter seeks a synthesis of basic information about fetal cerebral development and recent technical advances in ultrasound imaging as a guide to structuring prenatal examination of the central nervous system.

The brain consists of an enormous number of electrically interactive neurons and their support cells, which moderate the chemical and immune environment of the entire system. Neurons are arranged with topographic precision into conscious and unconscious modules that subsume perception, memory, learning, action and physiological control. The finest detail resolution of ultrasound imaging is (considerably) grosser than the scale of neuronal organization. Pure ultrasonic, anatomical evaluation of the fetal central nervous system is limited to major malformations, although subtle aspects of behavior can be inferred from dynamic observations, analogous to determining the function of a 'black box' with the tools of systems analysis without knowing anything about the components of the box itself. In the clinical realm we are concerned with the genetic pattern of brain development and with the interactions of that scheme and intrauterine, intrafetal and intracranial environments. This chapter emphasizes the problem of evaluating a maturing brain that appears normal anatomically at the millimeter scale of ultrasonic visualization.

TECHNICAL FACTORS

There have been three advances in ultrasound imaging during the past decade, which are relevant to mapping fetal cerebral features *in utero*. The earliest was the advent of large-aperture, multielement, electronically scanned array transducer technology, which achieves low-noise viewing of small anatomical regions displayed in a magnified format[4]. The second series of advances extended the performance features of magnification imaging for transabdominal viewing, including the ancillary use of pulsed, one- and two-dimensional Doppler processing. This series of improvements included transducer materials and fabrication techniques, pulse-shaping and beam-forming methods, signal processing and display characteristics. The third area has been the incorporation of all of these advances in an endovaginal array transducer, which has the highest theoretical performance for viewing fetal structures adjacent to the cervix, because this transmission path eliminates the degrading effects of reverberant noise from layers of skin, fat, fascia and muscle. 'Theoretical' is an important distinction, because ultrasound wave propagation is very complicated, the modules of the imaging chain do not have stable equilibria or optima, and specific implementations of commercial equipment vary greatly in performance.

Spatial resolution relates to the smallest structure that can be seen or the smallest distance between reflectors that can be separated unambiguously. Diffraction limits the best resolution to slightly more than a one-wavelength spacing[5]. For fetal brain viewing under optimal conditions, spatial resolution should be between 0.5 and 1.0 mm. Contrast resolution is an even more important consideration for diagnostic work, since it relates to the ability to distinguish structures or materials. A minute calcification can be identified anywhere within the brain, because it has a large contrast gradient with surrounding tissue. Conversely, a large region of leukomalacia might not be visible, if its inherent contrast (vs. normal tissue) were too low under some set of imaging conditions. Contrast relates in a complicated way to the bulk moduli of elasticity of the target and surrounding material as well as to the physical arrangement of the two regions, their population densities of reflectors and the statistics of their spacing, orientation, roughness, motion and temperature. Contrast depends upon the frequency spectrum of the interrogating acoustic pulse and appears to exhibit peaks and minima in simulations. Unfortunately, frequency content cannot be 'tuned' during an examination, nor are transmission paths or intervening tissue fields consistent between patients. The operator may, however, optimize perceived contrast by adjusting signal amplification factors, imposing image filters and altering perceived contrast with selected intensity maps and pseudocoloration[6].

Ultrasonic assessment of cerebral function involves inferences from observing and characterizing motion, which depends upon temporal resolution performance of the imaging device. Ultrasonic pulses are generated repetitively. The interval between pulses is usually set to be slightly longer than the round-trip transit time between the probe and the furthest site from which echoes may be received. Each pulse represents the potential data line. The repetition rate in pulses per second encompasses the number of lines per image and the number of images per second (the frame rate). In order to identify motion, the target must change its position by at least a few pixels between successive frames. Image magnification improves the ratio of display pixels to tissue distance, optimizing temporal resolution for whatever the combination of frame rate and line spacing. Interframe registration and beam positioning were additional concerns with mechanical scanning systems that have been obviated with electronic scanning.

Conventional, pulsed Doppler selects a window along the beam path and determines the frequency shift of the reference pulse within that zone. The frequency shift is proportional to the velocity of movement within that window along the beam axis. For blood flow in fetal cerebral and other vessels and ultrasound in the low megahertz range, the frequency shift is in the audible range of sound, and it is usually presented both as a sound and as a graph. Color Doppler involves mapping the Doppler shift as sampled and distributed over an area, a two-dimensional sampling. The original type of color Doppler mapped the amplitude of the frequency shift and preserved information about the direction of motion relative to the probe. New forms of Doppler imaging map a descriptor based on the squared magnitude of the frequency shift, which is related to signal energy. This technique results in a great improvement in sensitivity, at the expense of information pertinent to signal phase or flow direction. Doppler sensing is applied clinically for the most part for displaying fluid flows, either blood within vessels or lung liquid in the respiratory tract or in amniotic fluid adjacent to the nose and mouth.

There is no difference in information content between Doppler frequency shift and direct measurement of target movement, although frequency shift methods are easier to implement technically for small-amplitude, high-velocity movements. Movements of lower velocity and larger amplitude can be observed directly. These include the motor repertory of the fetus, i.e. neuromotor 'behavior'. Movements may be spontaneous or provoked. Those movements that occur principally within a plane can be characterized fully by ultasound. Evaluation may be descriptive or involve quantitation of velocity, displacement, or temporal statistics. Ultrasound observations of movements tend to be regional, since all current devices are configured for a single field of view.

Early array imaging devices with mechanical switching, high voltage and shock excitation of transducer elements generated an enormous amount of audible noise at the transducer excitation repetition rate, around 2500 Hz. Later in pregnancy, noise in this frequency range can provoke changes in fetal behavior and heart rate, which can be misinterpreted as an effect of ultrasound itself. Modern electronic probes tend to be noiseless, although there may be some combinations of dual Doppler and B-mode imaging that may generate noise. The issue of biological safety of ultrasound itself seems to have been resolved satisfactorily for the case of clinical fetal imaging with devices using higher power levels than are the current standard. In addition, there is always enough movement between the hand-held probe and the target (as well as pulse dispersion) to preclude standing wave and constructive interference, energy concentration, effects. We do, however, try to minimize scanning time and consequently exposure with transfontanelle viewing of a later fetus when, presumably, calvarial ossification has proceeded to a point that multiple intracranial reverberations might occur.

CEREBRAL CORTEX AND CORPUS CALLOSUM

We suggest the following simple model for organizational purposes when an ultrasound examination is structured. Neurons proliferate in the germinal matrix, a region that may be nourished primarily in early pregnancy by passive diffusion of substances conveyed by cerebrospinal fluid. The first phase of neuronal proliferation seems to occur at around 10–12 weeks after conception. Neurons begin to migrate centripetally at around 12–14 weeks, progressively thickening the cortex and forming histologically distinct layers[7]. Glial cells begin to proliferate after neuronal migration has commenced, further thickening the cortex. Radial glial cells positioned in the germinal matrix provide guides for subsequent neuronal migrations through pre-existent layers. These migrations continue until at least the fourth decade of life[8]. There is an overproduction of neurons, which compete for interconnections. There is a profound decrease in those neurons which fail to connect 'properly'; however, cerebral size continues to increase as myelination progresses.

Brain development is sequential, apparently following an exact timetable. Any abnormality sufficiently gross for ultrasound detection in early pregnancy can be expected to have catastrophic functional consequences, if there is survival. The embryological events have been traced for a number of genetic forms of dysmorphic brain development. By and large, these will be amenable to prenatal detection. An injury confined to the germinal matrix, destroying neurons before migration or killing radial glial cells (that will disarray years of timed migrations) can have serious functional consequences, even though the anatomical injury may escape detection *in utero*. This is a clinical concern with exposure to drugs, toxic agents or infectious diseases.

Throughout the remainder of this chapter, developmental time will be referenced to gestational age, equal to conceptual age plus two weeks. Ultrasound views of the cranium at 8–9 weeks already show paired choroid glomi. The predominant feature in early examination is the telencephalic vesicle. The choroid glomi are relatively massive by 12 weeks, when there is the barest outlining of cerebral cortex peripheral to the margins of the lateral ventricles. The brainstem is seen posteriorly; the cerebellum is defined by 13.0 weeks, when the transverse diameter is 10 mm and the fourth ventricle relatively capacious. All of the major vessels are present and positioned anatomically (Color Plates G and I). The gross pattern of the cerebral cortex and cerebellum become evident within the next two weeks. Coronal transfontanelle views show the cortex well from the mid-second trimester, with rudimentary

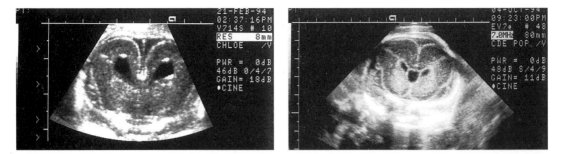

Figure 1 Progressive thickening of the cortex in the second trimester. The faint striae within the cortex, conforming to the ventricular margin, are vascular channels that appear when individual neuronal layers develop. The left image is an anterior, coronal section near the start of cortical development with wide interhemispheric fissure and lateral ventricular continuity

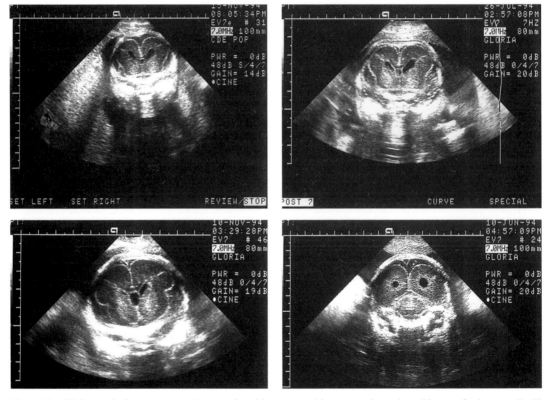

Figure 2 Mild ventricular asymmetry is normal and becomes evident as early as the mid-second trimester. Dr T. Naidich (Miami, personal communication) believes that symmetry, which is present in about 10% of cases, predicts left-handedness

subdivision of the cortex corresponding to, or at least coincident with, layering visible from 18 weeks onwards (Figure 1). Slight to moderate asymmetry of the lateral ventricles (without cortical mantle asymmetry) is common around 5 months (Figure 2). This appears to be a normal finding, which might be associated with the subsequent pattern of handedness. Temporal lobe asymmetries found in anatomical specimens has been related to language acquisition[9].

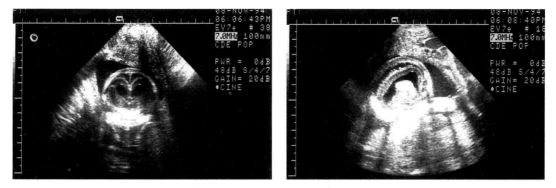

Figure 3 Trisomy 21 at 17.4 weeks' gestational age. Ventriculomegaly results from delayed cortical growth and may diminish after 5 months as glial cells proliferate

The choroid glomi produce cerebrospinal fluid, biochemically similar to the production of urine by the kidneys. It is possible that the type of hydrocephalus that is identified in the second trimester is due to a biochemical defect in choroid function, with undernutrition or starvation of proliferating cells in the germinal matrix. Most cases recognized early have an exceptionally thin cortical mantle and relatively small choroid that gravitates dependently within cerebrospinal fluid (implying relatively decreased fluid specific gravity). Obstructive forms of hydrocephalus appear to be late pregnancy or postnatal events. It is essential to visualize and evaluate the cortex before entertaining a diagnosis of hydrocephalus. We have seen many instances of alleged ventriculomegaly with low-performance equipment or attempted viewing through the calvarium (especially from a transabdominal portal) in which the choroid glomi were thought to float or be suspended within a capacious fluid space, whereas transfontanelle viewing showed the hyporeflective cortical mantle. True ventriculomegaly in the mid-second trimester is pathological. Spina bifida and aneuploidy are typical etiologies. It is possible that a biochemical transport deficit of the choroid occurs with trisomy 21, similar to the as yet unclassified placental transport deficit underlying alterations in maternal serum α-fetoprotein level. We have observed profuse choroidal vascularity with energy Doppler imaging in three recent cases of trisomy 21 at 17.4, 19 and 27.8 weeks, with moderate ventriculomegaly (Figures 3 and 4;

Color Plate H). The 19-week case also had numerous small choroidal cysts.

Growth of the brain in the third trimester involves a massive increase in surface area with sulcation. Jouandet and Deck[10] reported an elegant computer analysis technique for unravelling surface features of the brain from photographs of whole brain slices of 25 fetuses of 25–42 weeks' gestational age. They noted correlations between brain surface area, volume, weight and gestational age and reported a surface area slowly increasing to about 40 cm^2 at 24 weeks, expanding afterwards to some 300 cm^2 at term. Sulci are easily appreciated in tangential transfontanelle views of a parietal lobe late in the third trimester (Figure 5). A shallow indentation of the callosomarginal sulcus is seen medially along each occipital lobe by the start of the third trimester in transverse views. Migrational disorders result in a smooth (agyria) or hyposulcated (polymicrogyria, pachygyria) brain, which is not identified ultrasonically until sulcation is well established in the mid-third trimester. Brain growth is a continuum. An abnormal ultrasound appearance conveys a poor developmental prognosis; however, a 'normal' appearance cannot exclude a problem that may be unmasked later in development. 'Microcephaly' is a descriptive term that includes a vast number of individual syndromes, some of which will be abnormal from the mid-second trimester and others of which may evolve postnatally.

Ultrasound does not display the entire cerebral cortex. The corpus callosum, however, is a graphic

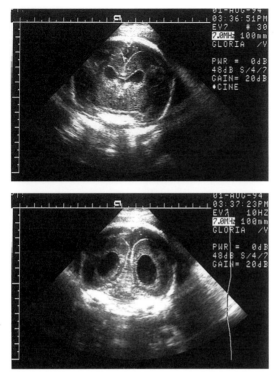

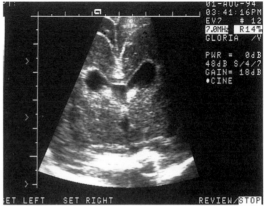

Figure 4 Persistent ventriculomegaly in the third trimester with trisomy 21 seems to imply clinical severity and is more often associated with extracerebral findings than when cortical thickness growth is better established. This case also had an atrioventricular canal defect

intracranial feature that appears to provide a global index of cortical development, being a collection of axons connecting isologous portions of neopallium (Figure 6). There may be as many as 800 million fibers at birth[11]. Callosal morphology has been related to brain mass, although interspecies comparisons suggest that the primary relationship is between callosal size and cortical neuronal density[12]. When the cortex is hypoplastic, the corpus callosum is small or absent; when there are focal injuries of the cortex, the fibers from that region atrophy and the corpus callosum becomes locally notched or pocked.

The embryological events preceding the formation of the corpus callosum have been established. One theory holds that a collection of cells derived from the lamina terminalis of the telencephalon, the massa communis, acts as a chemical attractor for axons to cross the midline[13]. Axons begin to cross between the hemispheres as neurons are migrating to their pre-determined layers. Crossing is patterned in time with frontal fibers initiating the process, occipital and temporal lobes being recruited later[14]. The cells of layer V that initiate crossing appear to be pre-determined before

migration and differ in their response to growth cone inducers from other cells of the same layer[15]. Genetic studies in mice have suggested several alleles contributing to callosal dysmorphology, operating through interference with growth cone guidance[16], and it is an ability of some cells to achieve crossing through alternate pathways (such as the bundle of Probst) that may account for the clinical heterogeneity of callosal agenesis (unassociated with other cortical abnormalities)[17]. The corpus callosum may also be absent because of a genetic midline defect (as with holoprosencephaly)

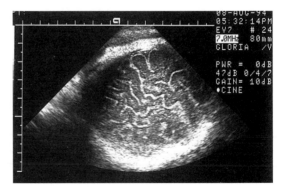

Figure 5 Tangential view of the parietal sulcal pattern in the mid-third trimester

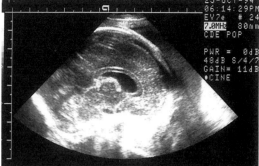

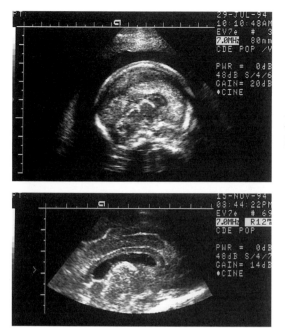

Figure 6 Midline sagittal views of the developing corpus callosum. Boundary definition, length, and the volume of the cavum increase with age; thickness variations emerge in the third trimester

or acquired from vascular injury of any or all of its three separate arteries. The commissural zone of the corpus callosum can be found at 13.0 weeks and becomes more distinct as a vertically orientated fragment, outlined by a short pericallosal artery, by the start of the 14th week (Color Plate I).

We have studied the maximal length of corpus callosum in a collection of some 600 clinically normal fetuses between 14 and 36 weeks. The variance of these data in each gestational age block is relatively low, which corresponds to the consistency in timing of brain development. These data fit with $CC^{0.5} = 7.564549 - 1287.3797/GA^2$ ($r^2 = 0.973$, $F = 21,243$, $SE = 1.45$), where GA is the gestational age in weeks and CC is the callosal length in mm. This can be used to generate a table of normal values. Growth is not linear. Peak velocity of elongation occurs at about 19.4 weeks (Figure 7). Velocity continues to diminish during the first year of life; low-velocity growth continues into adulthood[18]. Some 40% of callosal axons may be lost in normal development[19]. It is unclear when the process of neuronal cell death and axon degeneration begins, although it appears to commence by the mid-third trimester. In the third-trimester case of trisomy 21 noted above, there was an unusually thick corpus callosum. Neuronal cell density may be higher than normal with mental retardation, because cell death is incomplete (and optimal 'wiring' patterns are not formed). We have also observed an unusually thick corpus callosum in a case of tuberous sclerosis (Figure 8).

During collection of these data, we observed callosal length significantly less than anticipated for gestational age in four of six cases of maternal Dilantin[R] use with ultrasound studies beteen 20 and 24 weeks. It has recently been shown that prenatal hydantoin drug exposure is associated with diminished intellectual function demonstrable in childhood[20]. We speculate that callosal length near the start of the third trimester may correlate with intellectual testing in childhood and urge that this be studied prospectively. Conversely, we suspect that a normal callosal length provides evidence of normal brain development to the stage of the examination. In this series, we were able to visualize the margins of the corpus callosum clearly in about 70% of routine cases between 14 and 36 weeks. We selected length as a simple, relatively unequivocal measurement that can be made without additional image processing and computational requirements, although availability of such resources will permit a more complete characterization of morphology, as has been done with postnatal nuclear magnetic resonance studies[21].

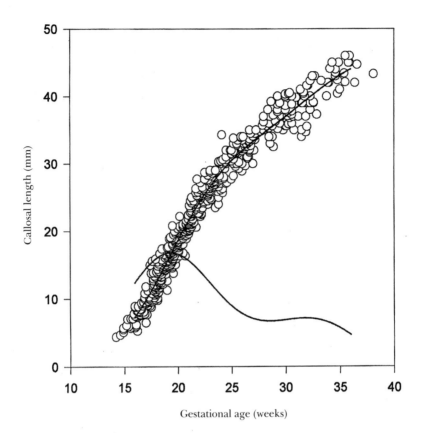

Figure 7 Corpus callosal length versus gestational age in some 600 cases. The line tracing represents velocity sampled at 1-day intervals with a peak at 19.4 weeks, just after the first phase of neuronal migration from the periventricular germinal matrix into the ipsilateral cortex

BLOOD FLOW AND ACQUIRED CONDITIONS

The distinction between inherent, embryological, or primary developmental disorders of the brain and acquired conditions tends to be arbitrary and vague. Primary causes of dysmorphic development are those that have been traced to early gestation, are without an obvious environmental cause, and have some sort of genetic predisposition. Acquired conditions are those for which some external agency explains the mechanism of malformation. The sequence of brain development is so complicated that it is to be expected that many different factors can have a similar morphological or functional outcome, blurring an understanding of malformation etiology. The neural tube defects, for example, have been traced very early in development to the time of neuropore closure and have about a 1.5% recurrence risk, which has been interpreted as implying a genetic component[22]. The mechanism of failed cell mass adhesion remains to be determined. Thermal stress has been implicated as a predisposing factor[23], and it has been suggested that folic acid deficiency accounts for the exceptionally high incidence of this condition in Wales, where pre-pregnancy vitamin supplementation has had an apparent impact upon the incidence of this condition[24].

The principal acquired abnormality in the perinatal period is hypoxic–ischemic injury, and it

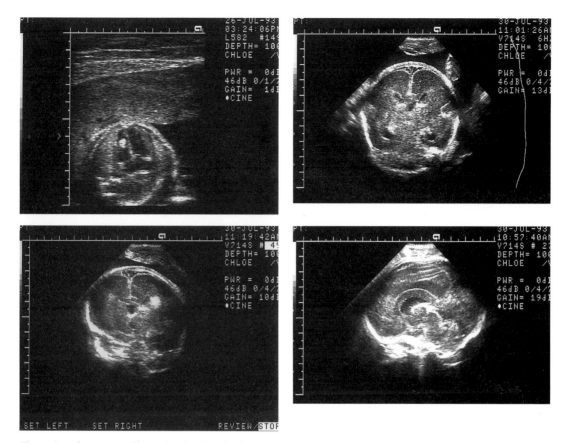

Figure 8 The corpus callosum is (abnormally) thick in a case of tuberous sclerosis from interference with the normal pattern cellular competition for interconnections and selective cell death of excessive neurons. Other findings are a periventricular reflective patch (lower right), thick cortex and elevated ventricles (upper right), and a cardiac rhabdomyoma (upper left)

is identification of risk for this condition that underlies the uses of intrapartum heart rate monitoring and prenatal 'biophysical' profiling. Periventricular hemorrhage is a common problem in premature infants (24–35 weeks), but prenatal instances are rare, tending to occur with conditions promoting venous thrombosis, such as maternal paroxysmal nocturnal hemoglobinuria and interruptions in cord flow. There is intense venous proliferation in both subependymal regions, beginning shortly after 5 months and regressing later in the third trimester, which can be visualized with the energy Doppler (Color Plate J). It is thought that hemorrhages in neonates occur from abrupt swings in central venous pressure, as with pneumothorax, and that hemorrhage within the

confined subependymal region compromises local venous flow from adjacent white matter, predisposing to associated periventricular hemorrhage. Prenatal vascular compromise of periventricular white matter presumably results from decreased flow within the endarterial watershed of that region, resulting in a morphologically identical sequence of lesions to venous infarction (although arterial hypotensive lesions are typically bilateral; venous lesions unilateral).

Agents such as cocaine cause infarcts by focal or diffuse arterial spasm. Injury sustained early in pregnancy may cause hydranencephaly or absence of all or most of a hemisphere. More typical stroke presentations occur in late pregnancy exposures, when placental abruption often overshadows the

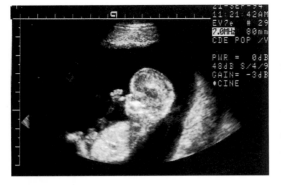

Figure 9 The rest position of the hands in early pregnancy is in front of the face. Hand–face contacts are frequent

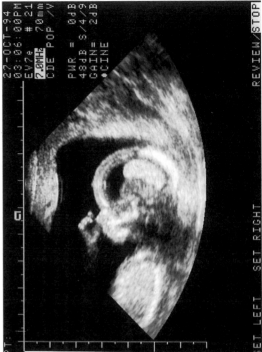

clinical presentation. We have seen two cases of perinatal stroke with an unusual placental architecture, raising the possibility that injury can also be sustained by intrafetal thromboembolism arising within the placental vascular bed. Major arterial and venous landmarks can be visualized throughout the second and third trimesters, whenever the anterior fontanelle can be accessed. Midline sagittal views show paired anterior cerebral arteries with an anterior trifurcation; the pericallosal artery within the pericallosal cistern outlines the corpus callosum. Magnification views may show the recurrent artery of Huebner (Color Plate K). The straight sinus and great vein are visible posteriorly. Anterior angled coronal views permit comparison of both middle cerebral arteries; the basal veins of Rosenthal form the dominant features in posterior angled views. Base planes identify the circle of Willis from lateral portals (Color Plate G) and the vertebrobasilar, pontine and medullary channels are seen through the posterior fontanelle. Posterior fossa venous flow is studied with the probe positioned at about shoulder level.

Some viral (and spirochete) infections will have an associated intracranial vasculopathy with progressive calcification of lenticulostriate vessels demonstrable ultrasonically[25], typically associated with mild dilatation of one or both lateral ventricles, thickening and hyperemia of the ventricular margin and intraventricular synechiae. Porencephaly represents a focal region of destruction of periventricular white matter, as does cystic encephalomalacia within the cortex.

FETAL BEHAVIOR

The developed central nervous system is the locus of physiological and neuromotor control. Demonstration of control implies something about functional maturation of the brain, and loss of control indicates an acute brain syndrome, which can be seen with hypoxia or sedative drug exposure. Control mechanisms are inferred from dynamics, which are, usually, classified subjectively. Movements that occur within a plane can be characterized completely from ultrasound observations.

Early speculations about fetal motor behavior included schemes of accruing progressively more complex movements from 'reflex' units (Figure 9). Observations on stimulus–response behaviors of live early pregnancy abortuses were reported by

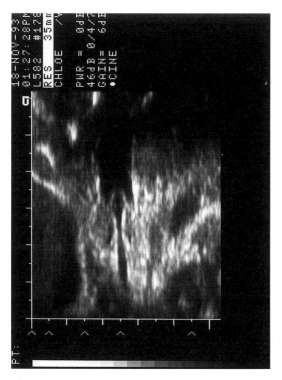

Figure 10 A coronal section of the neck demonstrates the tracheal fluid column. Deep valleculae emphasize the epiglottis, which projects into the hypopharynx. There is slight narrowing of the fluid column at the glottis

Hooker, Humphries and their students, 30–40 years ago[26], reinforcing an interpretive notion of reflex assimilation. Ultrasound permits detailed observations of a range of movements, under physiological conditions. Chronologies of movement patterns were reported soon after the introduction of electronic scanning[27,28], which attempted to build upon those earlier theories of development. Ultrasound experience suggests that a new and more sophisticated notion of fetal neuromotor development is necessary, with emphasis on central activity rather than on peripheral effectors. Spontaneous movements are already identified a month after conception, movements are more frequent than had been appreciated earlier (with mothers perceiving only a small percentage of activity after quickening) and a complex repertory of individual motor activities is possible by mid-pregnancy, even though prolonged observations may be required to identify specific activities or to align the observation window with fetomaternal environmental conditions.

The following sequence is proposed as an organizational model for ultrasound observations. A capability for making some kind of movement appears relatively early in development; fatigue effects limit 'practicing'; the incidence is sporadic, relatively uncommon. Mechanisms of central inhibition, specific to the movement pattern, develop (almost like an antigen–antibody complex), and the movement seems to disappear. Then it reappears, becoming progressively smoother in execution and coordinated with other motor activities. Bursts of diaphragm excursions (breathing) are seen between 13 and 15 weeks, vanishing during the next month, and increasing progressively in incidence throughout the third trimester. Breathing is most readily studied with the color flow Doppler, which demonstrates plumes or jets of fluid through the nasopharynx, ejected into amniotic fluid. Before 18 weeks, fluid flows are primarily through the mouth; between 18 and 24 weeks, flows tend to be by nose and mouth, and there is progressive increase in preferential nose breathing afterwards. Breathing also involves movements of the larynx and epiglottis, which are independent before the fifth month, but which become coordinated with diaphragm activity after that time[29]. Swallowing also involves a complex series of movements involving tongue oropharyngeal walls, pharynx, valleculae, epiglottis and esophagus, which can be observed in magnification views of the region of the neck (Figure 10). Swallowing and breathing remain separate until about 32 weeks, which is the stage at which a newborn infant can suckle and breathe at the same time without aspiration. The appearance, inhibition and reappearance sequence can be compressed or prolonged, and it is reiterated for the motor milestones that are sought in physical examinations of infants.

The notion of 'behavioral state' or an operant level for the nervous system was developed as an explanation for differences in peripheral reflex behavior, depending on whether an infant is awake, in active sleep, or deep sleep[30]. Other physiological factors also vary, including regional blood flow in the brain[31]. Specific behavioral states are defined as particular combinations of findings.

We do not subscribe to current attempts at identifying individual behavioral states antenatally. It is not practical to make multiple simultaneous fetal measurements with the restriction of cross-sectional imaging. Behavioral states underspecified by a few observational features appear to have such frequent transitions and evident lack of stability that it is difficult to assign a clinical value to their occurrence or absence, particularly before the final month of pregnancy. Observations can be standardized by altering the 'state' externally, by such means as a startling or oreintating form of stimulation.

The 'hardware' for auditory perception may be present near the end of the first trimester, but motor responses to stimulation are a feature of the third trimester. Decremental behavior, or at least some form of habituation, is demonstrated for repetitive stimuli after 28 weeks, which may be taken as a type of learning. There are preliminary reports of discriminatory responses to complex stimuli (mostly auditory) in the third trimester[32].

As oxygen delivery from the placenta diminishes, the fetus will attempt to compensate by increasing venous return to the heart, redistributing blood flow to the heart, brain and adrenals, and conserving energy in the short term by decreasing motor activity and over a longer timecourse by diminishing the somatic growth rate (by decreasing elaboration of growth factors from the gut). The practical issue for the examiner is to distinguish energy conservation from a sleep state, both of which involve centrally mediated inhibition of movements. The normal response to repetitive (loud) auditory stimulation is a startle, which becomes inhibited within 1–3 signal repeats after 28 weeks. As control is lost, the fetus appears to be irritable, with exaggerated, irregular and inconsistent responses. As compromise becomes more profound, a pre-terminal, coma-like state ensues, with a flaccid, immobile and unresponsive fetus, having bradycardia. A deaf fetus will have no response to a purely auditory stimulation; however, there will be responses to other forms of stimulation, including vibration. A motor response to manual compression of the uterus was described as a test of wellness about two centuries ago[33].

Fluid flows through the nose should be demonstrable in brief viewing segments sometime during each third-trimester examination. There is variability in the Doppler waveform from breath to breath, which is equivalent exactly to beat-to-beat heart rate variability. The timing of respiratory and cardiac events is influenced by the brainstem, which receives afferent information from a variety of pressure- and chemistry-sensitive receptors. Heart rate control operates through the sinoatrial pacemaker, but oscillatory circuits for respiration are situated in the brainstem itself. In both cases, it is the interplay of multiple sensors and effectors becoming activated within individual beat or breath intervals that results in variability, a type of stochastic or unstable equilibrium. There is a sequence of effects similar to auditory response behavior with progressive hypoxia, with short-term variability effects becoming erratic before they are abolished. An additional manifestation of progressive hypoxia is changed in the breathing pattern itself, with inspiration becoming shorter in duration and higher in peak velocity, and expiration taking on a passive recoil quality rather than being an active expulsion of fluid. Both ultrasonically observed respiratory activity and fetal electrocardiography can be applied as objective and quantitative signs of midbrain oxygenation and function.

The signs of distress that are applied clinically represent disordered control at the level of the brainstem. Presumably, disordered cortical mentation might identify lesser degrees of hypoxia. We believe that some information about cortical level function, including the extrinsic influence of the intrauterine environment, might be interpreted from facial expressions[34]. Anthropology research suggests that there are 'universal' expressions found in every society, which may be presumed to be innate. The face is an organ of communication with an enormous range of potential expressions. We presume that an infant tests a number of expressions, some of which are reinforced, presumably by the same resonance effects that seem to underlie verbal language acquisition. Facial observations can be made *in utero*, including a subjective determination of 'mood', which is a multivariate perceptual task accomplished subconsciously in human communication (Figure 11). In our preliminary experience we believe we have associated an appearance of serenity with well-

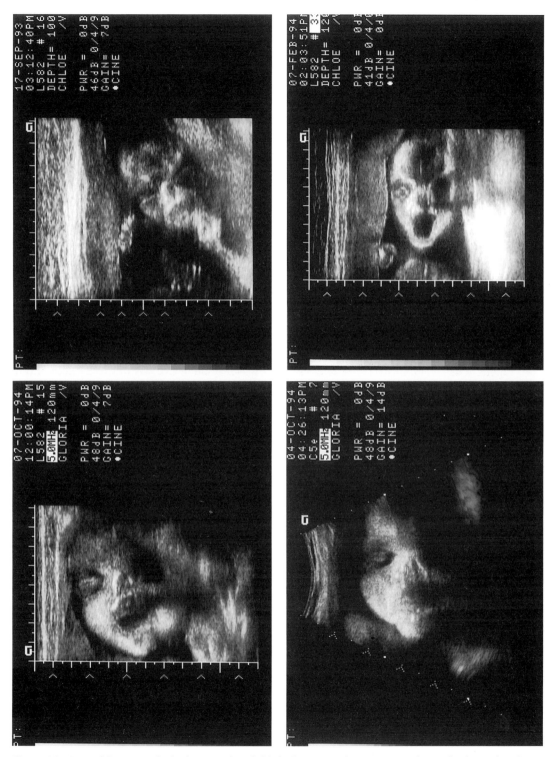

Figure 11 Frontal face portraits in the second and third trimesters. Observer perception and subconscious interpretation of facial expressions result in a feeling or emotive color to these views. The lower right image is the case of trisomy 21 of Figure 4

being, and persistent frowning and grimacing with placental failure. Increased suckling behavior represents an analog of hunger and is seen with growth retardation (primary intrauterine malnutrition) and with fetuses large for gestational age, in whom nutritional requirements are increased, perhaps beyond a level of satisfaction. Maternal nutritional factors may influence fetal behavior acutely via glucose level variations and chronically via lack of excess of trace elements[35].

CONCLUSION

Gross aspects of the morphological development of the brain can be monitored with ultrasound from the mid-first trimester through parturition. At some point, the complexity of neuronal interconnections initiates the mind, which exhibits central physiological control of most vital processes and perhaps begins to acquire awareness and an ability to learn. Information about the functional operations of the mind are inferred from ultrasound observations of dynamics, such as breathing, swallowing, spontaneous limb and torso movements, or specific responses to sensory stimulation. Consequently, evaluation of the developing central nervous system is integrative and involves observations of the entire fetus and of its supply line, including placenta, cord and mother. Although there have been significant improvements in neurobiological sophistication and in ultrasound imaging technology during the last few years, prenatal studies should be entered into with a profound respect for the enormous complexity of the brain and a constant appreciation of the limitations of the ultrasound technique.

Examination of the structural development of the brain is prompted by well-established incidence values of aneuploidy, neural tube defects and dysmorphic syndromes. Evaluation of central function is driven clinically by the problem of identifying distress prior to an irreversible cerebral injury, so that the fetus can be removed to a more supportive environment. As ultrasound imaging technology has advanced, primary epidemiological and prognostic applications of the technique have emerged. Study of external maternal conditions at the time of onset of a malformation or during a critical phase of organogenesis may reveal preventable causes of these lesions. Eventually, we may be able to design studies to determine those intrauterine conditions that might enhance intellectual, personality, or emotional development later in life.

References

1. Donald, I. and Brown, T.G. (1961). Demonstration of tissue interfaces within the body by ultrasonic echo sounding. *Br. J. Radiol.*, **34**, 539–46
2. Campbell, S., Johnstone, F.D., Holt, E.M. and May, P. (1972). Anencephaly: early ultrasonic diagnosis and active management. *Lancet*, **2**, 1226–7
3. Birnholz, J.C. (1983). Evolution of the ultrasound examination. *J. Clin. Ultrasound*, **13**, 83–5
4. Maslak, S. (1985). Computed sonography. In Sauders, R. (ed.) *Ultrasound Annual.* (New York: Raven Press)
5. Rayleigh, L. and Strutt, J.W. (1894). *The Theory of Sound*, Vol. 1. (New York: Dover Press). Reprinted 1945
6. Birnholz, J.C. (1990). The art of ultrasound. Ultrasound Q., 8, 267–90
7. Berry, M. (1986). Neurogenesis and gliogenesis in the human brain. *Fd. Chem. Toxic*, **24**, 79–89
8. Sarnat, H.B. (1987). Disturbances of late neuronal migrations in the perinatal period. *Am. J. Dis. Child.*, **141**, 969–80
9. Wittleson, S.F. and Pallie, W. (1973). Left hemisphere specialization for language in the newborn. *Brain*, **96**, 641–6
10. Jouandet, M.L. and Deck, M.D.F. (1993). Prenatal growth of the human cerebral cortex: brainprint analysis. *Radiology*, **188**, 765–74
11. Koppel, H. and Innocenti, G.M. (1983). Is there a genuine exuberancy of callosal projections in development? A quantitative electron microscopic study in the cat. *Neurosci. Lett.*, **41**, 33–40
12. Tarpley, R.J. and Ridgway, S.H. (1994). Corpus callosum size in delphinid cetaceans. *Brain Behav. Evol.*, **44**, 156–65
13. Rakic, P. and Yakovlev, P.I. (1968). Development of the corpus callosum and cavum septi in man. *J. Comp. Neurol.*, **132**, 45–72
14. Ozaki, H.S. and Wahlsten, D. (1992). Prenatal

formation of the normal mouse corpus callosum: a quantitative study with carbocyanine dyes. *J. Comp. Neurol.*, **323**, 81–90

15. Koester, S.E. and O'Leary, D.D. (1993). Connectional distinction between callosal and subcortically projecting cortical neurons is determined prior to axon stension. *Dev. Biol.*, **160**, 1–14

16. Wahlsten, D. and Bulman-Fleming, B. (1994). Retarded growth of the medial septum: a major gene effect in acallosal mice. *Dev. Brain Res.*, **77**, 203–14

17. Ozaki, H.S. and Wahlsten, D. (1993). Cortical axon trajectories and growth cone morphologies in fetuses of acallosal mouse strains. *J. Comp. Neurol.*, **336**, 595–604

18. Pujol, J., Vendrell, P., Junque, C., Marti-Vilata, J.L. and Capdevila, A. (1993). When does human brain development end? Evidence of corpus callosum growth up to adulthood. *Ann. Neurol.*, **34**, 71–5

19. LaMantia, A.S. and Rakic, P. (1990). Axon overproduction and elimination in the corpus callosum of the developing rhesus monkey. *J. Neurosci*, **10**, 2156–75

20. Scolnik, D., Nulman, T., Rovent, D., Gladstone, D., Czuchta, D., Gardner, H.A., Gladstone, R. *et al.* (1994). Neurodevelopment of children exposed *in utero* to phenytoin and carbamazepine therapy. *J. Am. Med. Assoc.*, **271**, 767–70

21. Gregory, B.A., Hesselink, J.R. and Jernigan, T.L. (1993). MR imaging of the corpus callosum. *Am. J. Roentgenol.*, **160**, 949–55

22. Holmes, L.B., Driscoll, S.G. and Atkins, L. (1976). Etiologic heterogeneity of neural tube defects. *N. Engl. J. Med.*, **294**, 365–9

23. Smith, D.W., Clarren, S.K. and Harvey, M.A. (1978). Hyperthermia as a possible teratogenetic agent. *J. Pediatr.*, **92**, 878–83

24. Laurence, K.M., James, N., Miller, M.H., Tennant, G.B. and Campbell, H. (1981). Double blind randomised controlled trial of folate treatment before conception to prevent recurrence of neural tube defects. *Br. Med. J.*, **282**, 1509–11

25. Ben-Ami,· T., Yousefzadeh, D., Backus, M., Reichman, B., Kessler, A. and Hammerman-Rozenberg, C. (1990). Lenticulostriate vasculopathy in infants with infections of the central nervous system: sonographic and Doppler findings. *Pediatr. Radiol.*, **20**, 575–9

26. Hooker, D. (1952). *The Prenatal Origin of Behavior*. (Lawrence: University of Kansas Press)

27. Birnholz, J.C., Stephens, J.C. and Faria, M. (1978). A possible means of defining neurologic developmental milestones *in utero*. *Am. J. Roentgenol.*, **138**, 537–40

28. DeVries, J.I.P., Visser, G.H.A. and Prechtl, H.F.R. (1982). The emergence of fetal behavior. I. Quantitative aspects. *Early Hum. Dev.*, **7**, 301–22

29. Isaacson, G. and Birnholz, J.C. (1991). Human fetal respiratory tract function as revealed by ultrasonography. *Ann. Otol. Rhinol. Laryngol.*, **100**, 743–7

30. Prechtl, H.F.R. (1974). The behavioral states of the newborn infant (a review). *Brain*, **76**, 1304–11

31. Shuto, H., Yasuhara, A., Sugimoto, T., Iwase, S. and Kobayashi, Y. (1987). Longitudinal determination of cerebral blood flow velocity in neonates with the Doppler technique. *Neuropediatrics*, **18**, 218–21

32. Shahidullah, S. and Hepper, P.G. (1994). Frequency discrimination by the fetus. *Early Hum. Dev.*, **36**, 13–26

33. Cazeau, P. (1871). In Bullock, W.R. (ed.) A *Theoretic and Practical Treatise on Midwifery*. (Philadelphia: Lindsay & Balkison)

34. Birnholz, J.C. (1995). The face. In Nielson, J.P. and Chambers, S. (eds.) *Obstetric Ultrasound*, vol. 2. (Oxford: Oxford University Press) in press

35. Golub, M.S., Tarantal, A.F., Gershwin, M.E., Keen, C.L. *et al.* (1992). Ultrasound evaluation of fetuses of zinc-deprived monkeys (Macaca mulatta). *Am. J. Clin. Nutr.*, **55**, 734–40

Fetal shunting for hydrocephalus

11

W. H. Clewell

INTRODUCTION

Congenital hydrocephalus, when it is severe, is a disfiguring and severely handicapping condition. In many cases, the severity of brain damage is related to the underlying cause of ventricular enlargement. In some cases, however, the degree of ventricular dilatation seems to determine the extent of brain damage. With the improved ability to diagnose fetal ventriculomegaly, physicians and families feel compelled to intervene to limit the degree of brain damage. In infants, children and adults, treatment of hydrocephalus by ventricular shunting is quite successful in preventing brain damage.

THE ASSUMPTIONS

In order to consider *in utero* ventricular decompression as a reasonable treatment option, one must assume that fetal ventriculomegaly is progressive and that the fetal brain is undergoing progressive damage during gestation. Oi and colleagues[1] have presented some observations which suggest that this hypothesis is correct. In their study, the longer the duration of hydrocephalus from diagnosis to delivery, the worse the developmental outcome. This was independent of the etiology or severity of the hydrocephalus at the time of diagnosis. As noted in other chapters, the cerebral ventricles change in size relative to the hemisphere with advancing gestation in normal fetuses. In hydrocephalus, they are larger than normal when the diagnosis is made and either do not decrease in size in a normal way or enlarge with advancing gestation. The concomitant decrease in cerebral mantle thickness correlates with the extent of fetal brain damage.

THE OPERATIONS

Animal studies

Teratogen-induced hydrocephalus in the monkey

In experimental fetal hydrocephalus, it has been shown that prenatal decompression of the ventricles reduces the severity of neurological injury. Using a rhesus monkey model of hydrocephalus, Michejda and Hodgen showed that with prenatal treatment the monkeys were born in anatomically and functionally better condition than untreated controls[2]. Administration of triamcinolone acetonide on days 21, 23 and 25 of pregnancy produced neural tube defects in 90% of monkey infants. A variety of abnormalities were produced, including hydrocephalus, encephalocele, meningocele and occipital bone hypoplasia. Fetal monkeys with hydrocephalus were treated by placement of a stainless steel valved shunt (hydrocephalic antenatal vent for intrauterine treatment or HAVIT) from the anterior horn of a lateral ventricle to the surface of the fetal skull. All treated infants had marked elevation of intraventricular pressure at the time of HAVIT placement. At birth, untreated control infants had growth retardation, severe hydrocephalus, progressive weakness and frequent seizures, and generally died within a few days of birth. Treated infants grew at near normal rates and demonstrated progressive physical dexterity. Magnetic resonance imaging and pathological examination of the brains of treated monkeys showed nearly normal brain anatomy[3]. At 6 months of age, the treated monkeys showed no neurobehavioral deficits.

Kaolin-induced hydrocephalus in the sheep and monkey

Kaolin injected into the cisterna magna of the fetus regularly results in obstructive hydro-cephalus[4]. Fetal monkeys and lambs with kaolin-induced ventriculomegaly were treated with *in utero* shunting of the ventricles at various intervals after kaolin injection. In the lamb fetus, shunting resulted in decreased ventricular size and improved survival compared to unshunted control animals. In the monkey fetus, shunting 2–3 weeks after kaolin injection resulted in little or no reduction in ventricular size. Shunted animals showed no further increase in ventricular size. The ventricles increased in size in unshunted animals and in several monkeys in which the shunts failed to function. In both animal models, there was extensive inflammatory reaction involving the meninges and the ventricles. While these results were encouraging, there were many complication of shunt treatments in these experiments. Subdural hematoma, subdural hydroma and shunt obstruction were frequently encountered. The severe and extensive inflam-matory response to the kaolin makes it difficult to interpret these results.

Neither triamcinolone nor kaolin induce fetal hydrocephalus is an ideal model. In both models the hydrocephalus is only part of a more extensive process leading to fetal brain damage. Both models showed, however, that shunting of the fetal ventricles reduced the severity of brain damage and improved survival of treated animals com-pared to untreated controls.

Human fetal operations

Serial ventriculocentesis

Ultrasound-guided serial fetal ventriculocentesis was reported by Birnholtz and Frigoletto as a treatment of hydrocephalus[5]. Subsequent to this first report, several other cases have been alluded to in the literature. In the case described by Birnholtz and Frigoletto, the fetus underwent ventricular aspirations at 25, 25.5, 27.5, 29, 30 and 31.5 weeks. In the first procedure, 40 ml of fluid

was removed. The amount aspirated increased to 180 ml in the last two aspirations. As the gestation advanced, it became more difficult to puncture the fetal head, due to increasing calcification of the fetal skull. The intracranial pressure measured at the time of aspiration rose with advancing gestation. Cesarean delivery was performed at 34 weeks' gestation. Postnatal evaluation showed asymmetric hydrocephalus, a posterior midline brain cyst and absence of the corpus callosum. The infant had a ventriculoperitoneal shunt placed shortly after birth. At 16 months of age, the infant was developmentally retarded and had been diagnosed with Becker's muscular dystrophy.

Limited experience makes the assessment of the efficacy of serial ventricular taps impossible. The fetus in the case described above had multiple associated anomalies that affected the develop-ment of the baby. The contribution of hydro-cephalus and its treatment to his developmental problems cannot be assessed. No other cases of serial ventriculocenteses have been described in detail. It seems unlikely that ventricular aspirations performed at the intervals described would be very effective. In newborn infants with acquired communicating hydrocephalus, serial spinal taps performed daily are marginally effective in relieving ventricular hypertension and preventing ventricular enlargement[6]. The ven-tricle must be continuously decompressed to achieve optimal benefit.

Ventriculo-amniotic shunts

Relief of intraventricular hypertension in the newborn by ventricular shunting is well estab-lished and generally accepted as effective treatment of hydrocephalus. These operations can be carried out in infants weighing as little as 500 g. The intent of such operations is to provide a controlled, continuous relief of elevated intraven-tricular pressure. In the cases of fetal hydro-cephalus, the intent is the same and the technique similar. A valved shunt is placed from a lateral ventricle of the fetal brain to drain away excessive fluid and pressure.

Placement of a ventriculo-peritoneal or ventriculo-atrial shunt would have required an

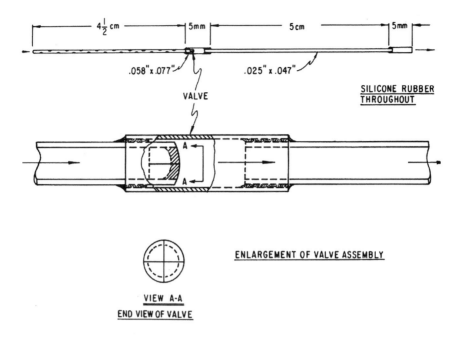

Figure 1 Diagram of the ventriculo-amniotic shunt, which is made from medical-grade silicone rubber. Dimensions on the tubing are the inside diameter by the outside diameter, in inches. Used with permission from reference 7

extensive hysterotomy and direct operation on the fetus. In the situation of uncertain fetal benefit, such an approach was deemed too risky for both the mother and the fetus. A technique was chosen that would place a shunt from the lateral ventricle to the amniotic space. This could be accomplished by a percutaneous ultrasound-guided approach under local anesthesia.

University of Colorado experience

A device was developed at the University of Colorado School of Medicine for shunting the lateral ventricle of the fetus to the amnion (Figure 1). This device was manufactured by Denver Biomaterials of Evergreen, Colorado. The device fit through a 13-gauge thin-walled needle (inside diameter 0.201 cm, outside diameter 0.244 cm). The first treated case has been described in detail[7]. Under local anesthesia and continuous ultrasound guidance, the needle was inserted into the uterus and directed to the posterior parietal area of the fetal skull. The needle was then pushed through the posterior parietal bone of the fetus and into the dilated lateral ventricle. Pressure measurements were taken in the amniotic fluid and the lateral ventricle. The amniotic fluid pressure was 160 cm of water. The lateral ventricle pressure was 225 cm of water. The difference, 65 cm of water, represented the pressure leading to ventricular dilatation. The shunt was then passed through the needle. The valve and proximal portion of the shunt were left in the lateral ventricle and the distal end in the amniotic space (Figure 2). Immediately after shunt placement, the ventricles decreased in size. The first patient treated had the shunt placed at 23 weeks' gestation. The ratio of lateral ventricle to hemisphere width (LVW/HW) was 0.87 prior to the operation and decreased to 0.76 by 6h after the operation. The lateral ventricle width decreased from 2.7 cm prior to the procedure to 2.2 cm 6h after. By 27 weeks' gestation, the LVW/HW ratio was 0.50, with a lateral ventricle width of 1.8 cm. At 34 weeks' gestation, the ventricles rapidly increased in size

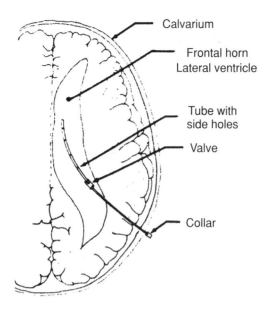

- Calvarium
- Frontal horn
  Lateral ventricle
- Tube with
  side holes
- Valve
- Collar

Figure 2 Diagram depicting the shunt from the lateral ventricle to the amnionic space. Used with permission from reference 10

(LVW/HW = 0.71, LVW = 3.2 cm) and shunt failure was suspected. The infant was delivered by Cesarean section. At birth, he was vigorous and had no significant respiratory problems. The ventriculoamniotic shunt was in place. The fetal fontanelles were full and no fluid was draining from the shunt. Shortly after birth, the baby was taken to the operating room for removal of the ventriculo–amniotic shunt and placement of a ventriculo-peritoneal shunt[7].

At birth, the infant was noted to have flexion contractures of both wrists and metacarpophalangeal joints. The distal phalanx of the left thumb was duplicated. The neonatal course was complicated by mild respiratory distress requiring continuous positive airway pressure and supplemental oxygen. He was discharged on the 28th hospital day. At discharge, his ventriculoperitoneal shunt was functioning well. He was responsive to his environment and had a normal EEG. He required some of his feedings by gavage. On follow-up at 2 years of age, the infant had a developmental quotient of less than 75.

Three other infants were treated with similar operations at the University of Colorado School of Medicine. All have had neonatal ventriculoperi-

toneal shunts placed and remain shunt-dependent. One of these had severe respiratory distress and hypoxia after birth, due to eventration of the diaphragm. He has severe handicap, but it is unclear how much of his disability is due to perinatal complications and how much is due to his central nervous system anomaly. The other two children have had nearly normal development. Recent contact with one of these patients at age 12 years finds him attending normal school. He has very mild motor and learning disability. *In utero*, he had severe and rapidly progressive ventricular enlargement. A ventriculoamniotic shunt was placed at 24 weeks. It resulted in immediate reduction in ventricular size. It was dislodged from the fetal head at 27 weeks and the ventricles rapidly enlarged again. A second shunt resulted in the ventricles returning to normal size and they remained so until 32 weeks, when the shunt was again dislodged from the fetal head and the ventricles enlarged (Figure 3). The baby was delivered by Cesarean section. He had mild respiratory distress and was discharged from the hospital after 28 days.

Between April 1981 and June 1984, 43 families with suspected fetal hydrocephalus were referred to the Program in Fetal Medicine and Surgery at the University of Colorado Health Sciences Center. All were evaluated as potential candidates for fetal treatment. Criteria for fetal surgery were: (1) progressive ventriculomegaly and thinning of the cortical mantle; (2) gestational age at the time of shunt placement less than 32 weeks; (3) singleton pregnancy; and (4) no significant other anomalies detected after a thorough evaluation. Five fetuses met the criteria for shunt placement and the families gave consent for the operation[8]. Twenty-five fetuses were excluded on the basis of these criteria. Thirteen cases met the criteria for shunt placement, but parents decided against the experimental operation. The outcomes in these cases are summarized in Table 1. Among these 13 fetuses, five had major anomalies found at birth, which had not been detected *in utero*. These do not constitute an ideal control group, since there was no randomization involved. The fact that the parents decided not to undergo the experimental procedure is undoubtedly related to the fact that four of these fetuses had cerebral decompression

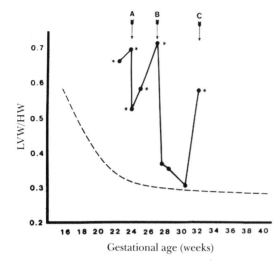

Figure 3 Plot of the ratio of ventricular width to hemisphere width (LVW/HW) as a function of gestational age. The broken line is the mean normal value. A and B indicate fetal shunt operations. C indicates delivery. Asterisks indicate points significantly above the normal range for gestational age. Used with permission from reference 8

Table 1 Outcome of the treatment of fetal hydrocephalus

	Fetal shunt	No shunt
Elective abortion	1	0
Stillbirth	0	5 (4)
Infant death	0	2
Neonatal death	0	3
Alive	4	3
normal development	2	2
mild handicap	0	1
severe handicap	2	0

during labor and were stillborn. One shunt candidate had an elective termination of pregnancy at 25 weeks. There were three neonatal deaths. One was due to extreme prematurity, one due to brain dysfunction and one due to shunt complications following surgery. There was one fetal demise with polymicrogyria. Two of the three survivors have ventriculoperitoneal shunts in place and initially had near-normal development. One survivor did not have a shunt placed until 1 year of age and has mild developmental delay. Comparison of this group with the babies treated *in utero* is difficult. The selection bias evident in the high rate of cerebral decompression and the high number of undiagnosed other anomalies further complicates comparison. The three survivors all seemed to have had relatively mild hydrocephalus compared to the fetal shunt group.

World experience

Fewer than 41 cases of *in utero* ventricular shunting have been reported to the International Fetal Surgery Registry. No cases appear to have undergone the operation since about 1985. The company that manufactured the Denver Shunt described above has stopped making it. In 1993 the reports to the Registry were summarized by Holzgreve and Evans[9]. There were 34 survivors from this experience. Four of seven deaths could be attributed to the procedure or preterm labor occurring immediately after it. Eighteen of the 34 survivors had severe handicaps. Fourteen survivors appeared to be developing normally at 1 year of age. The remainder showed some degree of compromise. The only intact survivors were those with simple aqueductal stenosis. The Registry experience also indicated that many treated fetuses had associated anomalies that were not identified prior to treatment. Some fetuses which were treated had anomalies that should have been identified, including abnormal karyotypes.

COMMENT

Fetal hydrocephalus can be a devastating problem. It is commonly accompanied by other malformations in the central nervous system and elsewhere, and in this circumstance the outcome is generally poor. When the condition is isolated and progressive, it appears that *in utero* shunting lessened the anatomic impact on the fetus. The operation of ultrasound-guided percutaneous shunt placement carried relatively low maternal and fetal morbidity and mortality risks. There were serious problems with shunt malfunction, usually related to dislodgement from the fetal skull. When adequate function was maintained, fetal brain injury seemed to be lessened and additional maturity attained.

At this time, no fetal ventricular shunts are being performed. It seems likely that with the improvement in ultrasound technology and interpretation that has occurred over the past decade, many of the missed diagnoses in this experience could now be avoided. This would allow better patient selection and presumably improve the outcome. There are probably a small number of cases with isolated, progressive hydrocephalus which would benefit from *in utero* treatment. If the procedure were to be undertaken, it would require a new device and should only be performed in selected centers.

References

1. Oi, S., Matsumoto, S., Katayama, K. and Mochizuki, M. (1990). Pathophysiology and postnatal outcome of fetal hydrocephalus. *Child's Nerv. Sys.*, **6**, 338–45

2. Michejda, M. and Hodgen, G.D. (1981). *In utero* diagnosis and treatment of non-human primate fetal skeletal anomalies: I. Hydrocephalus. *J. Am. Med. Assoc.*, **426**, 1093–7

3. Michejda, M. (1989). Neurobehavioral development of *in utero* treated hydrocephalic monkeys. *Z. Kinderchir.*, **44**, 52

4. Nakayama, D.G., Harrison, M.R., Berger, M.S., Chinn, D.H., Halks-Miller, M. and Edwards, M.S. (1983). Correction of congenital hydrocephalus *in utero*. The model: intracisternal kaolin produces hydrocephalus in fetal lambs and Rhesus monkeys. *J. Pediatr. Surg.*, **18**, 331–8

5. Birnholtz, J.C. and Frigoletto, F.D. (1981). Antenatal treatment of hydrocephalus. *N. Engl. J. Med.*, **303**, 1021

6. Papile, L.-A., Burstein, J., Burstein, R., Koffler, H., Koops, B.L. and Johnson, J.D. (1980). Post hemorrhagic hydrocephalus in low-birth weight infants: treatment by serial lumbar punctures. *J. Pediatr.*, **97**, 273–7

7. Clewell, W.H., Johnson, M.L., Meier, P.R., Newkirk, J.B., Zide, S.L., Hendee, R.W., Bowes, W.A., Hecht, F., O'Keeffe, D., Henry, G.P. and Shikes, R.H. (1982). A surgical approach to the treatment of fetal hydrocephalus. *N. Engl. J. Med.*, **306**, 1320–5

8. Clewell, W.H., Meier, P.R., Manchester, D.K., Manco-Johnson, M.L., Pretorius, D.H. and Hendee, R.W. (1985). Ventriculomegaly: evaluation and management. *Semin. Perinatol.*, **9**, 98–102

9. Holzgreve, W. and Evans, M.I. (1993). Nonvascular needle and shunt placements for fetal therapy. *West. J. Med.*, **159**, 333–40

10. Johnson, M.L., Pretorius, D., Clewell, W.H., Meier, P.R. and Manchester, D. (1983). Fetal hydrocephalus: diagnosis and management. *Semin. Perinatol.*, **7**, 83–9

Cephalocentesis

12

F. A. Chervenak and L. B. McCullough

Destructive procedures have played a central role in the history of obstetrics[1]. Before safe Cesarean delivery became available, fetal dismemberment with subsequent vaginal delivery was a life-saving intervention for the pregnant woman. Today, fetal dismemberment is not utilized, even in the instance of a fetal demise, because of the safety of Cesarean delivery and the maternal morbidity associated with extensive intrauterine manipulation.

One destructive procedure, however, still has a limited but important role in modern operative obstetrics: cephalocentesis, the drainage of an enlarged head caused by hydrocephalus[2]. Fetal hydrocephalus is caused by obstruction of cerebrospinal flow and is diagnosed by such sonographic signs as dilatation of the atrium or body of the lateral ventricles[3]. In the third trimester, macrocephaly often accompanies ventriculomegaly. In addition, sonography can diagnose hydrocephalus in association with gross abnormalities suggestive of poor prognosis. These include hydranencephaly, microcephaly, encephalocele, alobar holoprosencephaly, or thanatophoric dysplasia with cloverleaf skull[3]. In the absence of defined anatomical abnormalities, however, diagnostic imaging is, at the present time, unable to predict the outcome. Although cortical mantle thickness can be measured with ultrasound, its value as a prognostic index is not established[3].

Before the development of surgical shunting of the dilated ventricular system caused by increased intracranial pressure, the outlook for the infant with hydrocephalus was generally poor. Although obstructive hydrocephalus can be slowly progressive or arrest spontaneously, massive head enlargement with blindness and mental retardation were common in undeveloped countries. In 1954, Feeny and Barry reported that of 93 liveborn infants with hydrocephalus, only ten survived to leave the hospital[4]. In 1962, Laurence

and Coates[5] reported that, among 182 patients with hydrocephalus for whom surgery was not performed, the newborn's chances of reaching adulthood were 20–23%. Of the survivors, only 38% had an IQ greater than 85. Further, it should be appreciated that this was a selected group. Therefore, these figures are probably optimistic when the prognosis is considered for all newborn babies with hydrocephalus. Titus[6] referred to the treatment of hydrocephalus, saying: 'The disproportion must be overcome without regard for the child. It is already doomed to death or idiocy as so much of its brain tissue has been compressed or destroyed by the accumultion of fluid within the ventricles'.

With the advent of surgical shunting, the prognosis for the infant with hydrocephalus has improved. This is illustrated by the experience in the early days of shunt therapy, when a prospective randomized trial comparing surgical shunting with conservative management in 30 infants was attempted by Lorber and Zachary[7]. The trial was terminated prematurely, when 11 of the 13 infants in the control group needed surgery to arrest neurological deterioration or rapidly increasing head circumference.

In another study, 200 consecutive infants with neonatal hydrocephalus at Children's Memorial Hospital in Chicago underwent shunt procedures. Of these, only five died. Intellectual development in the survivors is related to the type of hydrocephalus, age at initial shunt placement, and shunt function, but not to the severity of the hydrocephalus or to the number of shunt revisions. For Caucasians with internal hydrocephalus, the mean IQ was 84 ± 25.8. Infants with other forms of hydrocephalus, such as those related to porencephaly or to Dandy–Walker cyst, had significantly lower mean IQs. In this series[8], those infants with congenital hydrocephalus were not clearly differentiated from those who developed hydrocephalus during the neontal period. At the University of Washington School of Medicine, 16 of 19 infants with congenital hydrocephalus who were treated achieved IQs of at least 80. Of 37 infants with congenital hydrocephalus and microcephaly managed at Georgetown University Medical Center, 32 survived. Of these survivors, 17 had an IQ above 80 and six had an IQ between 65 and 80[9].

Others have corroborated the finding that well-treated infants without associated congenital malformations have an excellent chance of achieving normal intelligence, irrespective of the initial severity of their hydrocephalus. At the University of Pennsylvania, ten neonates were followed after computed tomography (CT) demonstrated virtual absence of the cerebral tissue. Two well-defined clinical entities were distinguished. Five infants with hydranencephaly showed absence of cortical activity on EEG and a CT picture of minimal occipital brain parenchyma. Although these infants received shunt therapy, no neurological or radiological improvement occurred with time. The remaining five infants had severe hydrocephalus, but retained minimal frontal cerebral mantle on CT and exhibited electrical activity on EEG. After shunting procedures, a remarkable increase in brain tissue was demonstrated in the latter group by serial CT scans, and neurological development was either normal or slightly delayed[10]. The probable reason for the retention of cerebral function with a markedly thinned cerebral cortex is that ventricular dilatation occurs at the expense of the white matter, whereas the gray matter on the convoluted surface of the cerebral cortex is unfolded and spread over a wider surface area, with no true damage initially to nerve cells. This is supported by the normal appearance of the brain by computed tomography following successful shunting in certain cases[11].

Lorber[12] has followed 56 infants with severe congenital hydrocephalus (cortex 10 mm or less) in Sheffield, England over 8 years. A total of 46 infants survived. Of these, five were of superior intelligence, 29 were of average to good intelligence, five were educationally subnormal, and six were profoundly retarded. Intellectual outcome was better when the shunting procedure was performed prior to 6 months of age. Lorber concluded that 'These results suggest that no case of primary congenital hydrocephalus should be considered hopeless and all should have the benefit of the best treatment, irrespective of the degree of hydrocephalus, because the majority will do well if treated in the first few months of life. Even the most extreme degrees of hydrocephalus are compatible with normal physical development and a normal-sized head and intelligence if operative treatment is not delayed'.

Several more recent papers have focused on the outcome of hydrocephalus diagnosed during the fetal period. In each of these series, most of the fetuses (59–85%) had major structural anomalies in addition to hydrocephalus and most died during the perinatal period[13–18]. The much higher death rate observed in these fetal studies as compared to studies of children with hydrocephalus is at least partly attributable to the high frequency of associated anomalies and obstetric trauma from cephalocentesis.

Cephalocentesis should be performed under simultaneous ultrasound guidance, so that needle placement into the cerebrospinal fluid is facilitated. An 18-gauge needle is used with collapse of the cranial bones, the endpoint for this procedure. Enough fluid is drained to permit reduction of the skull diameters so that passage through the birth canal is possible. Cephalocentesis can be performed under ultrasound guidance either transabdominally or transvaginally. A local anesthetic may be used, but maternal sedation is not necessary[18, 19] (Figures 1–3).

Cephalocentesis is a potentially destructive procedure. Perinatal death following cephalocentesis has been reported in over 90% of cases[2]. The sonographic visualization of intracranial bleeding during cephalocentesis, and the demonstration of this hemorrhage at autopsy, further emphasize the morbid nature of the procedure. However, if decompression is performed in a controlled manner, the mortality may be reduced[20].

It should be obvious that cephalocentesis, a potentially destructive procedure in a term fetus, requires careful justification to avoid its inappropriate use. We believe that the language of ethics is essential to this justification for the following

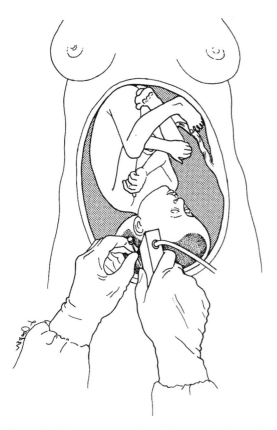

Figure 1 Demonstration of cephalocentesis with guidance by abdominal ultrasound. Reprinted with permission from reference 18

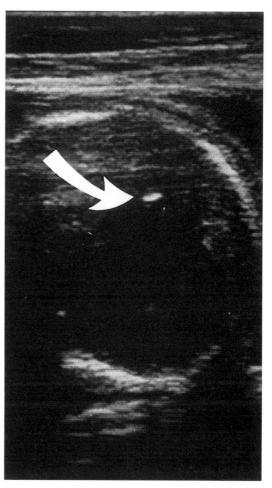

Figure 2 Sonogram demonstrating tip of cephalocentesis needle in dilated ventricle. Reprinted with permission from reference 18

reasons. First, the use of a virtually destructive procedure is directly at odds with one of the goals of obstetric care: protecting and promoting the fetal patient's interests. Cephalocentesis therefore requires ethical justification. Second, ethical analysis of clinical information permits the clinician to consider the significance of disease severity and the prognosis of hydrocephalus in the decision process. Finally, ethical analysis helps to identify clearly the appropriate management strategies for this continuum of disease severity. These strategies are essential for managing conflicts that may occur between pregnant women and their physicians[21,22].

Before we can address the clinical and ethical justification of cephalocentesis, we define obstetric ethics and two ethical principles and on this basis discuss when the fetus is a patient. In our view, the clinical performance of cephalocentesis without

first addressing these ethical dimensions would be incomplete and inadequate.

OBSTETRIC ETHICS AND TWO ETHICAL PRINCIPLES

Obstetric ethics

Ethics is the disciplined study of morality. Morality concerns both right and wrong behavior, i.e. what one ought and ought not to do, and good and bad character, i.e. virtue and vice. The fundamental question that ethics addresses is, 'What ought

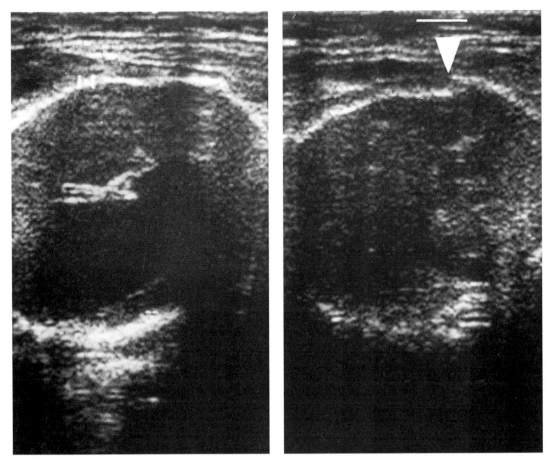

Figure 3 Left: macrocephaly due to hydrocephalus before cephalocentesis. Right: fetal head after cephalocentesis. Note reduction in size of head as well as overlapping of the cranial sutures (arrowhead). Reprinted with permissions from reference 18

morality to be?' This question involves two further questions, 'What ought our behavior to be?' and 'What virtues ought to be cultivated in our moral lives?' Ethics in obstetric practice deals with these same questions, focusing on what morality ought to be for obstetricians[22].

The basis for what morality ought to be in clinical practice has for centuries been the obligation to protect and promote the interests of the patient. This general ethical obligation needs to be made more specific if it is to be clinically useful. This can be accomplished by attending to two perspectives in terms of which the patient's interests can be understood: that of the physician and that of the patient[22].

Two ethical principles: beneficence and respect for autonomy

The most ancient of these two perspectives on the interests of patients in the history of medical ethics is a rigorous clinical perspective. Based on scientific knowledge, shared clinical experience and a careful, unbiased evaluation of the patient, the physician is able to identify those clinical strategies that will be most likely to serve the health-related interests of the patient and those that will not. The health-related interests of the patient include preventing premature death and preventing, curing, or at least managing disease, injury, handicap, or unnecessary pain and suffering. These matters are constitutive of any patient's health-related interests as a function of the competencies of medicine as a social institution. The identification of a patient's interests is not a function of the personal or subjective outlook of a particular physician, but rather of rigorous clinical judgment about the fetal patient's condition.

The ethical principle of beneficence structures this clinical perspective on the interests of the patient, because it obliges the physician to seek the greatest balance of goods over harms in the consequences of the physician's behavior for both the pregnant woman and the fetal patient. On the basis of rigorous clinical judgment, physicians should identify those clinical strategies that are expected to result in the greater balance of goods, i.e. the protection and promotion of health-related interests, over harms, i.e. impairments of those interests. The principle of beneficence has an ancient pedigree in Western medical ethics, at least back to the time of Hippocrates[23].

The principle of beneficence in obstetrics must be very carefully distinguished from the ethical principles of non-maleficence, commonly known as *primum non nocere* or 'first, do no harm'. Contrary to the belief of many physicians, *primum non nocere* does not appear in the Hippocratic Oath or in the texts that accompany the Oath. Instead, the principle of beneficence was the primary consideration of the Hippocratic writers. For example, in *Epidemics*, the text reads 'As to diseases, make a habit of two things – to help or to at least do no harm'.[24] Indeed, the historical origins of *primum non nocere* remain obscure.

There are more than historical reasons to be skeptical about *primum non nocere* as a principle of obstetric ethics. Virtually all medical interventions involve unavoidable risks of harm. If *primum non nocere* were the primary principle of obstetric ethics, virtually all of obstetric practice would be unethical. *Primum non nocere* is therefore essentially superseded in obstetric ethics by the principle of beneficence. The latter is sufficient to alert the physician to those circumstances in which a clinical intervention has the potential to harm the patient. When a clinical intervention is *on balance* harmful to a patient, it should not be employed. That is, *primum non nocere*, as a corollary of beneficence, makes it obligatory not to act in a way that is only

harmful. As Strong puts it, there is a powerful beneficence-based prohibition against killing[25]. This is obviously of direct relevance to the ethical evaluation of cephalocentesis in beneficence-based clinical judgment.

The physician's perspective on the interests of the patient is not the only legitimate perspective on those interests. The perspective of the patient on the patient's interests is at least equally worthy of consideration by the physician. Each patient has developed a set of values and beliefs according to which she is surely capable of making judgments about what will and will not protect and promote her interests. It is a commonplace that in other aspects of her life the patient regularly makes such judgments concerning matters of considerable complexity, e.g. choosing a professional calling, rearing children, entering into contracts and writing a will of property. Despite the complexity of these decisions, she is rightly assumed to be competent to make them, with the burden of proof on anyone who would challenge her competence.

The same is true about health care decisions made by the pregnant woman. She must be assumed by her physician to be competent to determine which clinical strategies serve her interests and which do not. It is important to note that, in making such judgments, the pregnant woman will utilize values and beliefs that can range far beyond the scope of health-related interests, e.g. religious beliefs or beliefs about how many children she wants to have. Beneficence-based clinical judgment, because it rests on the competencies of medicine, has no competence to assess the worth or meaning to the patient of the patient's non-health-related interests. These are matters solely for the patient to determine. Those values and beliefs help shape the patient's perspective on her interests.

The ethical significance of this perspective is captured by the ethical principle of respect for autonomy. This principle obliges the physician to respect the integrity of the patient's values and beliefs, to respect her perspective on her interests, and to implement only those clinical strategies authorized by her as the result of the informed consent process.

Respect for autonomy is thus put into clinical practice by the informed consent process. This process is usually understood to have three elements: (1) disclosure by the physician to the patient of adequate information about the patient's condition and its management; (2) understanding of that information by the patient; and (3) a voluntary decision by the patient to authorize or refuse clinical management[26].

There are obviously beneficence-based and autonomy-based obligations to the pregnant patient[22]. The physician's perspective on the pregnant woman's interests provides the basis for beneficence-based obligations owed to her. Her own perspective on those interests provides the basis for autonomy-based obligations owed to her. Because of an insufficiently developed central nervous system, the fetus cannot meaningfully be said to possess values and beliefs. Thus, there is no basis for saying that a fetus has a perspective on its interests. There can therefore be no autonomy-based obligations to any fetus[27,28]. Hence the language of fetal rights has little or no meaning in obstetric ethics, despite its popularity in public and political discourse. Obviously, the physician has a perspective on the fetus's health-related interests and the physician can have beneficence-based obligations to the fetus, *but only when the fetus is a patient*. Because of its importance for obstetric ethics generally and the ethics of destructive procedures in obstetrics, the topic of the fetus as patient requires detailed consideration.

THE FETUS AS PATIENT

The concept of 'the fetus as patient' has recently developed, largely as a consequence of developments in fetal diagnosis and management strategies to optimize fetal outcome[7-11] and has become widely accepted[29-31]. This concept has considerable clinical significance because, when the fetus is a patient, directive counselling, i.e. recommending a form of management, for fetal benefit would seem to be appropriate and, when the fetus is not a patient, non-directive counselling, i.e. offering but not recommending a form of management, would seem to be appropriate. However, these apparently straightforward roles for directive and non-directive counselling are often difficult to apply in actual obstetric practice, because of

uncertainty about when the fetus is a patient. One approach to resolving this uncertainty would be to argue that the fetus is or is not a patient in virtue of personhood[25,32], or some other form of independent moral status[33-35]. We will show that this approach fails to resolve the uncertainty and we will therefore defend an alternative approach that does resolve the uncertainty.

The independent moral status of the fetus

A prominent approach for establishing whether or not the fetus is a patient has involved attempts to show whether or not the fetus has independent moral status. The notion of independent moral status for the fetus means that one or more characteristics that the fetus is thought to possess in and of itself and, therefore, independently of the pregnant woman or any other factor, generate and therefore ground obligations to the fetus on the part of the pregnant woman and her physician.

A striking variety of intrinsic characteristics has been nominated for this role in the history of the debate on the moral status of the fetus, including moment of conception, implantation, central nervous system development, quickening, and the moment of birth[36-38]. It should come as no surprise that, given the variability of proposed characteristics, there have been and still are markedly varied views about when the fetus acquires independent moral status. Some take the view that the fetus has independent moral status from the moment of conception or implantation[39,40]. Others believe that independent moral status is acquired in degrees, thus resulting in 'graded' moral status[33,35]. Still others hold, at least by implication, that the fetus never has independent moral status so long as it is *in utero*[34].

Despite a continuing and voluminous theological and philosophical literature on this subject, there has been no closure on a single authoritative account of the independent moral status of the fetus[41] (and Roe vs. Wade, 1973). This is not a surprising outcome because, given the absence of a single methodology that would be authoritative for all of the markedly diverse theological and philosophical schools of thought involved in this endless debate, closure is impossible. For closure ever to be possible, debates about such a final authority within and between theological and philosophical traditions would have to be resolved in a way satisfactory to all. This is an inconceivable event. It is best therefore to abandon futile attempts to understand the fetus as patient in terms of independent moral status of the fetus and turn to an alternative approach that makes it possible to identify ethically distinct senses of the fetus as patient and their clinical implications for obstetric practice.

Beneficence-based obligations to the fetal patient

This alternative approach begins with the recognition that being a patient does not require that one possesses independent moral status. Rather, being a patient means that one can benefit from the applications of the clinical skills of the physician. Put more precisely, a human being without independent moral status is properly regarded as a patient when two conditions are met: that a human being (a) is presented to the physician (b) for the purpose of applying clinical interventions that are reliably expected to be efficacious, in that they are reliably expected to result in a greater balance of goods over harms for the human being in question[22, 31].

The authors have argued elsewhere that beneficence-based obligations to the fetus exist when the fetus can achieve independent moral status[22]. That is, the fetus is a patient when the fetus is presented for medical interventions, whether diagnostic or therapeutic, that reasonably can be expected to result in a greater balance of goods over harms later, when the fetus achieves independent moral status. The ethical significance of the concept of the fetus as patient, therefore, depends on links that can be established between the fetus and later achievement of independent moral status.

One such link is viability, introducing the first ethical sense of the fetus as patient. Viability is not, however, an intrinsic property of the fetus, because viability must be understood in terms of both biological and technological factors[30, 42] (and Roe vs. Wade, 1973). It is only in virtue of both factors that a viable fetus can exist *ex utero* and thus later achieve independent moral status. Moreover, these

two factors do not exist as a function of the autonomy of the pregnant woman. When a fetus is viable, i.e. when it is of sufficient maturity so that it can survive into the neonatal period and become a child given the availability of the requisite technological support, and when it is presented to the physician, the fetus is a patient. The fetus at term is a patient when the pregnant woman presents herself to the hospital for obstetric services.

Viability exists as a function of biomedical and technological capacities, which are different in different parts of the world. As a consequence, there is, at the present time, no world-wide, uniform gestational age to define viability. In the United States, the authors believe that viability at present occurs at approximately 24 weeks of gestational age[43]. It follows directly from this sense of the fetus as patient that destructive procedures on the at-term fetal patient must be ethically justified, a task to which we turn in the next section.

The only possible link between the pre-viable fetus and its later achieving independent moral status is the pregnant woman's autonomy, introducing the second ethical sense of the fetus as patient. This is because technological factors cannot result in the pre-viable fetus later achieving independent moral status. This is simply what pre-viable means. The link, therefore, between a fetus and later achieving independent moral status can be established, when the fetus is pre-viable, only by the pregnant woman's decision to confer the status of being a patient on her pre-viable fetus. The pre-viable fetus, therefore, has no claim to the status of being a patient independently of the pregnant woman's autonomy. The pregnant woman is free to withhold, confer, or having once conferred, withdraw the status of being a patient on or from her pre-viable fetus according to her own values and beliefs. The pre-viable fetus is presented to the physician solely as a function of the pregnant woman's autonomy. This has important ethical implications for a range of ethical issues in obstetrics, including antenatal diagnosis and abortion[22].

Clinical and ethical justification for cephalocentesis

Because fetal hydrocephalus is the product of varied etiologies having varied outcomes, ethical

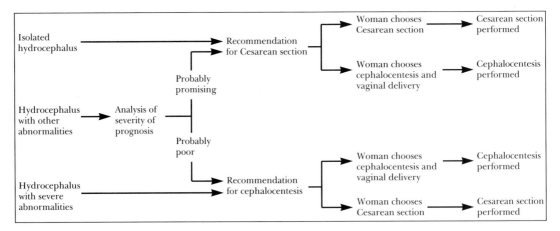

Figure 4 Management strategies for resolution of conflicts in the intrapartum management of hydrocephalus with macrocephaly

analysis must be carried out by respecting the heterogeneity of this condition[3]. Therefore, we consider resolution clinical management strategies for two extremes of the continuum between isolated fetal hydrocephalus and fetal hydrocephalus with severe associated abnormalities (those incompatible with postnatal survival or those characterized by the virtual absence of cognitive function). We then consider fetal hydrocephalus with milder associated abnormalities as a middle ground on the continuum (Figure 4). The proposed analysis of each of these situations takes place in the following steps. First, we identify the beneficence-based and autonomy-based obligations of the physician to the pregnant woman and the fetal patient. Second, we identify the conflicts that can occur among these obligations. Third, we weigh these obligations against each other in an attempt to arrive at a balance among conflicting obligations.

Isolated fetal hydrocephalus

We begin the clinical and ethical analysis of isolated fetal hydrocephalus by noting that there is considerable potential for normal, sometimes superior, intellectual function for fetuses with even extreme, isolated hydrocephalus[8–10, 12]. However, as a group, infants with isolated hydrocephalus experience a greater incidence of mental retardation and early death than the general population.

In addition, associated anomalies may go undetected, and a fetus may be incorrectly diagnosed as having isolated hydrocephalus[18]. One thing is clear in obstetric ethics: a viable fetus with isolated hydrocephalus is a fetal patient.

There are compelling ethical reasons, well founded in beneficence, for concluding that continuing existence of fetuses with isolated hydrocephalus is in their interests. Beneficence directs the physician to avoid mortality and morbidity for the fetal patient. Beneficence also directs the physician to clinical interventions that ameliorate handicapping conditions such as mental retardation. The probability of mental retardation does not diminish the interests of the fetal patient with isolated hydrocephalus in continuing existence, because (1) it is impossible to predict which fetuses with isolated hydrocephalus will have mental retardation, and (2) the degree of mental retardation cannot be predicted in advance.

In light of this ethical analysis of the at-term fetal patient's interests, the beneficence-based obligation of the physician caring for the fetus is to perform a Cesarean delivery, because this clinical intervention clearly involves the least risk of mortality, morbidity and handicap for the fetus, compared with cephalocentesis to permit subsequent vaginal delivery. Even when performed under maximal therapeutic conditions (i.e. under sonographic guidance), cephalocentesis cannot reasonably be regarded as protecting or promoting

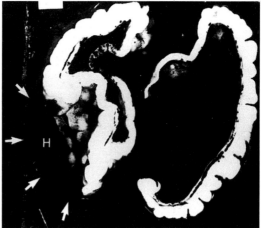

Figure 6 Coronal section of brain demonstrating a large subarachnoid hemorrhage (H) resulting from cephalocentesis. Reprinted with permission from reference 18

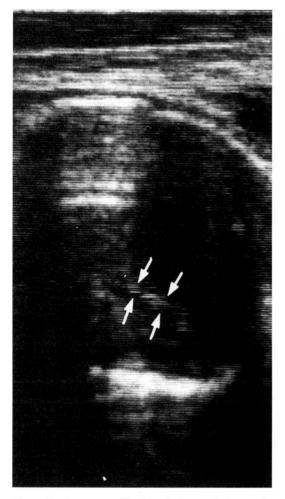

Figure 5 Sonogram of fetal head after cephalocentesis, with arrows outlining stream of blood. Reprinted with permission from reference 18

the interests of the fetal patient with isolated hydrocephalus. This procedure is followed by a high rate of perinatal mortality, fetal heart rate deceleration, and pathological evidence of intra-cranial bleeding[18] (Figures 5–8). As a consequence, cephalocentesis cannot reasonably be construed as an ethically justifiable mode of management, insofar as it is inconsistent with beneficence-based obligations to avoid increased mortality and mor-bidity risks for the fetal patient. Cephalocentesis, employed with a destructive intent, is altogether antithetical to these beneficence-based prohibi-tions against killing.

Complete ethical analysis requires that benef-icence-based obligations to the fetal patient be balanced against beneficence-based and autonomy-based obligations to the pregnant woman. First, the physician has a beneficence-based obligation to avoid performing a Cesarean delivery, because the possibility of morbidity and mortality for the woman is higher than that associated with vaginal delivery. Respect for autonomy obliges the physi-cian to undertake only those interventions or forms of treatment to which the woman has given voluntary, informed consent. Informed consent is grounded in an autonomy-based right of the pregnant woman to control what happens to her body. In particular, the woman has the right to authorize or refuse operative interventions – those that are, as well as those that are not, consistent with the physician's beneficence-based obligations[22].

We are now in a position to consider the full complexity of the management of the fetal patient with isolated hydrocephalus. Beneficence-based and autonomy-based obligations to the pregnant woman, as well as beneficence-based obligations to the fetal patient, must be considered. If, with informed consent, the woman authorizes Cesarean delivery, there is no conflict among these obliga-tions. The autonomy-based obligation to act on informed consent over-rides the beneficence-

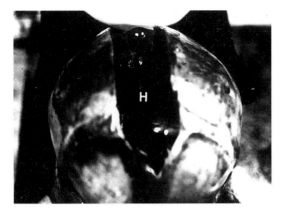

Figure 7 Section of brain demonstrating intraventricular hemorrhage (H) resulting from cephalocentesis. Reprinted with permission from reference 18

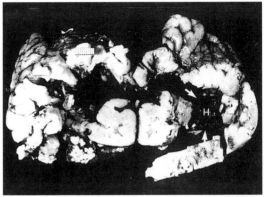

Figure 8 Subdural hematoma (H) resulting from cephalocentesis. Reprinted with permission from reference 18

based obligations to the pregnant woman that were identified earlier.

In contrast, her physician faces a significant conflict, indeed a genuine moral dilemma, if the woman refuses Cesarean delivery. Two clinical interventions, each with substantial ethical justification in beneficence-based and autonomy-based clinical judgment, can be employed in intrapartum management. On the one hand, the physician has an autonomy-based obligation to the pregnant woman to perform cephalocentesis followed by vaginal delivery. On the other hand, cephalocentesis violates beneficence-based obligations to the fetal patient.

This conflict should be resolved in favor of the beneficence-based obligations to the fetal patient. These obligations properly over-ride beneficence-based and autonomy-based obligations to the woman, because the harm to the fetal patient is final, namely, death, and will occur with high probability. Moreover, if the fetal patient survives (death is not guaranteed by cephalocentesis), it is likely to be more damaged due to intracranial hemorrhage than if Cesarean delivery is performed. Morbidity and mortality of the pregnant woman are both minimal, and are therefore risks that she ought to accept, to protect the fetal patient's interest[22]. Such ethical conflict should be prevented by employing the preventive ethics strategies of informed consent as an ongoing dialogue, negotiation, respectful persuasion and the proper use of ethics committees[22,44].

If these preventive ethics strategies fail and the pregnant woman continues to refuse Cesarean delivery, the physician confronts tragic circumstances. If neither Cesarean delivery nor cephalocentesis is performed, the woman is at risk for uterine rupture and death, and the fetal patient is at risk for death. This logic of beneficence-based obligations is to avoid such total and irreversible harm. Therefore, we believe that, because of the grave nature of possible consequences for the woman and the fetal patient, because of the dangers for the woman of performing a surgical procedure on a resistant patient, and because of the pitfalls of attempted legal coercion, the physician should act on beneficence-based obligations to the woman in such an extreme circumstance. In addition, to fail to respect an unwavering, voluntary and informed refusal of a Cesarean delivery would count as a fundamental assault on the woman's autonomy. The fetal patient is at high risk for death under either alternative. The woman's death, at least, can be avoided. Serious beneficence-based obligations to the fetal patient on the part of both the physician and the pregnant woman will probably be violated and a needless death will most probably result, however, by performing cephalocentesis. Herein lies the tragedy of these circumstances. To avoid this tragedy, redoubled efforts of preventive ethics should be undertaken. In one author's (FAC) experience, carefully explaining the fact that cephalocentesis does not guarantee death and may produce a worse outcome is very powerfully persuasive. In those rare cases in which this effort at respectful persuasion fails, cephalocentesis should be performed in the least destructive way possible or an appropriate referral made.

Hydrocephalus with severe associated abnormalities

Some abnormalities that occur in association with fetal hydrocephalus are severe in nature for the child afflicted with them. We define 'severe' abnormalities as those that are (1) incompatible with continued existence, e.g. bilateral renal agenesis or thanatophoric dysplasia with cloverleaf skull; or (2) compatible with survival in some cases but result in virtual absence of cognitive function, e.g. trisomy 18 or alobar holoprosencephaly[18,45]. Because there is no available intervention to prevent postnatal death in the first group, beneficence-based obligations of the physician and the pregnant woman to attempt to prolong the life of the fetal patient are nonexistent. No ethical theory obliges anyone to attempt the impossible. For the second group, beneficence-based obligations of the physician and the pregnant woman to sustain the life of the fetal patient are minimal, because the handicap imposed by the abnormality is severe. In these cases the potential for cognitive development – and therefore the achievement of other 'goods' for the child, e.g. relationships with others – are virtually absent. Such fetuses are fetal patients to which there are owed only minimal beneficence-based obligations.

In these circumstances, the woman is therefore released from her beneficence-based obligations to the at-term fetal patient to place herself at risk, because no significant good can be achieved by Cesarean delivery for the fetal patient. There remain only the autonomy-based and beneficence-based obligations of the physician to the pregnant woman. After the preceding analysis of these obligations, we conclude that the physician's overriding moral obligations are to the pregnant woman's voluntary and informed decision about employment of cephalocentesis.

Because there are no weighty beneficence-based obligations to the fetal patient in such clinical and ethical circumstances, the physician may justifiably recommend a choice between Cesarean delivery and cephalocentesis to enable vaginal delivery. Cesarean delivery permits women who wish to do so to have a live birth and satisfy religious convictions or help with the grieving process. A Cesarean delivery performed in this clinical setting is best viewed as an autonomy-based maternal indication. The strategy of offering a choice also avoids the potential negative consequences for maternal health of Cesarean delivery. Because the prognosis for infants with hydrocephalus associated with severe anomalies is poor, we believe that intrapartum fetal death resulting from cephalocentesis would not be a tragic outcome as it might be in the death of a fetal patient with isolated hydrocephalus.

Hydrocephalus with other associated anomalies

On the continuum between the extreme cases of isolated hydrocephalus and hydrocephalus with severe associated abnormalities, there is a variety of cases of hydrocephalus associated with other abnormalities with varying degrees of impairment of cognitive physical function. They range from hypoplastic distal phalanges to spina bifida to encephalocele[18,22]. Because these conditions have varying prognoses, it would be clinically inappropriate and therefore, ethically misleading to treat this third category as homogeneous. Therefore, we propose a working distinction between different kinds of prognoses. The first we call 'probably promising', by which we mean that there is a significant possibility that the child will experience cognitive development with learning disabilities and physical handicaps that perhaps can be ameliorated to some extent. The second we call 'probably poor'. By this phrase, we mean that there is only a limited possibility for cognitive development, because of learning disabilities and physical handicaps that cannot be ameliorated to a significant extent. We propose these definitions as tentative, so they are subject to revision as clinical and ethical investigation of such associated anomalies continues. As a consequence, our ethical analysis of these two categories cannot be carried out as extensively as those in the previous two sections. In essence, we propose that the clinical continuum in these cases is paralleled by an ethical continuum or progressively less weighty, beneficence-based obligations to the fetus. Such at-term fetuses are indeed fetal patients.

When the prognosis is 'probably promising', e.g. isolated arachnoid cyst, there are serious beneficence-based obligations to the fetal patient. However, they are not necessarily of the same order as those that occur in cases of isolated hydrocephalus. (It has been suggested that any associated anomaly may increase the possibility of a poor outcome[18].) Therefore, in such cases with a prognosis of 'probably promising', we propose that the physician recommend Cesarean delivery, although perhaps not as vigorously as in cases of isolated hydrocephalus. A pregnant woman's informed refusal of Cesarean delivery should therefore be respected.

In cases when the prognosis, even though uncertain, is 'probably poor', e.g. encephalocele, beneficence-based obligations to the fetal patient are less weighty than those owed to the fetal patient with a promising prognosis. These cases, then, resemble ethically those of hydrocephalus with severe anomalies, with the proviso that some, albeit limited, benefits can be achieved for the fetal patient by Cesarean delivery and aggressive perinatal treatment. Nonetheless, the physician may in these cases justifiably accept an informed voluntary decision by the woman for cephalocentesis followed by vaginal delivery. However, the physician cannot assume an advocacy role for such a decision with the same level of ethical confidence that he or she can in cases of hydrocephalus associated with severe anomalies.

In conclusion, the technique of cephalocentesis is a relatively simple component of operative obstetrics. The more complex but essential challenge for the obstetrician is to understand the ethical justification for this procedure before implementing it in clinical practice.

References

1. Douglas, R.G. and Strome, W.B. (1976). *Embryology in Operative Obstetrics*, 3rd edn, pp. 690–715. (New York: Appleton-Century-Crofts)

2. Chervenak, F.A. and Romero, R. (1984). Is there a role for fetal cephalocentesis in modern obstetrics? *Am. J. Perinatol.*, **1**, 170–3

3. Chervenak, F.A., Isaacson, G. and Campbell, S. (1993). Anomalies of the cranium and its contents. *Textbook of Ultrasound in Obstetrics and Gynecology*, pp. 825–52. (Boston: Little, Brown)

4. Feeny, J.K. and Barry, A.P. (1954). Hydrocephaly as a cause of maternal mortality and morbidity. *J. Obstet. Gynaecol. Br. Emp.*, **61**, 652

5. Laurence, K.M. and Coates, S. (1962). The natural history of hydrocephalus. *Arch. Dis. Child.*, **37**, 345

6. Titus, P. (1940). *The management of obstetric difficulties*, p. 519. (St Louis: C.V. Mosby)

7. Lorber, J. and Zachary, R.B. (1968). Primary congenital hydrocephalus: long-term results of controlled therapeutic trial. *Arch. Dis. Child.*, **43**, 516

8. Raimondi, A.J. and Soare, P. (1974). Intellectual development in shunted hydrocephalic children. *Am. J. Dis. Child.*, **127**, 664

9. McCulough, D.C. and Balzer-Martin, L.A. (1982). Current prognosis in overt neonatal hydrocephalus. *J. Neurosurg.*, **57**, 378

10. Sutton, L.N., Bruce, D.A. and Schut, L. (1980). Hydranencephaly versus maximal hydrocephalus: an important clinical distinction. *Neurosurgery*, **6**, 35

11. Rubin, R.C., Hochwald, G. and Liwnicz, B. (1972). The effect of severe hydrocephalus on size and number of brain cells. *Dev. Med. Child. Neurol.*, **14**, 118

12. Lorber, J. (1968). The results of early treatment on extreme hydrocephalus. *Med. Child. Neurol.* (Suppl.), **16**, 21

13. Nyberg, D.A., Mack, L.A., Hirsch, J., Pagon, R.O. and Shepard, T.H. (1987). Fetal hydrocephalus: sonographic detection and clinical significance of associated anomalies. *Radiology*, **163**, 187

14. Hudgins, R.J., Edwards, M.S.B., Goldstein, R., Callen, P.W., Harrison, M.R., Filley, R.A. and Golbus, M.S. (1988). Natural history of fetal ventriculomegaly. *Pediatrics*, **82**, 692

15. Drugan, A., Krause, B., Canady, A., Zador, I.E., Sacks, A.J. and Evans, M.I. (1989). The natural history of prenatally diagnosed cerebral ventriculomegaly. *J. Am. Med. Assoc.*, **261**, 1785

16. Glick, P.L., Harrison, M.R., Nakayama, D.K., Edwards, M.S.B., Filly, R.A., Chinn, D.H., Callen, P.W., Wilson, S.L. and Golbus, M.S. (1984). Management of ventriculomegaly. *J. Pediatr.*, **105**, 97

17. Pretorius, D.M., Davis, K., Manco-Johnson, M.L., Manchester, D., Meiet, P.R. and Clewell, W.H. (1985). Clinical course of fetal hydrocephalus: 40 cases. *Am. J. Neuroradiol.*, **6**, 23

18. Chervenak, F.A., Berkowitz, R.L., Tortora, M. and Hobbins, J.C. (1985). Management of fetal hydrocephalus. *Am. J. Obstet. Gynecol.*, **151**, 933–42

19. Clark, S.L., DeVore, G.R. and Platt, L.D. (1985). The role of ultrasound in the aggressive management of obstructed labor secondary to fetal malformations. *Am. J. Obstet. Gynecol.*, **152**, 1042–4

20. Birnholz, J.C. and Frigoletto, F.D. (1981). Antenatal treatment of hydrocephalus. *N. Engl. J. Med.*, **104**, 1021

21. Chervenak, F.A. and McCullough, L.B. (1987). Ethical challenges in perinatal medicine: the intrapartum management of pregnancy complicated by fetal hydrocephalus with macrocephaly. *Semin. Perinat.*, **11**, 232–9

22. McCullough, L.B. and Chervenak, F.A. (1994). *Obstetric Ethics*. (New York: Oxford University Press)

23. Beauchamp, T.L. and Childress, J.F. (1989). *Principles of Biomedical Ethics*, 3rd edn. (New York: Oxford University Press)

24. Jones, W.H.S. (trans.) (1923). Hippocrates. *Epidemics*, i:xi. *Loeb Classical Library*, vol. 147. (Cambridge, MA: Harvard University Press)

25. Strong, C. (1987). Ethical conflicts between mother and fetus in obstetrics. *Clin. Perinatol.*, **14**, 313–28

26. Faden, R.R. and Beauchamp, T.L. (1986). *A History and Theory of Informed Consent*. (New York: Oxford University Press)

27. Chervenak, F.A. and McCullough, L.B. (1985). Perinatal ethics: a practical method of analysis of obligations to mother and fetus. *Obstet. Gynecol.*, **66**, 442–6

28. Chervenak, F.A. and McCullough, L.B. (1990). Does obstetric ethics have any role in the obstetrician's response to the abortion controversy? *Am. J. Obstet. Gynecol.*, **163**, 1425–9

29. Harrison, M.R., Golbus, M.S. and Filly, R.A. (1984). *The Unborn Patient*. (New York: Grune & Stratton)

30. Fletcher, J.C. (1981). The fetus as patient; ethical issues. *J. Am. Med. Assoc.*, 246, 772–3

31. Chervenak, F.A. and McCullough, L.B. (1991). The fetus as patient: implications for directive versus nondirective counseling for fetal benefit. *Fetal Diagn. Ther.*, **6**, 93–100

32. Engelhardt, H.T. Jr (1986). *The Foundations of Bioethics*. (New York: Oxford University Press)

33. Dunstan, G.R. (1984). The moral status of the human embryo. A tradition recalled. *J. Med. Ethics*, **10**, 38–44

34. Elias, S. and Annas, G.J. (1987). *Reproductive Genetics and the Law*. (Chicago: Year Book Medical Publishers)

35. Evans, M.I., Fletcher, J.C., Zador, I.E., Newton, B.W., Quigg, M.H. and Struyk, C.D. (1988). Selective first-trimester termination in octuplet and quadruplet pregnancies: clinical and ethical issues. *Obstet. Gynecol.*, **71**, 289–96

36. Curran, C.E. (1978). Abortion: contemporary debate in philosophical and religious ethics. In Reich, W.T. (ed.) *Encyclopedia of Bioethics*, pp. 17–26. (New York: Macmillan)

37. Noonan, J.T. (ed.) (1970). *The Morality of Abortion*. (Cambridge, MA: Harvard University Press)

38. Hellegers, A.E. (1970). Fetal development. *Theol. Stud.*, **31**, 3–9

39. Noonan, J.T. (1979). *A Private Choice. Abortion in America in the Seventies*. (New York: The Free Press)

40. Bopp, J. (ed.) (1984). *Restoring the Right to Life: The Human Life Amendment*. (Provo: Brigham Young University)

41. Callahan, S. and Callahan, D. (eds.) (1984). *Abortion: Understanding Differences*. (New York: Plenum Press)

42. Fost, N., Chudwin, D. and Walker, D. (1980). The limited moral significance of fetal viability. *Hastings Cent. Rep.*, **10**, 10–13

43. Hack, M. and Fanaroff, A.A. (1989). Outcomes of extremely-low-birth-weight infants between 1982 and 1983. *N. Engl. J. Med.*, **321**, 1642–7

44. Chervenak, F.A. and McCullough, L.B. (1990). Clinical guides to preventing ethical conflicts between pregnant women and their physicians. *Am. J. Obstet. Gynecol.*, **162**, 303–7

45. Chervenak, F.A. and McCullough, L.B. (1990). An ethically justified, clinically comprehensive management strategy for third-trimester pregnancies complicated by fetal anomalies. *Obstet. Gynecol.*, **75**, 311–16

Genetics of central nervous system anomalies

13

Z. Papp, Zs. Ádám and M. Smith-Levitin

INTRODUCTION

Central nervous system (CNS) anomalies are among the most commonly diagnosed fetal anomalies. They frequently have a severe prognosis, which impacts on survival, appearance and future function in society. They are also a source of many questions regarding prenatal diagnosis and genetic counselling. In many cases, CNS anomalies have a genetic background which enable estimation of recurrence risk. Central nervous system anomalies can be classified as either neural tube defects or other malformations, including hydrocephalus. Each anomaly can occur as an isolated defect or as a part of a multiple malformation syndrome. Although the majority have a multifactorial basis, most of the anomalies can also be the result of chromosomal disorders, Mendelian disorders, or teratogen exposure[1-13].

A multifactorial trait is one in which environmental factors act on a polygenic predisposition to cause abnormal neural development. 'Polygenic' implies that a number of genes rather than a single pair of genes is responsible for the predisposition to the disease. The threshold model can be employed for better understanding of the concept of multifactorial inheritance. The genetic predisposition to a disease is greater as the number of defective genes increases. The distribution curve also more closely approximates a Gaussian distribution as the number increases. This determines the 'genetic threshold'. Above the genetically determined threshold, a wide range of mild environmental factors can precipitate disease: at levels below the genetic threshold, induction requires more violent environmental effects. The extremes can occur, in which individuals who are genetically very susceptible can develop pathological conditions in a seemingly normal environment, and individuals who are genetically resistant can develop anomalies in a highly harmful or damaging environment. Alterations inherited in this way can be quantitative or qualitative in nature. The severity of a given anomaly will also be influenced by the genetic predisposition and the environment. Examples of central nervous system anomalies that are multifactorial are listed in Table 1[1-13].

Chromosomal disorders that are involved in central nervous system anomalies are often aneuploidies (numeric abnormalities), which are the result of errors that occur during meiosis. Examples are non-disjunction, anaphase lag and polyploidy. Duplications, deletions, inversions, translocations and ring chromosomes can also occur during meiosis, resulting in gametes with unbalanced chromosomal constitutions. The fetuses that develop from fertilization of these gametes frequently have CNS anomalies. Table 2 lists some examples[1-13].

Mendelian disorders are single-gene phenotypes that follow Mendel's laws of segregation and independent assortment. Careful pedigree analysis can assist in the determination of the genetic transmission for a given phenotype. Autosomal dominant, autosomal recessive, sex-linked recessive, and sex-linked dominant inheritance have been demonstrated in CNS anomalies. Some examples, listed by mode of inheritance, are seen in Table 3[1-13].

Teratogens are agents or factors that can cause abnormalities in the form or function of an exposed fetus. In the case of CNS anomalies, they act by interfering with a vital step in neuromorphogenesis: either by causing cell death beyond the recuperative capacity of the fetus, by impairing cellular differentiation, or by inhibiting cell migration. Teratogens can have an effect at any gestational age because the development of the CNS is a continuous process. Examples of CNS anomalies that are associated with specific teratogens are listed in Table 4[1-13].

Table 1 Central nervous system anomalies that are multifactorial

Anencephaly
Exencephaly
Spina bifida
Encephalocele
Iniencephaly
Hydrocephalus

ETIOLOGY OF NEURAL TUBE DEFECTS

Neural tube defects are qualitative anomalies of variable severity. They are manifest as three separate anomalies: anencephaly/exencephaly, spina bifida and encephalocele. In the majority of cases, neural tube defects are isolated anomalies inherited as multifactorial traits. Major chromosomal alterations do not play an important role in their etiology. An exception to this is trisomy 13 (Patau's syndrome), which is frequently associated with holoprosencephaly.

Although the etiology of neural tube defects is poorly understood, various factors, such as nutritional deficiencies, physical effects, and environmental teratogens have been implicated[1-13].

Anencephaly/exencephaly

Failure of closure of the cranial pole of the neural tube results in a malformation, termed anencephaly, which is incompatible with life. This cranial defect may continue downwards along the whole spine (craniorachischisis), or it may be accompanied by a separate closure defect of the lumbar spine. Exencephaly is an almost complete absence of the calvaria with a large amount of protruding cerebral tissue. It, too, is always lethal. Inheritance of these severe anomalies is usually multifactorial. Certain monogenic syndromes (Table 5) and external factors (Table 4) can result in anencephaly in a small fraction of cases. There is a gender-dependent difference in multifactorial inheritance: anencephaly is found twice as often in female fetuses. The incidence varies widely, depending on geographical area. For example, the incidence is 1/1000 births in the United States and 6.7/1000 in the United Kingdom[1-14].

Table 2 Central nervous system anomalies that are the result of chromosomal errors

Chromosome deletions
Microcephaly (1q, 4p, 5p, 6q, 7p, 9r, 10q, 18p, 18q, 21q)
Holoprosencephaly (13q, 18p)

Chromosome duplications
Anencephaly (1q)
Holoprosencephaly (1q)
Hydrocephaly (7p, 7q, 9p)
Microcephaly (2q, 3q, 4p, 4q, 6q, 9p, 9q, 10q, 11q, 14q, 17q, 19q)
Dandy–Walker (5p)
Agenesis of the corpus callosum (8p)

Ring chromosomes
Microcephaly

Translocations
Agenesis of the corpus callosum (9/11)

Trisomy
Agenesis of the corpus callosum (8)
Holoprosencephaly (13)
Microcephaly (13, 14, 21, 22)
Hydrocephaly (13, 18, 21)
Dandy–Walker (13, 18)

Tetrasomy
Hydrocephaly (9)

Monosomy
Dandy–Walker (45,X)

Triploidy
Holoprosencephaly
Hydrocephaly
Neural tube defects

Tetraploidy
Microcephaly

Spina bifida

Spina bifida is a result of defective neural tube closure along the vertebral column. There are three anatomical variations of spina bifida. The most common, and most serious, is spina bifida occulta, in which there is no fusion of the halves of the vertebral arch. Spina bifida cystica includes meningoceles, in which there is herniation of the meninges through the defect, and the more common meningomyeloceles, in which there is herniation of the cord as well as the meninges through the defect. The third type of spina bifida is myeloschisis, which occurs in the lumbar region

Table 3 Central nervous system anomalies with Mendelian inheritance

Autosomal recessive
True microcephaly
Dandy-Walker
Encephalocele
Hydrocephalus
Holoprosencephaly
Anencephaly
Spina bifida
Agenesis of the corpus callosum

Autosomal dominant
True microcephaly
Encephalocele
Holoprosencephaly
Spina bifida
Agenesis of the corpus callosum

X-linked recessive
Hydrocephalus (cerebellar agenesis and aqueductal stenosis)
Holoprosencephaly
Anencephaly
Spina bifida
Agenesis of the corpus callosum

X-linked dominant
Holoprosencephaly
Spina bifida

Table 4 Central nervous system anomalies in teratogenic syndromes

Fetal alcohol syndrome
Holoprosencephaly/arhinencephaly

Fetal aminopterin/methotrexate syndrome
Anencephaly/craniorachischisis
Hydrocephaly
Spina bifida occulta

Fetal carbamazepine syndrome
Microcephaly
Spina bifida occulta

Fetal cocaine syndrome
Hydranencephaly/porencephaly
Meningocele/meningomyelocele
Microcephaly
Posterior encephalocele/meningocele

Fetal influenza syndrome
Anencephaly/craniorachischisis
Holoprosencephaly/arhinencephaly
Hydrocephaly
Spina bifida occulta

Fetal rubella syndrome
Anterior encephalocele/meningocele
Microcephaly

Fetal thalidomide syndrome
Meningocele/meningomyelocele
Spina bifida occulta

Fetal valproate syndrome
Anencephaly/craniorachischisis
Meningocele/meningomyelocele
Microcephaly

Fetal vitamin A syndrome
Holoprosencephaly/arhinencephaly
Hydranencephaly/porencephaly
Hydrocephaly
Meningocele/meningomyelocele
Microcephaly

Fetal warfarin syndrome
Hydrocephaly
Microcephaly
Posterior encephalocele/meningocele

Maternal diabetes syndrome
Anencephaly/craniorachischisis
Holoprosencephaly/arhinencephaly
Meningocele/meningomyelocele
Microcephaly

Maternal hyperthermia syndrome
Anencephaly/craniorachischisis
Meningocele/meningomyelocele
Microcephaly
Posterior encephalocele/meningocele
Spina bifida occulta

only, and is the result of a failure of the neural tubes to meet and fuse, thus exposing the neural plate to the surface. Inheritance in all types is usually multifactorial. However, monogenic inheritance (Table 6) and teratogenic factors (Table 4) may play a role as well. The incidence ranges from 0.4 to 4.0/1000 births [15–30].

Encephalocele

Encephalocele accounts for only 5% of neural tube defects. It refers to a hernia-like protrusion of meninges and brain tissue through a bone lesion of the cranial vault. In these cases, 75% involve the occipital region, but they can also be parietal, frontal, or nasopharyngeal. The frontoethmoidal form is the most common in Thailand. Isolated cases are inherited in a multifactorial way. When encephalocele is accompanied by other anomalies, monogenic inheritance (Table 7) and teratogenic factors (Table 4) can be involved in the etiology [15–30].

Table 5 Anencephaly/exencephaly as a part of mono-genically inherited multiple malformation syndromes

---

Autosomal recessive inheritance
Acrocallosal – agenesis of the corpus callosum; mental retardation; polydactyly (McKusick 200990)

X-linked recessive inheritance
X-linked neural tube defects (McKusick 301410)

ETIOLOGY OF NON-NEURAL TUBE MALFORMATIONS

Hydrocephalus

Of all hydrocephalus cases 10% are isolated and result from a primary defect, such as agenesis, hypoplasia, or malformation of one of the openings within the ventricular system. Inheritance is monogenic (X-linked recessive or autosomal recessive) in one-third of cases and multifactorial in the remainder. Of all cases of uncomplicated hydrocephalus, 2% are secondary to a sex-linked recessive aqueductal stenosis.

Hydrocephalus seen at birth is secondary to some other pathology in 90% of cases. The primary abnormality can be a neural tube defect, an intracranial hemorrhage, a choroid plexus papilloma, or the result of an intrauterine infection such as toxoplasmosis, cytomegalovirus, or listeriosis. The genetic etiology depends on the primary abnormality. The overall incidence of hydrocephalus at birth is 0.11–3.5/1000 births, depending on geographic location[31–48].

Dandy–Walker malformation

A complete or partial absence of the cerebellar vermis and a posterior fossa cyst that is continuous with the fourth ventricle constitutes a Dandy–Walker malformation. It is often associated with hydrocephalus. It may have a genetic background in some instances, as familial cases have been observed. For example, it is part of the Joubert syndrome which is inherited as an autosomal recessive. Chromosomal disorders also play a role[1–3].

Table 6 Spina bifida as a part of monogenically inherited multiple malformation syndromes

---

Autosomal recessive inheritance
Alar clefts – Hypertelorism (McK 203000)
Camptodactyly type Guadalajara (McK 211910)
Jarcho–Levin (Spondylothoracic dysplasia) (McK 277300)
Juberg–Hayward – clefting; radial defects; mental retardation (McK 216100)
Neu–Laxova syndrome (McK 250520)
Spondylocostal dysostosis (McK 277300)
Three-M slender-boned dwarfism (McK 273750)
Winter (1968) – renal, genital and middle-ear anomalies (McK 267400)

Autosomal dominant inheritance
Arteriohepatic dysplasia (Alagille) (McK 118450)
Cleidocranial dysostosis (McK 119600)
Duane anomaly – radial defects (McK 126800)
Familial cervical dysplasia (McK 118005)
Femoral hypoplasia – unusual facies (McK 134780)
Juvenile polyposis (McK 174900)
Osteopathia striata – cranial sclerosis (McK 166500)
Sacral agenesis – spina bifida (McK 182940)
Spondylocostal dysostosis (McK 277300)

X-linked recessive inheritance
Hydrocephaly with features of Vater
X-linked neural tube defects (McK 301410)

X-linked dominant inheritance
Frontometaphyseal dysplasia (Gorlin) (McK 305620)
Otopalatodigital (Taybi) syndrome (McK 311300)

Dysgenesis of the corpus callosum

Incomplete closure of the anterior neuropore results in defective formation of the corpus callosum. It can be isolated, but it is frequently seen in association with other CNS anomalies, such as holoprosencephaly. Most cases are sporadic, with unknown etiology. Some may be autosomal dominant, autosomal recessive, or sex-linked[1–3].

Hydranencephaly

An early occlusion or developmental defect of both internal carotid or cerebral arteries leads to a major hemisphere deficiency termed hydranencephaly. Those parts of the brain receiving their blood supply through the posterior circulation (brainstem, cerebellum, midbrain, basal ganglia

Table 7 Encephalocele as a part of monogenically inherited multiple malformation syndromes

Autosomal recessive inheritance
Craniotelencephalic dysplasia (McK 218670)
Frontofacionasal dysplasia (McK 229400)
Hydrolethalus syndrome (McK 236680)
Joubert–cerebellar vermis aplasia plus other anomalies (McK 213300)
Meckel–Gruber syndrome (dysencephalia splanchnocystica) (McK 249000)
Oculoencephalohepatorenal syndrome (McK 213010)
Oral–facial–digital syndrome type II (McK 252100)
Porphyria, homozygous acute intermittent
Roberts (pseudothalidomide) syndrome (McK 268300)
Rolland–desbuquois – dyssegmental dysplasia (McK 224400)
Warburg – hydrocephalus; agyria; eye anomalies; encephalocele (HARD±E) (McK 236670)

Autosomal dominant inheritance
Apert – acrocephalosyndactyly type I (McK 101200)
Goldenhar (facio–auriculo–vertebral) syndrome/hemifacial microsomia (McK 164210)
Weissenbacher–Zweymuller syndrome (McK 108300)

Table 8 Holoprosencephaly as a part of monogenically inherited multiple malformation syndromes

Autosomal recessive inheritance
Bowen syndrome–glaucoma; flexion contractures of fingers (McK 211200)
Camptomelic dysplasia (McK 211970)
Holoprosencephaly
Hydrolethalus syndrome (McK 236680)
Meckel–Gruber syndrome (dysencephalia splanchnocystica) (McK 249000)
Mohr–Majewski syndrome (McK 258860)
Smith–Lemli–Opitz syndrome type II (severe lethal form) (McK 268670)
Váradi–Papp–oral–facial–digital syndrome type VI (McK 277170)

Autosomal dominant inheritance
Aase–Smith–hydrocephalus: cleft palate: joint contractures (McK 147800)
Clefting–premaxilla agenesis (McK 157170)
DiGeorge syndrome (McK 188400)
Goldenhar (facio–auriculo–vertebral) syndrome/ hemifacial microsomia (McK 164210)
Holoprosencephaly
Velocardiofacial syndrome (McK 192430)

X-linked recessive inheritance
Ichthyosis–hypogonadism–mental retardation (X-linked) (McK 308200)
Kallmann syndrome

X-linked dominant inheritance
Aicardi syndrome (McK 304050)

and posterior part of the occipital lobe) are well developed, but the cerebral hemispheres are reduced to a gliomatous membrane filled with cerebrospinal fluid. Hydranencephaly occurs only as an isolated, sporadic anomaly with no known specific etiology. The incidence is less than 0.1/1000 births[1–3].

Holoprosencephaly

Failure of prechordial mesoderm migration leads to incomplete cleavage of the primitive prosenchephalon. As a consequence, structures that normally arise from the forebrain, such as the cerebral hemispheres, thalamus and hypothalamus, do not develop properly. Some of the manifestations include a common cerebral ventricle, a single cortex and thalamus, and absent or abnormal olfactory tracts and optic bulbs. When multiple anomalies occur as a consequence of a primary defect (in this case the migration problem of prechordial mesoderm), the alterations are denoted as a sequence. The holoprosencephaly sequence involves midline facial defects, such as cyclopia, proboscis, premaxillary agenesis, and

cleft lip and palate, in addition to the cerebral abnormalities. The etiology is heterogeneous. Most cases are sporadic with no increased risk of recurrence. There is one major chromosomal defect that is frequently associated with holoprosencephaly: trisomy 13 or Patau's syndrome. Some teratogenic factors, especially maternal hyperglycemia, can be involved in the etiology (Table 4). Holoprosencephaly may also arise as a part of a multiple malformation syndrome such as the Váradi–Papp syndrome (McKusick 277170) (Table 8)[49–54].

Microcephaly

Microcephaly may appear as an isolated defect or as a part of multiple malformation syndromes. It is usually the product of an underdeveloped brain, which can be the result of many factors. For example, teratogens play a significant role (Table 4) in the etiology of microcephaly. Infective agents such as rubella, toxoplasma, herpes and cyto-megalovirus have been particularly implicated. The majority of chromosomal errors are also accompanied by growth failure of the CNS leading to microcephaly of varying degrees. Furthermore, microcephaly is frequently seen in relation to multiple malformation syndromes with different types of Mendelian inheritance. True microcephaly without associated anomalies can also be inherited monogenically as an autosomal recessive (McK 251200) trait or as an autosomal dominant (McK 156580) trait with incomplete penetrance. The overall incidence of microcephaly is estimated to be between 1/6200 and 1/8500 births[55–58].

Iniencephaly

Iniencephaly is a developmental defect of the skull in the occipital region (the Greek word inion meaning 'occiput') that leaves the brain exposed. The cervical and some of the thoracic vertebrae are usually incomplete, irregularly fused, or absent, and there is also disorganization of the underlying nervous tissue (an open spina bifida). As a consequence of these anomalies, the head is in a 'stargazing' position. Iniencephaly is usually sporadic with no specific known etiology. It does occur more frequently in families with other neural tube defects. There is a gender-dependent difference in the incidence of this disease: it occurs more frequently in female fetuses[59, 60].

RECURRENCE RISK OF CNS ANOMALIES

We know that chromosomal errors, teratogens, monogenic disorders and multifactorial inheritance are involved in the etiology of some of the CNS anomalies. This enables us to establish four different counselling strategies. Assigning a general recurrence risk to CNS anomalies is not possible due to their heterogeneous etiology.

The recurrence risk for anomalies that are the result of chromosomal errors is mainly age-dependent. The risk increases with increasing age.

A young woman under the age of 35 has a recurrence risk that is equivalent to the risk for a woman of similar age in the general population who has no prior history. There are, however, some chromosomal errors that are the result of rare inheritable chromosomal rearrangements. If one of the parents carries such a rearrangement, the recurrence risk may be significant. Obtaining a careful family history may help to identify these couples.

The recurrence risk for CNS anomalies that are the result of exposure to teratogens depends on the nature of the involved agent. For drug or radiation exposures, the recurrence risk will approach zero if the patient can prevent exposure to the same agent in the next pregnancy. For teratogens such as glucose, the recurrence risk can be minimized by optimal preconceptional and antenatal management of maternal diabetes, but it cannot be entirely eliminated.

Central nervous system anomalies that are the result of monogenic disorders are infrequent, yet they have a high recurrence risk. Autosomal recessive traits carry a 25% recurrence risk, while auto-somal dominant and X-linked disorders (for male fetuses) carry a 50% risk. Proper embryopatho-logical or neonatological examinations are required to establish a correct diagnosis of these uncommon syndromes. Computer-aided syndrome identification can also be of value.

Isolated cases of CNS anomalies are generally inherited as multifactorial traits. The risk of recurrence is established by survey data. It is primarily influenced by the number of affected relatives, and by the pathoanatomical severity of the disease. In the majority of cases, the same type of anomaly tends to recur. For a healthy couple who have already had a child with an isolated neural tube defect, the risk for having a subsequent affected child is approximately 3%. The risk increases to 10–20% if there have been two or more affected children[1, 2, 3, 7, 10, 17, 19, 20, 28, 34, 61].

PREVENTION OF CNS ANOMALIES

Much of the attention given to CNS anomalies has been focused on prenatal diagnosis. The widespread use of maternal serum α-fetoprotein at 14–21 weeks' gestation as a screening test, combined with the improvements in sonographic equipment and skills, have made it easier to diagnose anomalies in the first and second trimesters. Progress in preventing CNS anomalies, however, has been slower due to their heterogeneous, and often unknown, etiologies.

There have been some advancements made in the prevention of recurrent neural tube defects. Studies in the early 1980s first suggested that low levels of folic acid might be closely associated with neural tube defects. A subsequent well-designed prospective, randomized study of folic acid supplementation demonstrated a significant reduction in the recurrence rate with daily 4-mg doses of folic acid, starting prior to conception and continuing through the first trimester. These promising results prompted the Committee on Obstetrics: Maternal and Fetal Medicine of the American College of Obstetricians and Gynecologists to recommend similar treatment for any patient who has had a previous fetus with a neural tube defect[62,63].

The data regarding prevention of first occurrences of neural tube defects are less clear. Certain patients, such as those with pre-gestational diabetes and those who are taking medications such as valproic acid or carbamazepine, are at higher risk of having an affected fetus. They may also benefit from pre-conceptional and early trimester folate supplementation. In the future, more information will be available that will guide recommendations for these patients as well as for low-risk patients[62,63].

References

1. Warkany, J., Lemire, R.J. and Cohen, M.M. (1981). *Mental Retardation and Congenital Malformations of the Central Nervous System*, pp. 13–100, 158–190, 224–243, 436–442. (Chicago: Year Book Publishers)

2. Chervenak, F.A., Isaacson, G.C. and Campbell, S. (eds.) (1993). Anomalies of the spine. In *Ultrasound in Obstetrics and Gynecology*, Vol. 2, pp. 883–92. (Boston: Little, Brown)

3. Chervenak, F.A., Isaacson, G.C. and Campbell, S. (eds.) (1993). Anomalies of the cranium and its contents. In *Ultrasound in Obstetrics and Gynecology*, Vol. 1, pp. 825–48. (Boston: Little, Brown)

4. Bauman, M.L. (1987). Neuroembryology. Clinical aspects. *Semin. Perinatol.*, **11**, 74–84

5. Bell, J.E. (1989). The pathology of central nervous system defects in human fetuses of different gestational ages. *Adv. Study Birth Defects*, **7**, 1–17

6. Carter, C.C., David, A. and Lawrence, K.M. (1968). A family study of major nervous system malformations in South Wales. *J. Med. Genet.*, **5**, 81–106

7. Carter, C.C. and Roberts, J.A.F. (1967). The risk of recurrence after two children with central nervous system malformations. *Lancet*, **1**, 306

8. Coalson, R.E. and Tomasek, J.J. (1992). *Embryology*, 2nd edn. (Berlin: Springer Verlag)

9. Icenogle, D.A. and Kaplan, A.M. (1981). A review of congenital neurologic malformations. *Clin. Pediatr.*, **20**, 565–75

10. Nevin, N.C. and Johnston, W.P. (1980). Risk of recurrence after two children with central nervous system malformations in an area of high incidence. *J. Med. Genet.*, **17**, 87–92

11. Papp, Z. (1990). *Obstetric Genetics*. (Budapest: Akadémiai Kradó)

12. Papp, Z., Csécsei, K., Lindenbaum, R.H., Szeifert, G.T., Tóth, Z. and Váradi, V. (1992). *Atlas of Fetal Diagnosis*. (Amsterdam: Elsevier)

13. Spirt, B.A., Oliphant, M. and Gordon, L.P. (1990). Fetal central nervous system abnormalities. *Radiol. Clin. N. Am.*, **28**, 59–73

14. Papp, Z., Csécsei, K., Tóth, Z., Polgár, K. and Szeifert, G.T. (1986). Exencephaly in human fetuses. *Clin. Genet.*, **30**, 440–4

15. Bamforth, S.J. and Baird, P.A. (1989). Spina bifida and hydrocephalus. A population study over a 35-year period. *Am. J. Hum. Genet.*, **44**, 225–32

16. Campbell, L.R., Dayton, D.H. and Sohal, G.S. (1986). Neural tube defects: a review of human and animal studies on the etiology of neural tube defects. *Teratology*, **34**, 171–87

17. Ayiomamitis, A. (1988). Birth prevalence and recurrence rates of neural-tube defects in Southern Alberta in 1970–81. *Can. Med. Assoc. J.*, **139**, 610–11

18. Baird, P.A. (1982). Neural tube defects and tracheo-oesophageal dysraphism. *Lancet*, **1**, 615

19. Cowchock, S., Ainbender, E., Greene, J., Crandall, B., Lau, L., Heller, R., Muir, W.A., Kloza, E., Feigelson, M., Mennuti, M. and Cederquist, L. (1980). The recurrence risk for neural tube defects in the United States: a collaborative study. *Am. J. Med. Genet.*, **5**, 309–14

20. Czeizel, A. and Métneki, J. (1984). Recurrence risk after neural tube defects in a genetic counselling clinic. *J. Med. Genet.*, **21**, 413–16

21. Hall, J.G., Friedman, J.M., Kenna, B.A., Popkin, J., Jawanda, M. and Arnold, W. (1988). Clinical, genetic, and epidemiological factors in neural tube defects. *Am. J. Hum. Genet.*, **43**, 827–37

22. Holmes, L.B., Driscoll, S.G. and Atkins, L. (1976). Etiologic heterogeneity of neural tube defects. *N. Engl. J. Med.*, **294**, 365–9

23. Khoury, M.J., Erickson, J.D. and James, L.M. (1982). Etiologic heterogeneity of neural tube defects. I. Clues from epidemiology. *Am. J. Epidemiol.*, **115**, 538–48

24. Khoury, M.J., Erickson, J.D. and James, L.M. (1982). Etiologic heterogeneity of neural tube defects. II. Clues from family studies. *Am. J. Hum. Genet.*, **34**, 980–7

25. Papp, Z., Tóth, Z., Török, O. and Szabó, M. (1987). Prenatal diagnosis policy without routine amniocentesis in pregnancies with a positive family history for neural tube defects. *Am. J. Med. Genet.*, **26**, 103–10

26. Seller, M.J. (1990). Neural tube defects. Are neurulation and canalization forms causally distinct? *Am. J. Med. Genet.*, **35**, 394–6

27. Simpson, J.L., Mills, J.L., Rhoads, G.G., Cunningham, G.C., Conley, M.R. and Hoffman, H.J. (1991). Genetic heterogeneity in neural tube defects. *Ann. Genet.*, **34**, 279–86

28. Toriello, H.V. and Higgins, J.V. (1983). Occurrence of neural tube defects among first-, second-, and third-degree relatives of probands: results of a United States study. *Am. J. Med. Genet.*, **15**, 601–6

29. Török, O. and Papp, Z. (1991). Are the neurulation and canalization forms of neural tube defects causally distinct? *Am. J. Med. Genet.*, **39**, 241

30. Wald, N.J. and Cuckle, H.S. (1982). Nomogram for estimating an individual's risk of having a fetus with open spina bifida. *Br. J. Obstet. Gynaecol.*, **89**, 598–602

31. Achiron, R., Schimmel, M., Achiron, A. and Mashiach, S. (1993). Fetal mild idiopathic lateral ventriculomegaly: is there a correlation with fetal trisomy? *Ultrasound Obstet. Gynecol.*, **3**, 89–92

32. Adams, C., Johnston, W.P. and Nevin, N.C. (1982). Family study of congenital hydrocephalus. *Dev. Med. Child Neurol.*, **24**, 493–8

33. Bruni, J.E., Delbigio, M.R., Cardoso, E.R. and Persaud, T.V.N. (1988). Hereditary hydrocephalus in laboratory animals and humans. *Exp. Pathol.*, **35**, 239–46

34. Burton, B.K. (1979). Recurrence risks for congenital hydrocephalus. *Clin. Genet.*, **16**, 47–53

35. Cochrane, D.D., Myles, S.T., Nimrod, C., Still, D.K., Sugarman, R.G. and Wittmann, B.K. (1985). Intrauterine hydrocephalus and ventriculomegaly: associated anomalies and fetal outcome. *Can. J. Neurol. Sci.*, **12**, 51–9

36. Cohen, T., Stern, E. and Rosenmann, A. (1979). Sib risk of neural tube defect: is prenatal diagnosis indicated in pregnancies following the birth of a hydrocephalic child? *J. Med. Genet.*, **16**, 14–16

37. Collmann, H., Sorensen, N., Krauss, J. and Muhling, J. (1988). Hydrocephalus in craniosynostosis. *Child. Nerv. Syst.*, **4**, 279–85

38. Habib, Z. (1981). Genetics and genetic counselling in neonatal hydrocephalus. *Obstet. Gynecol. Surv.*, **36**, 529–34

39. Imaizumi, Y. (1989). Concordance and discordance of congenital hydrocephalus in 107 twin pairs in Japan. *Teratology*, **40**, 101–3

40. Nyberg, D.A., Mack, L.A., Hirsch, J., Pagon, R.O. and Shepard, T.H. (1987). Fetal hydrocephalus: sonographic detection and clinical significance of associated anomalies. *Radiology*, **163**, 187–91

41. Teebi, A.S. and Naguib, K.K. (1988). Autosomal recessive nonsyndromal hydrocephalus. *Am. J. Med. Genet.*, **31**, 467–70

42. Váradi, V., Csécsei, K., Szeifert, G.T., Tóth, Z. and Papp, Z. (1987). Prenatal diagnosis of X linked hydrocephalus without aqueductal stenosis. *J. Med. Genet.*, **24**, 207–9

43. Váradi, V., Tóth, Z., Török, O. and Papp, Z. (1988). Heterogeneity and recurrence risk for congenital hydrocephalus (ventriculomegaly). A prospective study. *Am. J. Med. Genet.*, **29**, 305–10

44. Willems, P.J. (1988). Heterogeneity in familial hydrocephalus. *Am. J. Med. Genet.*, **31**, 471–72

45. Willems, P.J., Dijkstra, I., Vanderau, B.J., Vits, L., Coucke, P., Raeymaek, P., Van Broeckhoven, C., Consalez, G.G., Freeman, S.B. and Warren, S.T. (1990). Assignment of X-linked hydrocephalus to Xq28 by linkage analysis. *Genomics*, **8**, 367–70

46. Williamson, R.A., Schauberger, C.W., Varner, M.W. and Aschenbrener, C.A. (1984). Heterogeneity of prenatal onset hydrocephalus: management and counselling implications. *Am. J. Med. Genet.*, **17**, 497–508

47. Zlotogora, J., Sagi, M. and Cohen, T. (1994). Familial hydrocephalus of prenatal onset. *Am. J. Med. Genet.*, **49**, 202–4

48. Chervenak, F.A., Berkowitz, R.L., Romero, R., Tortora, M., Mayden, K., Duncan, C. and Mahoney, M.J. (1983). The diagnosis of fetal hydrocephalus. *Am. J. Obstet. Gynecol.*, **147**, 703–16

49. Berry, S.M., Gosden, C., Snijders, R.J. and Nicolaides, K.H. (1990). Fetal holoprosencephaly: associated malformations and chromosomal defects. *Fetal Diag. Ther.*, **5**, 92–9

50. Cohen, M.M. (1982). An update on the holoprosencephalic disorders. *J. Pediatr.*, **101**, 865–9

51. Lemire, R.J., Cohen, M.M., Beckwith, J.B., Kokich, V.G. and Siebert, J.R. (1981). The facial features of holoprosencephaly in anencephalic human specimens. I. Historical review and associated malformations. *Teratology*, **23**, 297–303

52. Munke, M. (1989). Clinical, cytogenetic, and molecular approaches to the genetic heterogeneity of holoprosencephaly. *Am. J. Med. Genet.*, **34**, 237–45

53. Verloes, A., Aymé, S., Gambarel, D., Gonzales, M., Lemerrer, M., Mulliez, N., Philip, N. and Roume, J. (1991). Holoprosencephaly polydactyly (pseudo-trisomy 13) syndrome. A syndrome with features of hydrolethalus and Smith–Lemli–Opitz syndromes. A collaborative multicenter study. *J. Med. Genet.*, **28**, 297–303

54. Holmes, L.B., Griscoll, S. and Atkins, L. (1974). Genetic heterogeneity of cebocephaly. *J. Med. Genet.*, **11**, 35–40

55. Persutte, W.H., Kurczynski, T.W., Chaudhury, K., Lenke, R.R. and Woldenberg, L. (1990). Prenatal diagnosis of autosomal dominant microcephaly and postnatal evaluation with magnetic resonance imaging. *Prenat. Diagn.*, **10**, 631–42

56. Pescia, G., Nguyen-The, H. and Deonna, T. (1983). Prenatal diagnosis of genetic microcephaly. *Prenat. Diagn.*, **3**, 363–5

57. Teebi, A.S., Alawadi, S.A. and White, A.G. (1987). Autosomal recessive nonsyndromal microcephaly with normal intelligence. *Am. J. Med. Genet.*, **26**, 355–9

58. Tolmie, J. L., McNay, M., Stephenson, J.B., Doyle, D. and Connor, J.M. (1987). Microcephaly. Genetic counselling and antenatal diagnosis after the birth of an affected child. *Am. J. Med. Genet.*, **27**, 583–94

59. Freeman, P.C. and Jeanty, P. (1991). Iniencephaly. *Fetus*, **1**, 7402–4

60. Mórocz, I., Szeifert, G.T., Molnár, P., Tóth, Z., Csécsei, K. and Papp, Z. (1986). Prenatal diagnosis and pathoanatomy of iniencephaly. *Clin. Genet.*, **30**, 81–6

61. Holmes-Siedle, M., Lindenbaum, R.H. and Galliard, A. (1992). Recurrence of neural tube defect in a group of at risk women. A 10 year study of Pregnavite forte-F. *J. Med. Genet.*, **29**, 134–5

62. ACOG Committee Opinion (1993). *Folic Acid for the Prevention of Recurrent Neural Tube Defects*, Number 120, March

63. MRC Vitamin Study Research Group (1991). Prevention of neural tube defects: results of the Medical Research Council Vitamin Study. *Lancet*, **338**, 131–7

Prognosis of fetal hydrocephalus

14

P. Kirkinen and M. Ryynänen

INTRODUCTION

Fetal hydrocephalus, the excessive accumulation of cerebrospinal fluid in the fetal ventricular or subarachnoid space, resulting in ventriculomegaly, complicates approximately 0.05–0.3% of pregnancies. Due to improved imaging methods, this etiologically heterogeneous condition can be diagnosed during the antepartum period. Antepartum imaging, combined with utilization of fetal blood sampling, chorion villus biopsy and amniocentesis, have facilitated increasingly exact etiological evaluation. The various etiologies, including cerebral malformations, infections, vascular accidents, tumors and single gene defects, and variable degrees of fetal neurological effects hamper exact assessment of fetal prognosis in this abnormality. The prognosis of fetal hydrocephalus diagnosed *in utero* is different from that of cases diagnosed neonatally[1-4]. Though the birth incidence of this condition seems to be decreasing, due to improved diagnosis in early pregnancy, fetal hydrocephalus in late pregnancy continues to be a difficult subject for assessment of appropriate strategies of perinatal care.

Because of scanty – and in many respects uncertain – results of long-term outcome as regards these fetuses, different opinions concerning ante- and peripartum therapy of fetal hydrocephalus have been put forward. Sufficient postpartum follow-up, etiological classification and exact antepartum estimation of the severity of the hydrocephalic process are parameters needed for comprehensive prognostic evaluation. In this chapter, we present a review and give some data from our own experience concerning prognostic aspects in fetal hydrocephaly.

DIAGNOSTIC METHODS FOR PROGNOSTIC ASSESSMENT

Table 1 presents the basic elements for prognostic evaluation of fetal hydrocephalus. Ultrasound is the main diagnostic method[5,6]. Imaging and the diagnostic criteria of ventriculomegaly are presented elsewhere in this book. The lateral ventricular index, the level of obstruction in fluid circulation and asymmetry of ventricular dilatation should be examined. The progress of ventricular dilatation during pregnancy is considered to show large individual variation. Our clinical impression is that there is rapid progress, particularly in late pregnancy, but documentation of relatively stable or even regressing processes in some fetuses has also been reported[3,7]. Associated intra- and extracerebral malformations are very important in diagnosis. The associated abnormalities found most often in the central nervous system are aqueductal stenosis, Dandy–Walker malformation, alobar holoprosencephaly and agenesis of the corpus callosum. The main etiology for communicating hydrocephaly is a spinal defect. The level and size of the spinal defect should be determined. Cardiac and renal malformations and conditions in the musculoskeletal system can also be associated. Cerebral macroanatomical changes can be well imaged by modern ultrasound techniques. Posterior fossa and medullary structures in a hydrocephalic head, however, are difficult objects for ultrasonic imaging, and there, sagittal magnetic resonance imaging is useful (Figures 1–3). Vaginal ultrasound scanning techniques are of great help, both in early and in late pregnancy, if the fetus is in a cephalic position and examination is possible through the large fontanelle.

Table 1 Diagnostic evaluation (diagnosis or exclusion) of hydrocephalic fetuses

(1) Ventricular size, lateral ventricular index, symmetry of dilatation, condition of ventricles III and IV
(2) Progress of ventricular dilatation
(3) Associated intracranial abnormalities (Dandy–Walker cyst, cerebellar agenesis, corpus callosum agenesis, holoprosencephaly, porencephalic cyst, hydranencephaly)
(4) Tissue characterization of the brain (calcification, hemorrhage, tumor, involvement of the plexus chorioideus)
(5) Associated spinal canal defect: size, type, location
(6) Associated malformations outside the central nervous system (heart, kidneys, musculoskeletal system)
(7) Fetal karyotype
(8) Examinations for infectious etiology
(9) Examinations of hemorrhagic diathesis in the fetus
(10) Fetal growth and well-being (dimensions, movements, cardiotocography)
(11) Obstetric parameters for delivery planning

An abnormal karyotype is associated with 10–30% of hydrocephalic cases, therefore fetal blood sampling or chorion villus biopsy is needed. Fetal musculoskeletal anatomy and activity (deformities, movements, swallowing, amniotic fluid) ought to be investigated.

An important aspect is evaluation of fetal well-being, including growth capacity and oxygenation. Increased intracranial pressure is proposed to be a reason behind decreased variability and increased incidence of decelerations in hydrocephalic fetuses. Sometimes, in addition, the heart rate baseline is decreased, and all these events can mask or simulate hypoxia in severe fetal hydrocephalus[8]. Trisomy or multiple malformations can cause severe growth retardation, as a sign of multiorgan involvement.

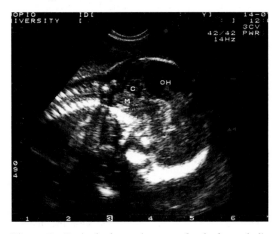

Figure 1 Sagittal ultrasonic scan of a hydrocephalic fetus. Cerebellum (C), medullar area (M) and dilated occipital horn (OH) can be visualized

An infectious etiology is investigated by antibody determinations in maternal and fetal blood, DNA/PCR techniques, amniotic fluid viral culture and imaging of neural tissue calcifications by ultrasonography. Some intracranial abnormalities are caused by intracranial hemorrhage or thrombotic processes, and therefore, for example, fetal hematological disturbances such as alloimmunothrombocytopenia, ought to be kept in mind. Embolization associated with twin-to-twin transfusion syndrome can sometimes disturb brain development and cause ventricular dilatation.

PROGNOSTIC FINDINGS

The outcome in neonatally detected and particularly surgically treated hydrocephaly is well documented. Long-term survival rates are 50–90%, and normal mental development is achieved in 30–60% of cases[9–12]. In contrast, much less information is available on long-term results in antepartum detection of hydrocephaly, and antepartum parameters affecting the prognosis.

There are sufficient data for a statement concerning mortality in fetal hydrocephalus; for all cases, mortality is 60–75%, and for isolated ventriculomegaly, mortality is 30–50%[2–4, 13]. The percentage of severe motor and cognitive handicap in long-term follow-up of surviving children is about 50–70%[2–4, 12, 14, 15]. On the other hand, in some cases normal or excellent mental development is possible[11]. Based on these reports, it is possible to list some parameters associated with definitively

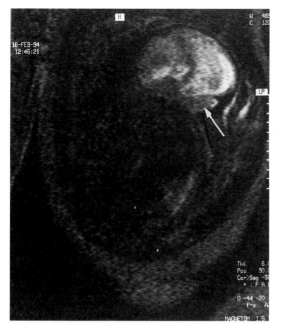

Figure 2 Sagittal magnetic resonance (proton density) image of a hydrocephalic fetus. The hypoplastic cerebellum (arrow) could not be imaged by ultrasound

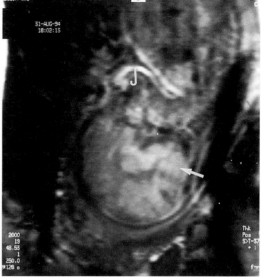

Figure 3 Proton-density-weighted magnetic resonance image of normal fetal head. Arrow, cerebellum; J, fetal jaw

poor prognosis (Table 2). The primary etiology of ventriculomegaly is the central prognostic factor, and mortality is mainly due to associated abnormalities. The majority of deaths occur during the periods of peri- or immediate postpartum.

Early diagnosis of hydrocephalus is usually an indicator of severe anatomical malformation (Figure 4). Thus, for example, Oi and colleagues[16,17] have reported that a long gestational period after hydrocephalus diagnosis worsens prognosis. We can expect severe progress and poor prognosis in most of these cases. Rapid progress in the third trimester is associated with many cases of isolated, obstructive ventriculomegaly and recognition of this development often leads to urgency in the decision on therapy. Intraventricular pressure first affects development of the white matter of the brain, and the gray matter is said to be protected for longer from permanent damage. However, no definitive information is available concerning the irreversibility of cortical damage. Not all types of hydrocephalus are associated with increased intracranial pressure.

Signs of acceptable or good prognosis for antepartum-detected hydrocephalus are more speculative. Minimal demands before deciding on a good prognosis are that careful imaging of intra- and extracerebral anatomy excludes severe associated malformations, chromosomal aberrations are excluded and associated complicating factors, such as intrauterine hypoxia, are taken into consideration. Two controversial questions arise in prognostic assessment:

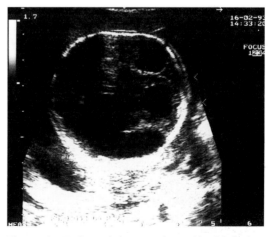

Figure 4 Hydrocephalus merging with the hydrolethalus syndrome. Transverse ultrasonic scan of a fetal head in the 17th gestational week. Ventricles are enlarged and irregular

Table 2 Signs of poor prognosis in fetal hydrocephalus

(1)	Multiple extracranial malformations
(2)	Associated chromosomal defect
(3)	Severe intracranial malformation or tumor
(4)	Disseminated signs of fetal infection (disseminated calcifications in the brain, hydrops, ascites)
(5)	Severe growth retardation
(6)	Retarded (microcephalic) cranial growth
(7)	Extreme ventriculomegaly (membranous cortex)
(8)	Large spinal canal defect associated with progressive hydrocephalus

(1) Is the thickness of the cerebral mantle a central prognostic factor?

(2) Can neurological damage and its irreversibility be evaluated by investigating fetal motor activity?

Some authors have reported that, in neonatal hydrocephaly and in optimal conditions, good shunting procedures cure an originally very thin cerebral mantle, resulting in favorable development[11,18] (Figure 5). However, extreme fetal ventriculomegaly with absent neonatal cortical activity results in a poor late outcome. In our own series of fetuses with hydrocephalus (mostly isolated cases), 24 surviving children were followed-up to 10 years of age. A poor outcome was significantly more often registered in the group with an increased biparietal diameter (>12 cm) or a markedly increased ventricular/hemispheric ratio ($>80\%$) (Figure 6). Similarly, Anhoury and colleagues[19] found that a fetal ventricular/hemispheric ratio more than 50% of normal indicated a poorer prognosis. Cortical mantle thickness served as a reasonable prognostic indicator in idiopathic aqueductal stenosis in a neonatally examined group of patients[20]. It can be concluded that the prepartum thickness of the fetal cerebral mantle (including the white and gray matter) – if cases with extreme dilatation are excluded – has some prognostic importance, but this factor is not as central as are associated abnormalities and the type and etiology of hydrocephalus. Extreme ventriculomegaly, however, can indicate a hydranencephalic condition, which has a hopeless prognosis. Most therapeutic recommendations stress the importance of early induction of delivery in isolated, progressive ventriculomegaly, before cerebral mantle thickening is too extreme.

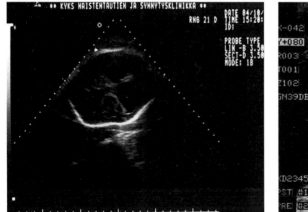

Figure 5 Moderate/severe ventriculomegaly and aqueductal stenosis. An ultrasound image of a fetal head in the 34th gestational week. This child was normally developed at the age of 9 years

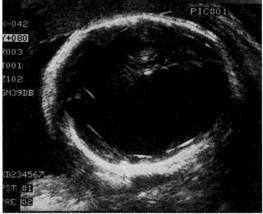

Figure 6 Severe ventriculomegaly imaged by ultrasound in the 32nd gestational week. This child was severely retarded at the age of 13 years

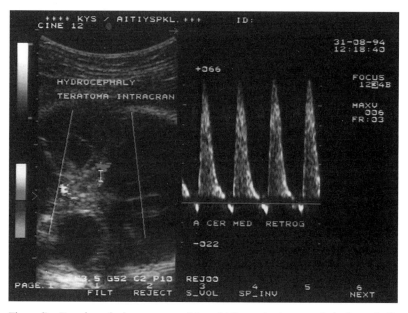

Figure 7 Doppler velocity spectrum of the middle cerebral artery of a hydrocephalic fetus. Increased vascular resistance with retrograde flow during diastole is evident

The investigation of fetal motor activity to evaluate the degree of neuronal impairment has received little attention. In large spinal defects, the absence of motor activity in the lower limbs has traditionally been seen as a bad sign, but precise data are lacking. Vintzileos and associates[14] published a study in which a low (<7) biophysical profile score in hydrocephalic fetuses pointed to fatal prognosis in spite of good umbilical pH levels. Severe effects on the musculoskeletal system are associated with some types of hydrocephalus, resulting in limb and muscle deformities and lack of movement. It can be concluded that markedly decreased fetal activity in hydrocephalus is a poor prognostic sign.

Doppler examinations of the cerebral circulation of hydrocephalic fetuses have been carried out in some studies[21,22] (Figure 7). Although increased vascular resistance or even retrograde pulsations seem to be associated with severe fetal ventriculomegaly, the prognostic importance of these findings is not definitive.

Table 3 presents a summary of long-term follow-up of hydrocephalic fetuses. Antepartum parameters pointing to good prognosis are much more speculative than those indicating fatal or very poor prognosis.

PROGNOSIS, THE ROUTE OF DELIVERY, POSTPARTUM ASPECTS

Vaginal delivery exposes ventriculomegalic fetuses and their mothers to mechanical trauma. Often, in addition, these fetuses are delivered in the breech position. Besides the mechanical damage, the increased pressure during uterine contractions could increase ischemic conditions in the brain tissue, as is considered to occur in spinal canal defects. On the other hand, there exists no evidence that ventriculomegalic fetuses with normal outer dimensions of the head would be additionally handicapped during vaginal birth. A spinal canal defect with mild-to-moderate hydrocephalus usually indicates elective Cesarean section. In fact, the effect of delivery method has been better evaluated by controlled studies in spinal canal defects than in isolated hydrocephalus[23,24]. Ventricular dilatation associated with a spinal canal defect can be less progressive than in other types of ventriculomegaly. Sometimes, however, rapid progress is evident, suggesting a poor prognosis and more conservative obstetric management. In fetal hydrocephalus with good prognostic assessment, elective Cesarean section ought to be liberally used in order to avoid

Table 3 Studies on long-term results in fetal hydrocephalus. Good outcome = normal or minimally retarded development. Most of the cases were the isolated, obstructive type of hydrocephalus with surgical postnatal treatment

| Authors | Follow-up | Good outcome | | Remarks |
		Number	%	
Vinzileos et al.[14]	18 months	4/9	44.4	
Drugan et al.[15]	28 months	8/26	30.8	
Anhoury et al.[19]	2 months	4/20	20.0	
Hanigan et al.[20]	18 months	4/14	28.6	all idiopathic aqueductal stenoses
Hudgins et al.[3]	3.5 years	13/22	59.1	non-progressive course in most cases during pregnancy
Rosseau et al.[4]	2.5–4 years	15/32	46.9	non-progressive course in most cases during pregnancy
Our series	10 years	9/24	37.5	

mechanical damage and labor-associated cerebral ischemia. In isolated and progressive hydrocephalus, this ought to be performed when lung maturity is achieved.

Some discrepancy between ante- and postpartum evaluation of a hydrocephalic process often exists. Ventricular dilatation at postpartum examinations often seems more severe than at antepartum examinations. One reason could be that antepartum amniotic fluid pressure and engagement of the head in the maternal pelvis opposes the effects of increased intracranial pressure.

Facilities for rapid and complete postnatal diagnosis, including an intensive care ward, must be provided before delivery. Urgent operation is needed for spinal canal defects. Thus, regionalization is necessary for optimal antepartum diagnosis, delivery planning and postnatal therapeutic procedures.

FAMILIAL PROGNOSIS IN FETAL HYDROCEPHALUS

Congenital hydrocephalus can be an isolated and primary phenomenon. The empirically documented recurrence risk in subsequent pregnancy is low: 1–2%[25]. The risk is 8% if two siblings are affected. However, some cases of hydrocephalus are due to genetic or chromosomal abnormalities or are associated with specific syndromes, and then the recurrence risk follows the mode of the specific syndrome. Up to 25% of aqueductal obstructions

in males may be the result of an X-linked recessive disorder. The risk to male siblings has been shown to be 5–10%[26].

Hydrocephalus occurs in association with several multiple malformation syndromes, many of which show single gene inheritance: syndromes of Beemer, Ertbruggen, Hard (or Warburg), Smith, Lemli and Opitz, FG syndrome and hydrolethalus. All these are extremely rare, but their recurrence risk is 25%. Some, for example the hydrolethalus syndrome can be seen in early pregnancy (Figure 4)[27].

Dandy–Walker anomaly may occur in several chromosome abnormalities, including triploidy and trisomies 9, 13 and 18, and in some single-gene disorders. Dandy–Walker with associated hydrocephalus can also be a manifestation of tendency to midline field defects, sometimes genetic in origin, and then the recurrence risk of siblings can rise to 7%[28].

The association of hydrocephalus with chromosomal anomalies has been observed in 10–29% of cases[29,30]. If parenteral translocations are excluded, the recurrence risk is the same as in isolated hydrocephalus, approximately 1–2%.

FUTURE ASPECTS IN PROGNOSTIC ASSESSMENT

Currently, when good imaging of fetal structures is possible, further investigation concerning the association of certain anatomical findings to long-term outcome is much needed. It is important that long-term outcomes in different etiological sub-

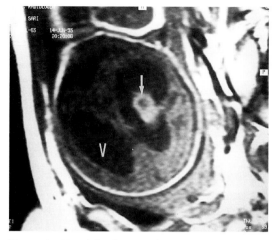

Figure 8 T$_1$-weighted magnetic resonance image of a hydrocephalic fetus with dilated ventricles (V). Intensive signal in the other plexus chorioideus (arrow), due to methemoglobin, indicated a recent hemorrhage in this area

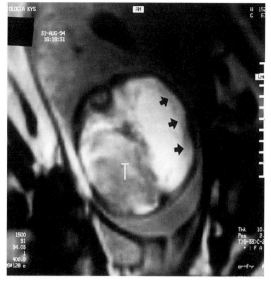

Figure 9 T$_2$-weighted magnetic resonance image of a fetus with large intracranial teratoma (T) and contralateral ventriculomegaly. The lateral wall of the ventricle is indicated by arrows

groups of fetal hydrocephalus be studied in a sufficient number of cases. Even more important is the development of methods for functional assessment of fetal neurological damage. These could be utilization of magnetic resonance imaging (Figures 8 and 9), for example for tissue characterization of the developing brain and its myelinization, or for examination of fetal brain metabolism *in vivo*. Fetal EEG, nowadays experimentally utilized during labor and delivery, would be of some use for assessment of fetal neurological function.

SUMMARY

In general, the prognosis in fetal hydrocephalus is poor. Mortality is 60–75%, due to the high fre-quency of serious associated abnormalities. More than half of the surviving children are retarded, in spite of intensive and long-lasting postnatal care. It is important to develop methods for accurate and early diagnosis and prognosis of fetal hydrocephalus, to optimize clinical management.

ACKNOWLEDGEMENTS

We thank K. Partenen, MD and P. Vainio, PhD from the Department of Radiology, University of Koupio, for the MR images in this chapter.

References

1. Holzgreve, E., Feil, R., Louwen, F. and Miny, P. (1993). Prenatal diagnosis and management of fetal hydrocephaly and lissencephaly. *Child's Nerv. Syst.*, **9**, 408–12
2. Serlo, W., Kirkinen, P., Jouppila, P. and Herva, R. (1986). Prognostic signs in fetal hydrocephalus. *Child's Nerv. Syst.*, **2**, 93–7
3. Hudgins, R., Edwards, M., Goldstein, R., Callen, P., Harrison, M., Filly, R. and Golbus, S. (1988). Natural history of fetal ventriculomegaly. *Pediatrics*, **82**, 692–7
4. Rosseau, G., McCullough, D. and Joseph, L. (1992). Current prognosis in fetal ventriculomegaly. *J. Neurosurg.*, **77**, 551–5
5. Chervenak, F., Isaacson, G. and Campbell, S. (1993). Anomalies of the cranium and its contents.

In Chervenak, F., Isaacson, G. and Campbell, S. (eds.) *Ultrasound in Obstetrics and Gynecology*, pp. 825–51. (Boston, Toronto, London: Little, Brown)

6. Kurjak, A., Gogolja, D., Kogler, A. and Rajhvajn, B. (1984). Ultrasound diagnosis and perinatal management of surgically correctable fetal malformations. *Ultrasound Med. Biol.*, **10**, 443–51

7. Tol, A. (1987). Spontaneous resolution of fetal ventriculomegaly in a diabetic patient. *J. Ultrasound Med.*, **6**, 37–8

8. Mooij, P., Nijhuis, J., Jongsma, H. and Menssen, J. (1992). Intracranial pressure and fetal heart rate in a hydrocephalic fetus during labor. *Eur. J. Obstet. Reprod. Biol.*, **43**, 161–5

9. O'Brien, M. and Harris, M. (1993). Long-term results in the treatment of hydrocephalus. *Neurosurg. Clin. N. Am.*, **4**, 625–32

10. Raimond, A. and Soare, P. (1974). Intellectual development in shunted hydrocephalic children. *Am. J. Dis. Child.*, **127**, 664–70

11. Lorber, J. (1968). The results of early treatment of extreme hydrocephalus. *Med. Child. Neurol.* (Suppl.), **16**, 21

12. Hirsch, J. (1992). Surgery of hydrocephalus: past, present and future. *Acta Neurochir. Wien*, **116**, 155–60

13. Chervenak, F., Berkowitz, R., Tortora, M. and Hobbins, J. (1985). The management of fetal hydrocephalus. *Am. J. Obstet. Gynecol.*, **151**, 933–42

14. Vintzileos, A., Campbell, W., Weinbraum, P. and Nochimson, D. (1987). Perinatal management and outcome of fetal ventriculomegaly. *Obstet. Gynecol.*, **69**, 5–11

15. Drugan, A., Krause, B., Canady, A., Zador, I., Sacks, A. and Evans, M. (1989). The natural history of prenatally diagnosed cerebral ventriculomegaly. *J. Am. Med. Assoc.*, **261**, 1785–8

16. Oi, S., Matsumoto, S., Katayama, K. and Mochizuki, M. (1990). Pathophysiology and postnatal outcome of fetal hydrocephalus. *Child's Nerv. Syst.*, **6**, 338–45

17. Oi, S., Yamada, H., Kimura, M., Ehara, K., Matsumoto, S., Katayama, K., Mochizuki, M., Uetani, Y. and Nakamura, H. (1990). Factors affecting prognosis of intrauterine hydrocephalus diagnosed in the third trimester. *Neurol. Med. Chir. Tokyo*, **30**, 456–61

18. Sutton, L., Bruce, D. and Schut, L. (1980). Hydranencephaly versus maximal hydrocephalus: an important clinical distinction. *Neurosurgery*, **6**, 35–9

19. Anhoury, P., Andre, M., Droulle, P., Czorny, A., Gilgenkrantz, S., Schweitzer, M. and Leheup, B. (1991). Dilatation of the cerebral ventricles diagnosed *in utero*. 85 case reports. *J. Gynecol. Obstet. Biol. Reprod. Paris*, **20**, 191–7

20. Hanigan, W., Morgan, A., Shaaban, A. and Bradle, P. (1991). Surgical treatment and long-term neurodevelopmental outcome for infants with idiopathic aqueductal stenosis. *Child's Nerv. Syst.*, **7**, 386–90

21. Kirkinen, P., Muller, R., Baumann, H., Briner, J., Lang, W., Huch, R. and Huch, A. (1988). Cerebral blood flow velocity waveforms in hydrocephalic fetuses. *J. Clin Ultrasound*, **16**, 493–8

22. Wladimiroff, J., Heydanus, R. and Stewart, P. (1993). Doppler colour flow mapping of fetal intracerebral arteries in the presence of central nervous system anomalies. *Ultrasound Med. Biol.*, **19**, 355–7

23. McCurdy, C. and Seeds, J. (1993). Route of delivery of infants with congenital anomalies. *Clin. Perinatal.*, **20**, 81–106

24. Luthy, D., Wardinsky, T. and Shurtleff, D. (1991). Cesarean section before the onset of labour and subsequent motor function in infants with meningomyelocele diagnosed antenatally. *N. Engl. J. Med.*, **324**, 662–6

25. Burton, B. (1979). Recurrence risks for congenital hydrocephalus. *Clin. Genet.*, **16**, 47–53

26. Holmes, L., Nash, A. and ZuRhein, M. (1973). X-linked aqueductal stenosis: clinical and neuropathological findings in two families. *Pediatrics*, **51**, 697–704

27. Hartikainen-Sorri, A.-L., Kirkinen, P. and Herva, R. (1983). Prenatal detection of hydrolethalus syndrome. *Prenat Diagn.*, **3**, 219–24

28. Murray, J., Johnson, J. and Bird, T. (1985). Dandy–Walker malformation: etiological heterogenity and empiric recurrence risks. *Clin. Genet.*, **28**, 272–83

29. Nyberg, A., Mark, L. and Hirsch, J. (1987). Fetal hydrocephalus: sonographic detection and clinical significance of associated anomalies. *Radiology*, **163**, 187–91

30. Pretorius, D., Davis, K., Manco-Johnson, M., Manchester, D., Meier, P. and Clewell, W. (1985). Clinical course of fetal hydrocephalus: 40 cases. *Am. J. Roentgenol.*, **144**, 827–31

Fetal and neonatal brain damage

15

K. Maeda, M. Utsu and M. Imanishi

INTRODUCTION

It has been argued that intrapartum electronic fetal monitoring (EFM) does not reduce the frequency of cerebral palsy[1,2]. In addition, there are many possible etiologies of cerebral palsy that may originate before or after the intrapartum period (Table 1). The incidence of cerebral palsy is dependent upon inclusion criteria[3,4]. This chapter reviews the mechanisms and criteria for diagnosis of fetal and neonatal brain damage[4].

HYPOXIC–ISCHEMIC INJURIES

Hypoxic–ischemic encephalopathy is diagnosed in the neonatal brain after hypoxic–ischemic damage. Two main mechanisms exist in hypoxic–ischemic injuries, which are closely related and may occur in combination. The first is neuronal necrosis, caused by general hypoxia or anoxia, and the second is caused by local ischemia due to circulatory collapse. General anoxia is related to selected neuronal necrosis, and general circulatory collapse with the necrosis of the neurons and/or white matter. Focal necrosis due to infarction is caused by the loss of perfusion, due to cerebral arterial obstruction.

Selective neuronal necrosis

Neuronal necrosis occurs in wide areas of the brain, in the cortex, diencephalon (thalamus, hypothalamus, lateral geniculate body), basal ganglia, midbrain, pons, medulla and cerebellum[4]. Neurological long-term sequelae include mental retardation, spastic quadriplegia, seizure disorder, ataxia, bulbar and pseudobulbar palsy, hyperactivity and impaired attention[4]. Neonatal

magnetic resonance imaging (MRI) shows high intensity of basal ganglia, atrophic changes and loss of myelination in the neonate after severe intrapartum asphyxia (Figures 1 and 2).

Neuronal necrosis can be caused by severe hypoxia or anoxia in the fetus or the newborn. Fetal damage can be caused by severe intrapartum acute anoxia, due to severe accidents, e.g. sudden placental separation or complete cord vessel occlusion. Fetal heart rate monitoring changes show sudden, severe and prolonged bradycardia. The fetuses under chronic or subacute hypoxia are detected by signs of fetal distress, e.g. severe variable decelerations or late decelerations. Rapid delivery may prevent severe brain damage. In our 10 year experience with universal intrapartum monitoring, the rate of cerebral palsy was reduced from 2.2 to 0.3 per 1000 births[3]. Therefore, the outcome for the fetuses was greatly improved. The reduction of cerebral palsy after introduction of widespread fetal monitoring was confirmed by pediatric neurologists[5]. The rare case of cerebral palsy that occurs at present is due to sudden, acute and severe anoxia. It is reported that delayed neuronal death is characteristic after severe anoxia, and that the process lasts for more than 10 h after the anoxic insult, but cannot be stopped by reoxygenation or reperfusion of the brain. Instead, there is the possibility of the treatment of delayed neuronal death by blockers of glutamate and the calcium ion, or the free radical scavenger[6,7]. These may be proven to be of value in postanoxic treatment in the future.

Although status marmoratus is described as one of the hypoxic–ischemic pathologies, the change will not be discussed in this chapter, because its appearance is limited in the later half of the first year[4].

Table 1 The causes of fetal and neonatal brain damage[4]

Hereditary impairment
Congenital anomaly
   gross anomalies
   minor anomalies
Hypoxic–ischemic injuries
   selective neuronal necrosis
   status marmoratus
   parasagittal ischemic injury
   periventricular leukomalacia
   focal (and multifocal) ischemic brain necrosis
Intraventricular hemorrhage
Unknown causes

Periventricular leukomalacia

This disorder is frequent in premature infants born in the 27–35th weeks of pregnancy. The origin of periventricular leukomalacia (PVL) is mainly ischemic necrosis of the paraventricular white matter fibers. MRI diagnosis is useful in the newborn. The initial change is high intensity on MRI, due to hypertrophic astrocytes and absent blood vessels. On ultrasound, the change appears as hyperechogenicity of the periventricular area. Bilateral occurrence is usual. PVL cysts are formed within 2 weeks of the insult (Figures 3

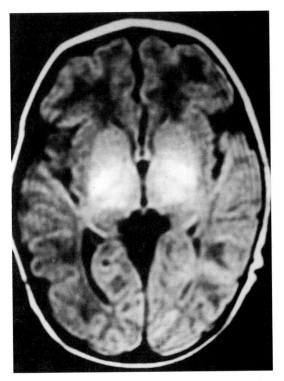

Figure 2 T1 magnetic resonance image, demonstrating high intensity of basal ganglia and atrophy in the brain of a neonate who showed quadriplegia after severe intrapartum hypoxia

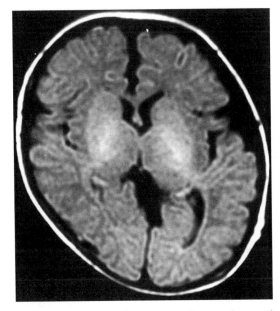

Figure 1 T1 magnetic resonance image of normal neonatal brain

and 4). If PVL cysts are formed, they will last for weeks. After the cyst resolves, the lateral ventricles dilate, and the lateral edges are grossly irregular, due to the atrophy and shrinkage of the necrotic periventricular tissue (Figures 5 and 6). Therefore, the diagnosis is made by three findings: bilateral high intensity (high echogenicity in ultrasound), formation of cysts, and ventricular dilatation with an irregular lateral wall.

The sequela of PVL is frequently cerebral palsy, and has been reported to occur in 86% of premature neonates with PVL[8]. The corticospinal tract, which originates from the motor cortex, passes the periventricular white matter where the PVL lesion occurs; hence spastic diplegia of the legs is frequent, and in widespread lesions, upper extremity function and intellectual function may also be affected[4]. PVL has been reported to develop even in the antepartum period[9]. The PVL cysts which are found immediately after birth strongly suggest its development at least 1 week

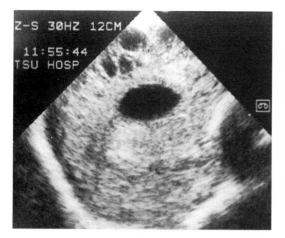

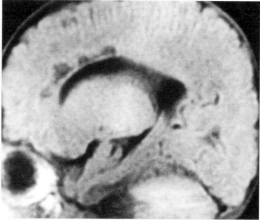

Figure 3 Periventricular leukomalacia (PVL) cysts in an infant of 4 months after a non-eventful neonatal stage. The coronal scan was obtained by 5-MHz sector scan transducer placed at the fontanelle. PVL cysts are observed close to the anterior horn of the left lateral ventricle. The ventricle is dilated, due to the atrophy of white matter

Figure 4 T1 magnetic resonance image, showing periventricular leukomalacia cysts in the parasagittal plane of a cerebral palsy patient of 2 months. The case was a very low birth weight infant

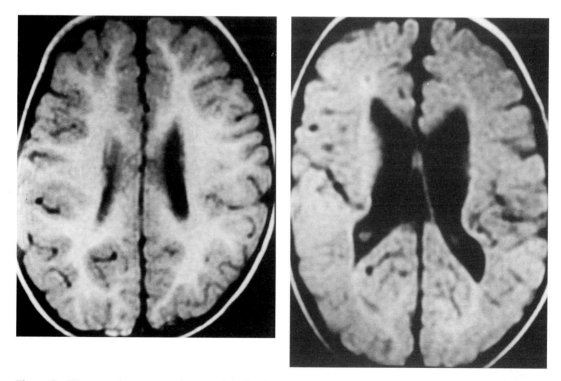

Figure 5 T1 magnetic resonance images of the brain. Left: normal infant of 8 months. Plenty of white matter is observed adjacent to the ventricle. Right: 4-month infant with periventricular leukomalacia. The ventricle is dilated, due to the atrophy of white matter

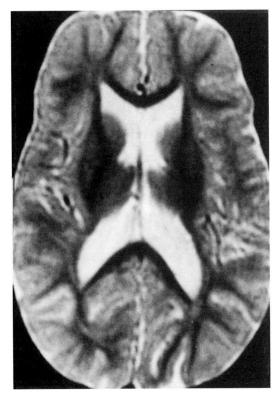

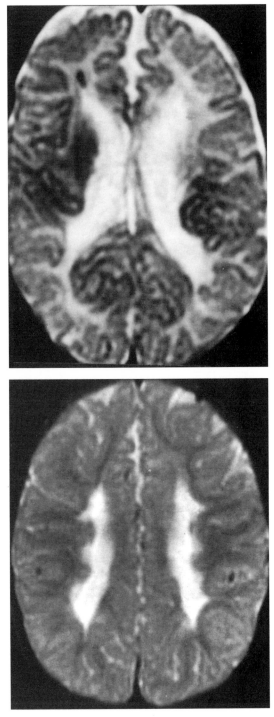

Figure 6 T2 magnetic resonance images of 2-year-old infants. Top left: normal infant. Plenty of white matter (dark) adjacent to the ventricle and well-developed myelination (dark). Top right: infant with periventricular leukomalacia (PVL). The pregnancy was 27 weeks and birth weight 1284 g. Irregularly deformed ventricle wall and no extended myelination. Bottom: Another infant with PVL. Dilated ventricle and irregularly deformed wall, due to atrophic contraction of the white matter

before the birth. Therefore, antepartum PVL development is diagnosed when the periventricular cysts are found within 1 week after the birth. Ultrasonic screening of the newborn is, therefore, important immediately after the birth of an infant with intrapartum asphyxia, particularly if it is premature infant.

There is a need for further investigation into the detection of fetal brain damage, including PVL, in the antepartum stage. High-risk factors for PVL are prematurity, vaginal hemorrhage, hypoxic event, asphyxia diagnosed by abnormal fetal heart monitoring, infection, endotoxin[4], and multiple pregnancy. In these cases, there should be intensive evaluation with morphological and behavioral examinations.

No successful antepartum diagnosis of PVL has been reported, but the diagnosis would be made by the same diagnostic criteria as in the neonate. We made efforts to detect signs of PVL in fetuses with abnormalities, and found periventricular hyperechogenicity in fetuses who suffered such conditions as suspected aneuploidy, growth retardation and renal agenesis. Most of the fetuses died, due to the underlying disorders.

Another diagnostic strategy is the study of cerebral blood flow in high-risk cases of PVL. We have examined intrapartum cerebral blood flow in normal term fetuses during labor. In addition, we have seen the reduction of ultrasonic Doppler diastolic flow on abdominal scan when the fetal head was compressed. After detection of middle cerebral arteries with color flow mapping in intrapartum transvaginal scan, Doppler flowmetry confirmed the reduction and reverse of diastolic flow during labor contractions. As the reduction of cerebral arterial blood flow should be found in the circulatory collapse in the developing process of PVL, ultrasonic color flow mapping and Doppler flowmetry should be further evaluated in the cerebral arteries of such high-risk cases. MRI angiography may be more effective, if it is available for the fetus.

It is postulated that the circulatory collapse is produced by accidental hypotension caused by bradycardia and cardiac failure in severe hypoxia. The threshold of such severe change is unknown, and should be further studied. Tissue characterization with use of ultrasonic gray-level histogram width[10] will be useful in quantitative estimation of periventricular echogenicity, and may be useful in PVL diagnosis in the future.

Parasagittal ischemic injury

Parasagittal injury is the bilateral necrosis of parasagittal cortical neurons and subcortical white matter, due to the impairment of circulatory perfusion in the watershed formed by anterior, middle and posterior cerebral arteries. It is characteristic that PVL appears frequently in premature babies, and parasagittal injury mostly in term infants[4]. Although the two major disorders are caused similarly by circulatory collapse in asphyxia, in parasagittal ischemic injury the damage usually occurs in developed vessels. The long-term clinical picture will be intellectual deficiency and impaired motor function, because of cortical and subcortical necrosis[4]. Successful

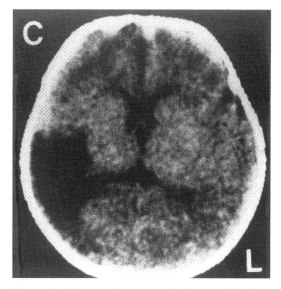

Figure 7 Computed tomography image of wedge-shaped brain infarction due to the obstruction of the middle cerebral artery

antepartum diagnosis has not been reported, but ultrasonic blood flow studies on cerebral arteries will be important in clarifying the mechanism of the disorder.

Focal (and multifocal) ischemic brain necrosis

Brain infarction, porencephaly and hydranencephaly usually occur before birth. Brain infarction appears as a high-intensity magnetic resonance image or echogenic ultrasound image in its initial state resulting from the gathering of astroglia or other cells appearing after the necrosis of brain tissue. The image usually evolves into a wedge-shaped low-intensity or low-echogenic image. This shows the progress of brain tissue necrosis after the obstruction of the cerebral artery due to vascular disease, emboli or thrombi of the artery[4]. The infarction appears usually unilaterally (Figure 7). Antepartum development is suspected when the classic low-intensity image is observed immediately after the birth. Ultrasonic screening of the newborn infant is important in every depressed neonate. Lastly, hydranencephaly is thought to be caused by bilateral obstruction of fetal carotid arteries.

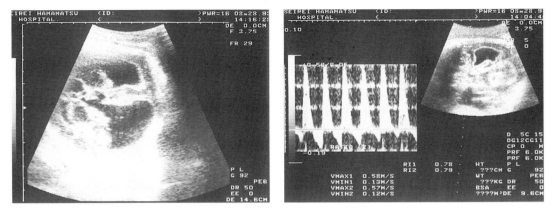

Figure 8 Left: antepartum ultrasound image of ventricular dilatation due to hemorrhage at 36 weeks of pregnancy. The hemorrhage was confirmed by magnetic resonance imaging after the birth. Right: reverse flow in the middle cerebral artery in a case of intraventricular hemorrhage and ventricular dilatation

INTRAVENTRICULAR HEMORRHAGE

Intraventricular hemorrhage detected immediately after birth is evidence of antepartum development[11]. An echogenic mass appears in the ventricle, filling it as the cast of the ventricle in advanced intraventricular hemorrhage. Many ultrasonic diagnoses of antepartum intraventricular hemorrhage have been reported. Usually, the condition is followed by ventricular dilatation (Figure 8). Ultrasonic screening for intraventricular hemorrhage should be performed, not only in the neonate, but also in the complicated pregnancy.

SUMMARY AND CONCLUSION

There are many causes of brain damage, due to hypoxic–ischemic injury. The fetus with a progressive hypoxic process is detected by signs of fetal distress, and damage can be minimized by rapid delivery. In most cases of intrapartum hypoxia, fetal damage can be prevented. In the premature fetus and the neonate whose cerebral vascular development is premature, local perfusion may collapse and local necrosis may develop. Hypoxia will be the main cause of cardiac and circulatory failure, and, in addition, hypoxia may directly produce brain damage. There are direct and delayed neuronal deaths due to severe anoxia in the fetus and newborn, and it is difficult to treat an anoxic insult effectively with oxygenation. New therapeutic methods may emerge with metabolic and pharmacological treatments in the future. These are needed particularly after severe accidental anoxia in a fetus, when delayed neuronal death may occur.

Antepartum brain damage should be more precisely studied to enable recognition of its characteristic changes. In the future, we may find effective ways to prevent or cure the fetus and newborn. Although current knowledge is limited, we expect improvement in the diagnosis and management of asphyxic fetal and neonatal brain damage.

References

1. Naeye, R.L., Peters, E.C., Bartholomew, M. and Landis, J.R. (1989). Origins of cerebral palsy. *Am. J. Dis. Child.*, **143**, 1154–61
2. McDonald, D., Grant, A., Sherikan-Perira, M., Boylan, P. and Chalmers, I. (1985). The Dublin randomized controlled trial of intrapartum fetal heart rate monitoring. *Am. J. Obstet. Gynecol.*, **152**, 524–39
3. Tsuzaki, T., Morishita, K., Takeuchi, Y., Mizuta, M., Minagawa, Y., Nakajima, K. and Maeda, K. (1990). The survey on the perinatal variables and the perinatal incidence of cerebral palsy for 12

years before and after the application of the fetal monitoring system. *Acta Obstet. Gynaecol. Jpn.*, **42**, 99–105

4. Volpe, J.J. (1981). Neurology of the newborn. In Schaffer, A.J. and Markowitz, M. (eds.) *Major Problems in Clinical Pediatrics*, Vol. 22, pp. 180–233. (Philadelphia: W.B. Saunders)

5. Takeshita, K., Ando, Y., Ohtani, K. and Takashima, S. (1989). Cerebral palsy in Tottori, Japan. *Neuroepidemiology*, **8**, 184–92

6. Espinoza, M.I. and Parer, J.T. (1991). Mechanisms of asphyxiated brain damage, and possible pharmacologic interventions, in the fetus. *Am. J. Obstet. Gynecol.*, **164**, 1582-91

7. Kochhar, A., Zivin, J.A., Lyden, P.D. and Mazzarella, V. (1988). Glutamate antagonist therapy reduces neurologic deficits produced by focal central nervous system ischemia. *Arch. Neurol.*, **45**, 148–53

8. Fujimoto, S. (1992). The outcome of PVL. *NICU*, **5**, 640–3

9. Bejar, R., Wozniak, P., Allard, M., Benirschke, K., Vaucher, Y., Coen, R., Berry, C., Schragg, P., Villegas, I. and Resnik, R. (1988). Antenatal origin of neurologic damage in newborn infants. I. Preterm infants. *Am. J. Obstet. Gynecol.*, **159**, 357–63

10. Maeda, K. (1992). Tissue characterization in obstetrics and gynecology: the present state and future possibilities. *Ultrasound Obstet. Gynecol.*, **2**, 75–6

11. Scher, M.S., Belfar, H., Martin, J. and Painter, M.J. (1991). Destructive brain lesions of presumed fetal onset: antepartum causes of cerebral palsy. *Pediatrics*, **88**, 898–906

Index